New Frontiers in Therapeutic Drug Monitoring of Biologics in Inflammatory Bowel Disease and Other Immune-Mediated Inflammatory Diseases

New Frontiers in Therapeutic Drug Monitoring of Biologics in Inflammatory Bowel Disease and Other Immune-Mediated Inflammatory Diseases

Editor

Konstantinos Papamichael

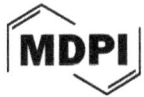

Basel • Beijing • Wuhan • Barcelona • Belgrade • Novi Sad • Cluj • Manchester

Editor
Konstantinos Papamichael
Beth Israel Deaconess
Medical Center, Harvard
Medical School
Boston, MA, USA

Editorial Office
MDPI
St. Alban-Anlage 66
4052 Basel, Switzerland

This is a reprint of articles from the Special Issue published online in the open access journal *Journal of Clinical Medicine* (ISSN 2077-0383) (available at: https://www.mdpi.com/journal/jcm/special_issues/Therapeutic_Drug_Monitoring_IBD_IMID).

For citation purposes, cite each article independently as indicated on the article page online and as indicated below:

Lastname, A.A.; Lastname, B.B. Article Title. *Journal Name* **Year**, *Volume Number*, Page Range.

ISBN 978-3-0365-9843-7 (Hbk)
ISBN 978-3-0365-9844-4 (PDF)
doi.org/10.3390/books978-3-0365-9844-4

© 2023 by the authors. Articles in this book are Open Access and distributed under the Creative Commons Attribution (CC BY) license. The book as a whole is distributed by MDPI under the terms and conditions of the Creative Commons Attribution-NonCommercial-NoDerivs (CC BY-NC-ND) license.

Contents

Byron P. Vaughn
A Practical Guide to Therapeutic Drug Monitoring of Biologic Medications for Inflammatory Bowel Disease
Reprinted from: *J. Clin. Med.* **2021**, *10*, 4990, doi:10.3390/jcm10214990 1

Mir Zulqarnain, Parakkal Deepak and Andres J. Yarur
Therapeutic Drug Monitoring in Perianal Fistulizing Crohn's Disease
Reprinted from: *J. Clin. Med.* **2022**, *11*, 1813, doi:10.3390/jcm11071813 11

Rodrigo Bremer Nones, Phillip R. Fleshner, Natalia Sousa Freitas Queiroz, Adam S. Cheifetz, Antonino Spinelli, Silvio Danese, et al.
Therapeutic Drug Monitoring of Biologics in IBD: Essentials for the Surgical Patient
Reprinted from: *J. Clin. Med.* **2021**, *10*, 5642, doi:10.3390/jcm10235642 23

Benjamin L. Gordon and Robert Battat
Therapeutic Drug Monitoring of Infliximab in Acute Severe Ulcerative Colitis
Reprinted from: *J. Clin. Med.* **2023**, *12*, 3378, doi:10.3390/jcm12103378 39

Mathilde Barrau, Xavier Roblin, Leslie Andromaque, Aurore Rozieres, Mathias Faure, Stéphane Paul and Stéphane Nancey
What Should We Know about Drug Levels and Therapeutic Drug Monitoring during Pregnancy and Breastfeeding in Inflammatory Bowel Disease under Biologic Therapy?
Reprinted from: *J. Clin. Med.* **2023**, *12*, 7495, doi:10.3390/jcm12237495 51

Sanket Patel and Andres J. Yarur
A Review of Therapeutic Drug Monitoring in Patients with Inflammatory Bowel Disease Receiving Combination Therapy
Reprinted from: *J. Clin. Med.* **2023**, *12*, 6577, doi:10.3390/jcm12206577 67

Robert D. Little, Mark G. Ward, Emily Wright, Asha J. Jois, Alex Boussioutas, Georgina L. Hold, et al.
Therapeutic Drug Monitoring of Subcutaneous Infliximab in Inflammatory Bowel Disease—Understanding Pharmacokinetics and Exposure Response Relationships in a New Era of Subcutaneous Biologics
Reprinted from: *J. Clin. Med.* **2022**, *11*, 6173, doi:10.3390/jcm11206173 79

Kathryn Demase, Cassandra K. Monitto, Robert D. Little and Miles P. Sparrow
The Role of Low-Dose Oral Methotrexate in Increasing Anti-TNF Drug Levels and Reducing Immunogenicity in IBD
Reprinted from: *J. Clin. Med.* **2023**, *12*, 4382, doi:10.3390/jcm12134382 97

Rochelle Wong, Lihui Qin, Yushan Pan, Prerna Mahtani, Randy Longman, Dana Lukin, et al.
Higher Adalimumab Trough Levels Are Associated with Histologic Remission and Mucosal Healing in Inflammatory Bowel Disease
Reprinted from: *J. Clin. Med.* **2023**, *12*, 6796, doi:10.3390/jcm12216796 117

Tina Deyhim, Adam S. Cheifetz and Konstantinos Papamichael
Drug Clearance in Patients with Inflammatory Bowel Disease Treated with Biologics
Reprinted from: *J. Clin. Med.* **2023**, *12*, 7132, doi:10.3390/jcm12227132 129

Rani Soenen, Christophe Stove, Alessio Capobianco, Hanne De Schutter, Marie Dobbelaere, Tahmina Mahjor, et al.
Promising Tools to Facilitate the Implementation of TDM of Biologics in Clinical Practice
Reprinted from: *J. Clin. Med.* **2022**, *11*, 3011, doi:10.3390/jcm11113011 141

Christian Primas, Walter Reinisch, John C. Panetta, Alexander Eser, Diane R. Mould and
Thierry Dervieux
**Model Informed Precision Dosing Tool Forecasts Trough Infliximab and Associates with Disease
Status and Tumor Necrosis Factor-Alpha Levels of Inflammatory Bowel Diseases**
Reprinted from: *J. Clin. Med.* **2022**, *11*, 3316, doi:10.3390/jcm11123316 . . . . **157**

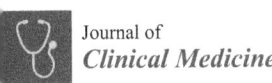

Review

A Practical Guide to Therapeutic Drug Monitoring of Biologic Medications for Inflammatory Bowel Disease

Byron P. Vaughn

Inflammatory Bowel Disease Program, Division of Gastroenterology, Hepatology and Nutrition, University of Minnesota, Minneapolis, MN 55455, USA; bvaughn@umn.edu

Abstract: Therapeutic drug monitoring (TDM) is a useful strategy to optimize biologic medications for inflammatory bowel disease not responsive to standard dosing regimens. TDM is cost effective for anti-tumor necrosis factor agents in the setting of loss of response (reactive TDM). Optimizing drug dosing when patients are in remission (proactive TDM) may be beneficial in certain circumstances. However, frequently the serum drug concentration in isolation becomes the focus TDM. Additionally, the lines of reactive and proactive TDM can quickly blur in many common clinical settings. Physicians employing a TDM based strategy need to place the drug concentration in context with the inflammatory status of the patient, the underlying pharmacokinetics and pharmacodynamics of the drug, the risk of immunogenicity, and the therapeutic goals for the patient. Physicians should understand the limits of TDM and feel comfortable making therapeutic decisions with imperfect information. The goal of this narrative review is to provide a framework of questions that physicians can use to employ TDM effectively in practice.

Keywords: infliximab; adalimumab; vedolizumab; ustekinumab; Crohn's disease; ulcerative colitis

Citation: Vaughn, B.P. A Practical Guide to Therapeutic Drug Monitoring of Biologic Medications for Inflammatory Bowel Disease. *J. Clin. Med.* **2021**, *10*, 4990. https://doi.org/10.3390/jcm10214990

Academic Editor: Konstantinos Papamichael

Received: 28 September 2021
Accepted: 20 October 2021
Published: 27 October 2021

Publisher's Note: MDPI stays neutral with regard to jurisdictional claims in published maps and institutional affiliations.

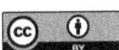

Copyright: © 2021 by the author. Licensee MDPI, Basel, Switzerland. This article is an open access article distributed under the terms and conditions of the Creative Commons Attribution (CC BY) license (https://creativecommons.org/licenses/by/4.0/).

1. Introduction

"What levels do you aim for?" This might be the most consistently asked question at any modern inflammatory bowel disease (IBD) conference. It is the wrong question. The goal of using biologic therapy in IBD is to suppress inflammation (i.e., pharmacodynamics or what the drug does to the body). Biologic therapies approved by the US FDA at the time of this writing include monoclonal antibodies to anti TNF-α (infliximab, adalimumab, certolizumab, and golimumab) along with their related biosimilars, agents targeting leukocyte trafficking (the anti-integrin α4β7 monoclonal antibody vedolizumab) and monoclonal antibodies binding the p40 subunit of the pro-inflammatory interleukins (IL)-12 and-23 (ustekinumab). All current biologic therapies have assays in clinical use to measure the serum drug concentration and anti-drug antibody (ADA) concentration. Overreliance on targeting a serum drug concentration (i.e., pharmacokinetics) without an accurate clinical and inflammatory context will leave providers confused and patients underserved. "Targeting a level" for clinical decision-making is similar to a platitude, a flat truth. On one level, it is an easy to measure endpoint; but focusing only on the concentration belies the difficult, complex decisions involving IBD therapy. Serum drug concentrations are one of many important data points. Using serum drug concentrations appropriately requires knowledge of drug mechanism, the risk of immunogenicity, the inflammatory status of the disease, and realistic therapy goals.

The fact that therapeutic drug monitoring (TDM) is complex, should not dissuade the provider from the practice. Rather, with a few well-posed questions, this strategy can be easily implemented in practice. There are a number of excellent reviews that summarize the literature on TDM in IBD [1,2]. The goal of this review is to provide a useful framework for implementing the literature in practice. Providers should ultimately feel more confident in a TDM based strategy and less confident in any specific serum concentration. If "what levels do you aim for?" is the wrong question, then what is the right question? This review sets out to outline the right question(s) to effectivity use TDM in practice.

2. Association versus Causation

Drug concentrations are inversely associated with inflammation. In almost all post-induction studies, serum drug concentrations are significantly higher in patients who are in remission [3–5]. Ongoing inflammation is associated with lower drug concentrations. One important reason for this association is the protein losing colopathy seen with severe intestinal inflammation [6,7]. As the molecules constituting biologic therapies are roughly the same size (100–150 kilodaltons), this phenomenon is likely true for biologics as a class of therapy. There are other mechanisms for increased biologic metabolism. In states of inflammation monoclonal antibodies undergo increased proteolytic degradation [8]. These effects occur with a number of proteins that are negatively associated with inflammation, albumin being the most common. Albumin likely acts as a surrogate marker for monoclonal antibody turnover.

Therefore, on a population level, any cross-sectional analysis will have a trend of higher drug concentrations with increased remission rates. Importantly, these do not provide insight into a threshold effect (i.e., a limit at which higher concentrations would not decrease inflammation further). It is appealing to identify of a threshold effect, but the study designs prohibit that type of interpretation. It is problematic to use population level associations as actionable data on an individual level. For a given individual, a biologic concentration threshold may exist; but population pharmacokinetic studies do not provide that information. For example, a given cohort of IBD patients, infliximab concentrations >4 µg/mL may be associated with remission. However, specific individuals in that cohort will vary. A given individual with severe penetrating Crohn's disease may only achieve remission once the infliximab concentration is >15 µg/mL. Or perhaps, infliximab is targeting the wrong inflammatory pathway in this that patient. Population association studies are important and hypothesis generating, but they should not be over-relied on to identify thresholds for individual patients in clinical practice.

3. What Is the Target?

The ideal target would directly inform the activity of the inflammatory pathway involved in the biologic mechanism of action. Rather than make changes based on a drug concentration, changes would be made based on a direct measure of the targeted inflammatory pathway. Some individuals would have pathway suppression at a low concentration, while some would require higher doses. However, the drug concentration itself is secondary to the measurement of the pathway. In this theoretical model, measurements of inflammatory pathways would also help guide biologic therapy choice.

Unfortunately, there is no current measurement in clinical practice of a specific inflammatory pathway. When considering TDM it is essential to first establish inflammation and use inflammation as the target over time [9,10]. While our measure of inflammation are not pathway specific, trends over time can aide in assessing a therapeutic response [11]. Low drug concentrations typically also predict who will respond to a dose intensification [12,13]. The combination of active inflammation and low drug concentration suggests that the inflammatory pathway is not saturated, and dose escalation is likely to capture or recapture a response. However, some biologic concentrations may be less predictive of response than others. Typically the cytokine based biologic therapies (anti-TNFs and anti-IL-12/23) have a high correlation between concentration and response to dose escalation [12,13], while the anti-integrins may not [14]. Other factors to consider in how helpful a drug concentration will be in predicting a response to dose intensification include the current dose/frequency, the underlying risk of immunogenicity, and if the patient had a primary response. An overview of key questions to consider with TDM is found in Figure 1.

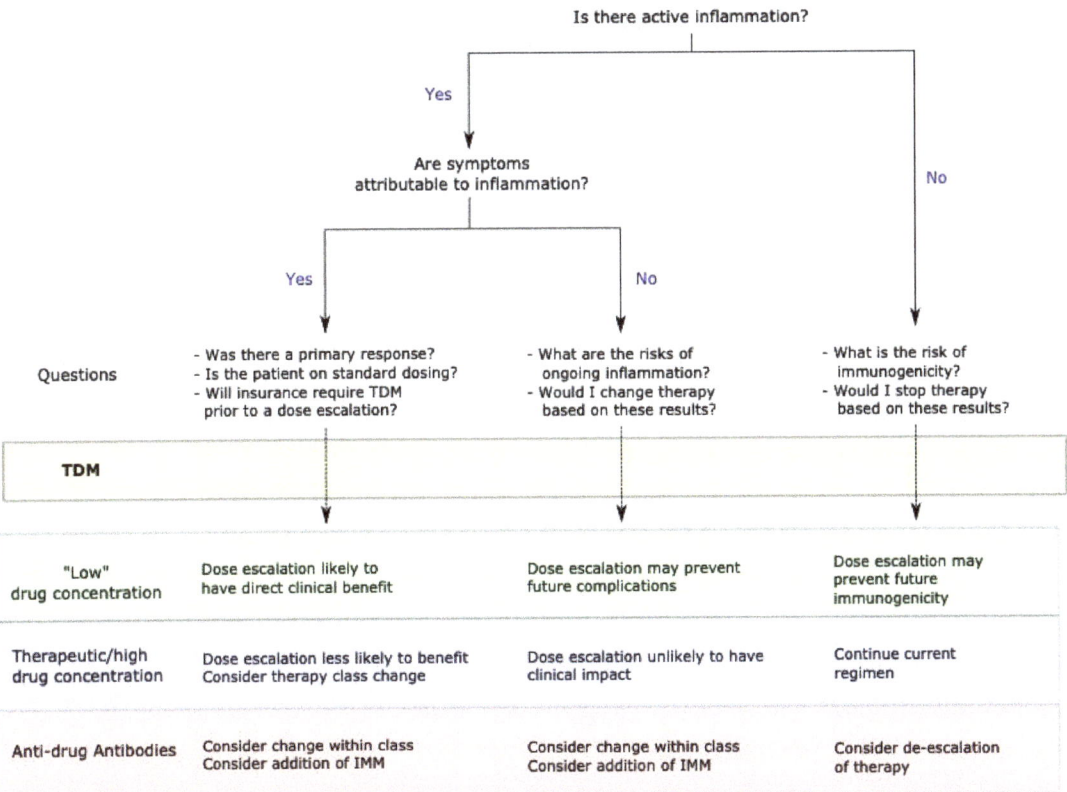

Figure 1. Algorithm of key questions to consider prior to implementing therapeutic drug monitoring (TDM) in clinical practice. Clinical benefit refers to immediate symptomatic improvement. Clinicians should have a clear understanding of the disease status prior to TDM and be able to articulate to the patient the benefit of a dose change in response to the natural history of the disease. In some cases of low-level antibodies, it may be appropriate to add an immunomodulator (IMM) to the current therapy to eliminate anti-drug antibodies. This choice should be individualized based on other available therapies and risks of dual immunosuppression for patient.

4. Reactive Therapeutic Drug Monitoring for Secondary Loss of Response in the Maintenance Phase of Biologic Therapy

Patients with an initial clinical response who then lose response in the maintenance phase with recurrence of inflammation are likely benefit from a therapeutic dose escalation in two settings: (1) lack of anti-drug antibodies (2) low serum trough concentrations.

4.1. Anti-Drug Antibodies

Anti-drug antibodies (ADAs) effectively eliminate a given biologic and can also lead to infusion or injection related reactions [15,16]. The reference range of ADA detection varies with different assays. Most assays in clinical use are drug intolerant, meaning ADAs are only detectable when low or absent serum drug concentration. Compared to drug intolerant assays, drug tolerant assays (i.e., assays that can detect ADAs in the presence of serum drug) appear to be more consistent in ADA detection [17]. Some ADAs are clinically significant, while other appear to be transitory [18]. Non-neutralizing ADAs may bind the drug without inhibiting the pharmacologic effect [19]. An ADA is likely neutralizing in the setting of high ADA concentrations with low/absent serum drug. If the measurement is a trough measurement and the drug concentration is low/absent with ADA, then the ADA is likely neutralizing the drug. A drug concentration of zero is clearly the easiest to interpret, although understanding the limitations of the specific assay being used remains important. My research group previously identified a subset of individuals with positive ADA to adalimumab and a drug concentration of zero who had a detectable drug concentration after dose escalation, even though ADAs persisted [20]. In these settings it is imperative to closely follow the clinical course for changes in inflammation and drug related side effects.

Low level ADAs, particularly if using a drug tolerant assay, are common and often disappear over time [21]. These likely represent clinically insignificant, non-neutralizing antibodies. Addition of an immunomodulator can eliminate these ADAs [22,23]. High antibody concentration with a non-low drug concentration may reflect lab error. In these cases, repeating the drug concentration and ADA with a different assay (e.g., drug tolerant) may provide more data. Ultimately, clinical context is still required. Table 1 summarizes the likelihood of neutralizing antibodies based on the serum drug and anti-drug antibody concentration.

Table 1. Framework for evaluating detectable biologic trough concentration and detectable anti-drug antibodies.

		Serum Drug Concentration	
		"High" concentration	"Low" concentration
Serum Anti-drug Antibody Concentration	"High" antibodies	• Neutralizing antibodies unlikely • Consider lab error • Consider repeating	• Neutralizing antibodies likely • Consider within class change
	"Low" antibodies	• Neutralizing antibodies unlikely • Consider repeating	• Neutralizing antibodies possible • Consider dose escalation or addition of IMM

IMM: Immunomodulator. Assuming trough concentrations at standard maintenance dosing, anti-drug antibodies in the presence of adequate or high serum drug concentration are unlikely to be neutralizing. Low serum drug concentrations increase the chance of neutralizing antibodies. Any antibody in the setting of probable drug mediated side effects may still be clinically significant.

In the setting of recurrent inflammation with low/absent serum trough concentrations, and high ADAs, the best choice is to stop the current therapy and proceed to another biologic. The provider must consider the future risk of anti-drug antibodies with another biologic therapy. Patients who develop ADAs to one biologic are more likely to develop repeat ADAs to another biologic [24]. Consideration should be given to adjunct therapy with an immunomodulator to prevent ADAs, [25] using a biologic with a baseline low immunogenicity rate, or using a non-biologic therapy to avoid the concern for ADAs all together.

4.2. Low Trough Concentrations

Active inflammation may improve with a biologic dose escalation in the presence of low serum trough concentrations. However, there is no universal definition of low. There is substantial variation in an individual's drug concentration-clinical response, making id challenging to identify universal concentration threshold values. The best data regarding a target concentration are from the TAXIT study, a randomized controlled trial of a TDM strategy versus empiric dose escalation for patients with Crohn's disease on infliximab. In the optimization phase, patients with Crohn's disease were more likely to be in remission after a dose escalation for infliximab trough concentrations under 3 µg/mL [26]. However, using other outcomes different infliximab cut-offs can be identified: 3–5 µg/mL for clinical disease, [27] 8–12 µg/mL for endoscopic remission, [28] and 18–20 µg/mL for fistula healing [29,30]. As noted above, low trough concentrations from population cohort studies are problematic as they do not inform an individual's inflammatory pathway activity. The concentration is not the target. The true target is suppression of an inflammatory pathway, which we cannot effectively measure. The appropriate clinical question is not *"what drug level should I aim for"*, but *"will this patient's inflammation regress with a dose escalation?"* There is no simple answer.

The main benefit to reactive-TDM is in the identification of ADAs. Sparing a patient any dose of a biologic that is no longer effective is beneficial and cost effective [31–33]. However, in the absence of ADAs it is unclear what the upper limit of a serum drug concentration should be. If on standard maintenance dosing without ADAs, dose escalation should strongly be considered. For patients already dose escalated, but with still low levels, there are little data to guide. Patients with concentrations under 10–12 µg/mL (for anti-TNFs) may still benefit from dose escalation. Some early data suggest that trough concentrations have little effect on predicting dose escalation to vedolizumab [14,34]. Ultimately, having objective measures of inflammation, and prespecified time points to assess a change in inflammation (6–12 weeks typically) are key to determining success or failure of a dose change.

4.3. Subclinical Inflammation

Until now, no distinction has been made between inflammation causing clinical symptoms and ongoing intestinal inflammation without any gastrointestinal symptoms, i.e., subclinical inflammation. In the setting of subclinical inflammation, therapy optimization based on trough concentrations can be quite helpful. This is essentially "reactive TDM", although with some important nuance. Consider the following scenario. Biologic A gets a patient into clinical remission, but the patient has ongoing endoscopic inflammation. The provider checks a trough concentration of biologic A, which returns in the "therapeutic" range. In typical reactive TDM (i.e., with clinical symptoms from inflammation), changing biologics to a different mechanism would be appropriate. However, in this case, presumably the clinical remission is due to biologic A. Changing to therapy B could lead to a clinical disease recurrence. This is not to say that changing biologic therapy is wrong. Changing to therapy B could lead to both clinical and endoscopic remission. Or increasing the dose of biologic A further could result in complete suppression of inflammation. In these situations, a discussion with the patient on the risks and benefits is essential. The decision should include how many other therapies have been tried, the risks of ongoing inflammation (e.g., colon cancer in the setting of PSC), and the patient's treatment goals. A holistic approach to an individual can help determine the need for treatment modification. For example, certain comorbidities (e.g., venous thromboembolism) or extra-intestinal manifestations of IBD (e.g., arthritis) may sway a provider to escalate or change a biologic despite the lack of GI symptoms. Managing subclinical inflammation does not lend itself well to an algorithm, and falls more into an art.

5. Reactive Therapeutic Drug Monitoring during Induction Therapy

The concept of "primary non-response" is simple on face value: A medication fails to control inflammation because it is not targeting the correct inflammatory pathway(s). Unfortunately, as noted previously, we do not have a measurement what inflammatory pathways are overactive in an individual patient; nor do we have a measure of if that pathway responded to a given therapy. Thus, two problems exist with primary non-response: (1) was the therapy underdosed and (2) was enough time given to see a benefit. TDM may help a provider determine if a primary non-responder is due to underdosing of a biologic therapy.

To date, drug trials in IBD use fixed dosing strategies for large, randomized placebo-controlled studies. For medications with reproducible pharmacokinetics, this process works well. However, with biologic therapy, there is wide individual variation in the serum concentration that is also dependent on the disease. In cases of acute-severe colitis, infliximab loss in the stool through a protein losing colopathy is well documented [6]. The disease process has a negative feedback loop on the drug itself. As such, there are observational data that accelerated induction dosing of infliximab for acute, severe ulcerative colitis decreases the early colectomy rates [35]. However, increasing all induction dosing is not likely to be an effective strategy. A recent study of high dose adalimumab versus standard dose adalimumab did not improve post induction remission rates for Crohn's disease or ulcerative colitis [36,37]. These are important studies, yet they are not evaluating TDM in induction. The goal of TDM in induction is to identify the subpopulation that is most likely to benefit from escalated induction dosing.

An induction TDM strategy presents some practical problems. First, and most importantly, there is a dearth of data on drug concentrations in the induction phase. An extensive review by Sparrow et al. thoroughly summarizes the post induction concentration data to date [38]. The authors note the current data are from observational studies and post-hoc analysis of clinical trials. While this is currently a knowledge gap, there exist several ongoing trials incorporating TDM into the induction period (e.g., NCT03029143). Second, the turnaround time for the results of drug concentration testing can make dose adjustments in the induction phase difficult. Most clinicians do not have "in-house" drug concentration assays and rely on a runaround time of a week or more for the information to return. Fortunately, ADAs are less common in the induction phase. Therefore, empiric dose escalation may be a more useful clinical strategy. Risk calculators or dashboards exist and are being developed (e.g., NCT04835506) aid in induction TDM decisions [39,40].

A recent trial of randomized controlled trial of proactive TDM dosed infliximab versus standard dosed infliximab in Norway (NOR-DRUM Part A) did not identify a benefit of clinical remission across a number of inflammatory conditions (including IBD) [41]. This trial highlights the importance of clinical context paired with TDM. The trial protocol had strict escalation and de-escalation criteria to achieve infliximab concentrations in a pre-set therapeutic range, regardless of inflammatory status. While "proactive", this approach is not "personalized". Strict therapeutic ranges without the context of the inflammatory status are not likely to be useful strategies.

Overall, reactive TDM in the induction phase is like TDM in the maintenance phase. On standard dosing, if a patient is not responding to a therapy, the goal of TDM is to identify anti-drug antibodies. Without anti-drug antibodies, it is likely that standard dosed biologic therapy should be escalated.

6. Therapeutic Drug Monitoring When a Patient Is in Deep Remission

In the absence of inflammation or a suspected antibody mediated side effect, TDM does not have a direct clinical benefit to a patient. Meaning the knowledge of the serum drug concentration and ADA status and subsequent therapeutic changes will not immediately improve a patient's quality of life. The most important role of TDM in this setting is the identification of anti-drug antibodies. Potentially 15% of patients with a stable clinical response or remission will have undetectable serum drug and positive ADAs to infliximab [26,27]. At this point the provider needs to determine if the patient should be de-escalated from biologic therapy completely or transition to a new therapy. The decision to perform TDM in deep should depend on the underlying risk of immunogenicity. If the risk of immunogenicity is quite small (no prior history of ADA, patient on combination therapy with immunomodulator, or using a biologic with low ADA rate), then the benefit of TDM is low. Likely the greatest benefit of TDM in deep remission is with anti-TNF monotherapy.

7. Special Situations

7.1. Reinduction of a Biologic Therapy

Re-starting a biologic runs the risk of inducing anti-drug antibodies [42]. The greatest risk of infusion reaction is with the second re-induction dose. Identification of anti-drug antibodies after the first dose can spare a patient an infusion reaction with the second dose [43]. A practical way to implement this strategy is to alter the induction dose for infusions. For infliximab, an induction schedule could be at week 0, 4, and 8. A serum drug concentration and antibody status at week 2 can inform the presence of antibodies and determine subsequent dosing. For self-injectable biologic therapies, it is not possible to alter the induction schedule in the same way. Obtaining a drug level 1–2 weeks after the first dose is helpful, but given the typical turnaround time, the information may not be back before administration of the second dose.

7.2. De-Escalation of Therapy

After a patient is in remission on combination therapy with a biologic therapy and immunomodulator, a provider may consider stopping the immunomodulator and continuing biologic monotherapy to maintain remission. This is a reasonable strategy to minimize long term side effects of dual immunosuppression. Immunomodulator cessation may reduce serum biologic concentrations. Obtaining a serum drug concentration while on combination therapy can help to guide de-escalation. The risk is the development of ADAs after stopping the immunomodulator. In the case of very low trough concentrations, providers may consider dose escalating the biologic prior to stopping the immunomodulator. Or at a minimum, repeating the serum drug concentration on monotherapy soon after de-escalation.

TDM may also aide in biologic de-escalation in the maintenance phase. Some patients can successfully de-escalate the dose of a biologic [44]. In the STORI trial, where patients on infliximab and a thiopurine stopped the infliximab, those with low trough concentrations (<2 mg/ul) were less likely to experience a clinical relapse [45]. Measuring both biologic and thiopurine concentration can help inform de-escalation. If one is "subtherapeutic" that may be the best to de-escalate [46]. Informing the patient on the potential long-term risks of therapy de-escalation is essential, and this strategy should be individualized with close follow-up.

7.3. Suspicion for Antibody Mediated Side Effects

ADAs can cause a number adverse clinical effects. Most common is disease recurrence in the setting of rapidly cleared drug. ADAs can also lead to infusion reactions, both acute and delayed [47]. Most data on TDM to guide dosing are based on trough concentrations. However, when the question pertains to a potential side effect, non-trough levels may be helpful. Knowledge of the drug and antibody assay is essential in these cases. As noted before, most assays in clinical practice can only detect ADAs when the serum drug concentration is very low or absent. In this case, drawing the drug concentration too early may fail to identify antibodies. For infusion-based biologics, waiting 4-weeks post infusion should be sufficient for clinically significant antibodies to clear the serum drug and be identified. For subcutaneous biologics, it is likely best to obtain a trough measurement. Alternatively, use of a TDM assay that can measure ADAs in the presence of circulating drug can circumvent this issue.

8. Conclusions

TDM is an extremely useful tool in the management of IBD patients on biologic therapies. However, TDM is only helpful in the context of the patient's inflammatory status and response to therapy. Population pharmacodynamic studies can identify helpful trends in serum drug concentrations but should not be mistaken for individual therapeutic thresholds. Practically, clinicians should always objectively measure inflammation at the time of TDM. Clinicians should also have a working understanding of the risk of immunogenicity of a given biologic therapy in a patient. Finally, clinicians using a TDM based strategy should understand what question they are trying to answer before a drug concentration is measured (Figure 1). TDM should be used as a form of personalized medicine incorporating the clinical inflammatory status, therapeutic options, and individual goals of care. Rather than focus too much on *reactive* or *proactive* TDM, we should focus on *personalized* TDM.

Funding: This research received no external funding.

Institutional Review Board Statement: Not applicable.

Conflicts of Interest: Vaughn has received consulting fees from Prometheus Laboratories and grant support from Genentech, Takeda, Celgene, and Diasorin. The funders had no role in the writing of this manuscript.

References

1. Argollo, M.; Kotze, P.G.; Kakkadasam, P.; D'Haens, G. Optimizing biologic therapy in IBD: How essential is therapeutic drug monitoring? *Nat. Rev. Gastroenterol. Hepatol.* **2020**, *17*, 702–710. [CrossRef] [PubMed]
2. Vermeire, S.; Dreesen, E.; Papamichael, K.; Dubinsky, M.C. How, When, and for Whom Should We Perform Therapeutic Drug Monitoring? *Clin. Gastroenterol. Hepatol.* **2020**, *18*, 1291–1299. [CrossRef]
3. Casteele, N.V.; Feagan, B.G.; Gils, A.; Vermeire, S.; Khanna, R.; Sandborn, W.J.; Levesque, B.G. Therapeutic Drug Monitoring in Inflammatory Bowel Disease: Current State and Future Perspectives. *Curr. Gastroenterol. Rep.* **2014**, *16*, 1–8. [CrossRef]
4. Chiu, Y.-L.; Rubin, D.T.; Vermeire, S.; Louis, E.; Robinson, A.M.; Lomax, K.G.; Pollack, P.F.; Paulson, S.K. Serum Adalimumab Concentration and Clinical Remission in Patients with Crohn's Disease. *Inflamm. Bowel Dis.* **2013**, *19*, 1112–1122. [CrossRef] [PubMed]
5. Osterman, M.T.; Rosario, M.; Lasch, K.; Barocas, M.; Wilbur, J.D.; Dirks, N.L.; Gastonguay, M.R. Vedolizumab exposure levels and clinical outcomes in ulcerative colitis: Determining the potential for dose optimisation. *Aliment. Pharmacol. Ther.* **2019**, *49*, 408–418. [CrossRef]
6. Brandse, J.F.; Brink, G.R.V.D.; Wildenberg, M.E.; van der Kleij, D.; Rispens, T.; Jansen, J.M.; Mathôt, R.A.; Ponsioen, C.Y.; Löwenberg, M.; D'Haens, G.R. Loss of Infliximab Into Feces Is Associated with Lack of Response to Therapy in Patients with Severe Ulcerative Colitis. *Gastroenterology* **2015**, *149*, 350–355.e2. [CrossRef]
7. Szántó, K.J.; Madácsy, T.; Kata, D.; Ferenci, T.; Rutka, M.; Bálint, A.; Bor, R.; Fábián, A.; Milassin, Á.; Jójárt, B.; et al. Advances in the optimization of therapeutic drug monitoring using serum, tissue and faecal anti-tumour necrosis factor concentration in patients with inflammatory bowel disease treated with TNF-α antagonists. *Expert Opin. Biol. Ther.* **2021**, *21*, 539–548. [CrossRef]
8. Ryman, J.T.; Meibohm, B. Pharmacokinetics of Monoclonal Antibodies. *CPT: Pharmacomet. Syst. Pharmacol.* **2017**, *6*, 576–588. [CrossRef]
9. Papamichael, K.; Cheifetz, A.S.; Melmed, G.Y.; Irving, P.M.; Casteele, N.V.; Kozuch, P.L.; Raffals, L.E.; Baidoo, L.; Bressler, B.; Devlin, S.M.; et al. Appropriate Therapeutic Drug Monitoring of Biologic Agents for Patients with Inflammatory Bowel Diseases. *Clin. Gastroenterol. Hepatol.* **2019**, *17*, 1655–1668.e3. [CrossRef]
10. Peyrin-Biroulet, L.; Sandborn, W.; Sands, B.E.; Reinisch, W.; Bemelman, W.; Bryant, R.V.; D'Haens, G.; Dotan, I.; Dubinsky, M.; Feagan, B.; et al. Selecting Therapeutic Targets in Inflammatory Bowel Disease (STRIDE): Determining Therapeutic Goals for Treat-to-Target. *Am. J. Gastroenterol.* **2015**, *110*, 1324–1338. [CrossRef] [PubMed]
11. Sorrentino, D.; Gray, J.M. Timely Monitoring of Inflammation by Fecal Lactoferrin Rapidly Predicts Therapeutic Response in Inflammatory Bowel Disease. *Inflamm. Bowel Dis.* **2021**, *27*, 1237–1247. [CrossRef] [PubMed]
12. Afif, W.; Loftus, E.; Faubion, W.A.; Kane, S.V.; Bruining, D.H.; Hanson, K.A.; Sandborn, W.J. Clinical Utility of Measuring Infliximab and Human Anti-Chimeric Antibody Concentrations in Patients with Inflammatory Bowel Disease. *Am. J. Gastroenterol.* **2010**, *105*, 1133–1139. [CrossRef] [PubMed]
13. Roblin, X.; Rinaudo, M.; Del Tedesco, E.; Phelip, J.M.; Genin, C.; Peyrin-Biroulet, L.; Paul, S. Development of an Algorithm Incorporating Pharmacokinetics of Adalimumab in Inflammatory Bowel Diseases. *Am. J. Gastroenterol.* **2014**, *109*, 1250–1256. [CrossRef]
14. Vaughn, B.P.; Yarur, A.J.; Graziano, E.; Campbell, J.P.; Bhattacharya, A.; Lee, J.Y.; Gheysens, K.; Papamichael, K.; Osterman, M.T.; Cheifetz, A.S.; et al. Vedolizumab Serum Trough Concentrations and Response to Dose Escalation in Inflammatory Bowel Disease. *J. Clin. Med.* **2020**, *9*, 3142. [CrossRef]
15. Nanda, K.S.; Cheifetz, A.S.; Moss, A.C. Impact of Antibodies to Infliximab on Clinical Outcomes and Serum Infliximab Levels in Patients with Inflammatory Bowel Disease (IBD): A Meta-Analysis. *Am. J. Gastroenterol.* **2013**, *108*, 40–47. [CrossRef]
16. O'Meara, S.; Nanda, K.S.; Moss, A. Antibodies to Infliximab and Risk of Infusion Reactions in Patients with Inflammatory Bowel Disease. *Inflamm. Bowel Dis.* **2014**, *20*, 1–6. [CrossRef]
17. Bloem, K.; van Leeuwen, A.; Verbeek, G.; Nurmohamed, M.T.; Wolbink, G.J.; van der Kleij, D.; Rispens, T. Systematic comparison of drug-tolerant assays for anti-drug antibodies in a cohort of adalimumab-treated rheumatoid arthritis patients. *J. Immunol. Methods* **2015**, *418*, 29–38. [CrossRef] [PubMed]
18. Sandborn, W.J.; Wolf, U.C.; Kosutic, G.; Parker, G.; Schreiber, S.; Lee, S.D.; Abraham, B.; Afzali, A.; Arsenescu, R.I.; Gutierrez, A.; et al. Effects of Transient and Persistent Anti-drug Antibodies to Certolizumab Pegol. *Inflamm. Bowel Dis.* **2017**, *23*, 1047–1056. [CrossRef]
19. Shankar, G.; Arkin, S.; Cocea, L.; Devanarayan, V.; Kirshner, S.; Kromminga, A.; Quarmby, V.; Richards, S.; Schneider, C.K.; Subramanyam, M.; et al. Assessment and Reporting of the Clinical Immunogenicity of Therapeutic Proteins and Peptides—Harmonized Terminology and Tactical Recommendations. *AAPS J.* **2014**, *16*, 658–673. [CrossRef]
20. Jasurda, J.S.; McCabe, R.P.; Vaughn, B.P. Adalimumab Concentration Changes after Dose Escalation in Inflammatory Bowel Disease. *Ther. Drug Monit.* **2021**, *43*, 645–651. [CrossRef]
21. Van Stappen, T.; Vande Casteele, N.; Van Assche, G.; Ferrante, M.; Vermeire, S.; Gils, A. Clinical relevance of detecting anti-infliximab antibodies with a drug-tolerant assay: Post hoc analysis of the TAXIT trial. *Gut* **2018**, *67*, 818–826. [CrossRef]
22. Ben–Horin, S.; Waterman, M.; Kopylov, U.; Yavzori, M.; Picard, O.; Fudim, E.; Awadie, H.; Weiss, B.; Chowers, Y. Addition of an Immunomodulator to Infliximab Therapy Eliminates Antidrug Antibodies in Serum and Restores Clinical Response of Patients with Inflammatory Bowel Disease. *Clin. Gastroenterol. Hepatol.* **2013**, *11*, 444–447. [CrossRef] [PubMed]

23. Colman, R.J.; Portocarrero-Castillo, A.; Chona, D.; Hellmann, J.; Minar, P.; Rosen, M.J. Favorable Outcomes and Anti-TNF Durability After Addition of an Immunomodulator for Anti-Drug Antibodies in Pediatric IBD Patients. *Inflamm. Bowel Dis.* **2021**, *27*, 507–515. [CrossRef]
24. Casteele, N.V.; Abreu, M.T.; Flier, S.; Papamichael, K.; Rieder, F.; Silverberg, M.S.; Khanna, R.; Okada, L.; Yang, L.; Jain, A.; et al. Patients with Low Drug Levels or Antibodies to a Prior Anti–Tumor Necrosis Factor Are More Likely to Develop Antibodies to a Subsequent Anti–Tumor Necrosis Factor. *Clin. Gastroenterol. Hepatol.* **2021**, *6*, S1542–S3565. [CrossRef]
25. Colombel, J.-F.; Adedokun, O.J.; Gasink, C.; Gao, L.-L.; Cornillie, F.J.; D'Haens, G.R.; Rutgeerts, P.J.; Reinisch, W.; Sandborn, W.J.; Hanauer, S.B. Combination Therapy with Infliximab and Azathioprine Improves Infliximab Pharmacokinetic Features and Efficacy: A Post Hoc Analysis. *Clin. Gastroenterol. Hepatol.* **2019**, *17*, 1525–1532.e1. [CrossRef]
26. Casteele, N.V.; Ferrante, M.; Van Assche, G.; Ballet, V.; Compernolle, G.; Van Steen, K.; Simoens, S.; Rutgeerts, P.; Gils, A.; Vermeire, S. Trough Concentrations of Infliximab Guide Dosing for Patients with Inflammatory Bowel Disease. *Gastroenterology* **2015**, *148*, 1320–1329.e3. [CrossRef] [PubMed]
27. Vaughn, B.P.; Martinez-Vazquez, M.; Patwardhan, V.R.; Moss, A.; Sandborn, W.J.; Cheifetz, A.S. Proactive Therapeutic Concentration Monitoring of Infliximab May Improve Outcomes for Patients with Inflammatory Bowel Disease: Results from a pilot observational study. *Inflamm. Bowel Dis.* **2014**, *20*, 1996–2003. [CrossRef] [PubMed]
28. Papamichael, K.; Rakowsky, S.; Rivera, C.; Cheifetz, A.S.; Osterman, M.T. Infliximab trough concentrations during maintenance therapy are associated with endoscopic and histologic healing in ulcerative colitis. *Aliment. Pharmacol. Ther.* **2018**, *47*, 478–484. [CrossRef] [PubMed]
29. Yarur, A.J.; Kanagala, V.; Stein, D.J.; Czul, F.; Quintero, M.A.; Agrawal, D.; Patel, A.; Best, K.; Fox, C.; Idstein, K.; et al. Higher infliximab trough levels are associated with perianal fistula healing in patients with Crohn's disease. *Aliment. Pharmacol. Ther.* **2017**, *45*, 933–940. [CrossRef] [PubMed]
30. Papamichael, K.; Casteele, N.V.; Jeyarajah, J.; Jairath, V.; Osterman, M.T.; Cheifetz, A.S. Higher Postinduction Infliximab Concentrations Are Associated with Improved Clinical Outcomes in Fistulizing Crohn's Disease: An ACCENT-II Post Hoc Analysis. *Am. J. Gastroenterol.* **2021**, *116*, 1007–1014. [CrossRef]
31. Negoescu, D.M.; Enns, E.A.; Swanhorst, B.; Baumgartner, B.; Campbell, J.P.; Osterman, M.T.; Papamichael, K.; Cheifetz, A.S.; Vaughn, B.P. Proactive Vs Reactive Therapeutic Drug Monitoring of Infliximab in Crohn's Disease: A Cost-Effectiveness Analysis in a Simulated Cohort. *Inflamm. Bowel Dis.* **2019**, *26*, 103–111. [CrossRef] [PubMed]
32. Velayos, F.S.; Kahn, J.G.; Sandborn, W.J.; Feagan, B.G. A Test-based Strategy Is More Cost Effective than Empiric Dose Escalation for Patients with Crohn's Disease Who Lose Responsiveness to Infliximab. *Clin. Gastroenterol. Hepatol.* **2013**, *11*, 654–666. [CrossRef] [PubMed]
33. Roblin, X.; Attar, A.; Lamure, M.; Savarieau, B.; Brunel, P.; Duru, G.; Peyrin-Biroulet, L. Cost savings of anti-TNF therapy using a test-based strategy versus an empirical dose escalation in Crohn's disease patients who lose response to infliximab. *J. Mark. Access Health Policy* **2015**, *3*, 29229. [CrossRef] [PubMed]
34. Ungar, B.; Malickova, K.; Hanžel, J.; Abu Arisha, M.; Paul, S.; Rocha, C.; Ben Shatach, Z.; Abitbol, C.M.; Natour, O.H.; Selinger, L.; et al. Dose optimisation for Loss of Response to Vedolizumab— Pharmacokinetics and Immune Mechanisms. *J. Crohn's Coliti* **2021**, *15*, 1707–1719. [CrossRef]
35. Gibson, D.J.; Heetun, Z.S.; Redmond, C.E.; Nanda, K.S.; Keegan, D.; Byrne, K.; Mulcahy, H.E.; Cullen, G.; Doherty, G. An Accelerated Infliximab Induction Regimen Reduces the Need for Early Colectomy in Patients with Acute Severe Ulcerative Colitis. *Clin. Gastroenterol. Hepatol.* **2015**, *13*, 330–335.e1. [CrossRef]
36. D'Haens, G.; Sandborn, W.; Loftus, E.; Hanauer, S.; Schreiber, S.; Peyrin-Biroulet, L.; Panaccione, R.; Panes, J.; Colombel, J.F.; Ferrante, M.; et al. High versus Standard Adalimumab Induction Dosing Regimens in Patients with Moderately to Severely Active Crohn's Disease: Results from the SERENE-CD Induction Study [UEG Week Abstract LB27]. *United Eur. Gastroenterol. J.* **2019**, *7*. Available online: https://ueg.eu/library/high-versus-standard-adalimumab-induction-dosing-regimens-in-patients-with-moderately-to-severely-active-crohns-disease-results-from-the-serene-cd-induction-study/208601 (accessed on 28 September 2021).
37. Panes, J.; Colombel, J.F.; D'Haens, G.; Schreiber, S.; Panaccione, R.; Peyrin-Biroulet, L.; Loftus, E.; Danese, S.; Louis, E.; Armuzzi, A.; et al. High versus Standard Adalimumab Induction Dosing Regimens in Patients with Moderately to Severely Active Ulcerative Colitis: Results from the SERENE-UC Induction Study [UEG Week Abstract OP216]. *United Eur. Gastroenterol. J.* **2019**, *7*. Available online: https://www.ecco-ibd.eu/publications/congress-abstracts/item/op01-higher-vs-standard-adalimumab-maintenance-regimens-in-patients-with-moderately-to-severely-active-ulcerative-colitis-results-from-the-serene-uc-maintenance-study.html (accessed on 28 September 2021).
38. Sparrow, M.P.; Papamichael, K.; Ward, M.G.; Riviere, P.; Laharie, D.; Paul, S.; Roblin, X. Therapeutic Drug Monitoring of Biologics During Induction to Prevent Primary Non-Response. *J. Crohn's Coliti* **2020**, *14*, 542–556. [CrossRef]
39. Strik, A.S.; Löwenberg, M.; Mould, D.R.; Berends, S.E.; Ponsioen, C.I.; Brande, J.M.H.V.D.; Jansen, J.M.; Hoekman, D.R.; Brandse, J.F.; Duijvestein, M.; et al. Efficacy of dashboard driven dosing of infliximab in inflammatory bowel disease patients; A randomized controlled trial. *Scand. J. Gastroenterol.* **2021**, *56*, 145–154. [CrossRef]
40. Dave, M.B.; Dherai, A.J.; Desai, D.C.; Mould, D.R.; Ashavaid, T.F. Optimization of infliximab therapy in inflammatory bowel disease using a dashboard approach—An Indian experience. *Eur. J. Clin. Pharmacol.* **2021**, *77*, 55–62. [CrossRef]

41. Syversen, S.W.; Goll, G.L.; Jørgensen, K.K.; Sandanger, Ø.; Sexton, J.; Olsen, I.C.; Gehin, J.E.; Warren, D.J.; Brun, M.K.; Klaasen, R.A.; et al. Effect of Therapeutic Drug Monitoring vs Standard Therapy During Infliximab Induction on Disease Remission in Patients with Chronic Immune-Mediated Inflammatory Diseases. *JAMA* **2021**, *325*, 1744–1754. [CrossRef]
42. Rutgeerts, P.; Feagan, B.G.; Lichtenstein, G.R.; Mayer, L.F.; Schreiber, S.; Colombel, J.F.; Rachmilewitz, D.; Wolf, D.C.; Olson, A.; Bao, W.; et al. Comparison of scheduled and episodic treatment strategies of infliximab in Crohn's disease. *Gastroenterology* **2004**, *126*, 402–413. [CrossRef] [PubMed]
43. Baert, F.; Drobne, D.; Gils, A.; Casteele, N.V.; Hauenstein, S.; Singh, S.; Lockton, S.; Rutgeerts, P.; Vermeire, S. Early Trough Levels and Antibodies to Infliximab Predict Safety and Success of Reinitiation of Infliximab Therapy. *Clin. Gastroenterol. Hepatol.* **2014**, *12*, 1474–1481.e2. [CrossRef]
44. Peris, M.A.; Bosó, V.; Navarro, B.; Marqués-Miñana, M.R.; Bastida, G.; Beltrán, B.; Iborra, M.; Sáez-González, E.; Monte-Boquet, E.; Poveda-Andrés, J.L.; et al. Serum Adalimumab Levels Predict Successful Remission and Safe Deintensification in Inflammatory Bowel Disease Patients in Clinical Practice. *Inflamm. Bowel Dis.* **2017**, *23*, 1454–1460. [CrossRef]
45. Louis, E.; Mary, J.; Vernier–Massouille, G.; Grimaud, J.; Bouhnik, Y.; Laharie, D.; Dupas, J.; Pillant, H.; Picon, L.; Veyrac, M.; et al. Maintenance of Remission Among Patients with Crohn's Disease on Antimetabolite Therapy After Infliximab Therapy Is Stopped. *Gastroenterology* **2012**, *142*, 63–70.e5. [CrossRef] [PubMed]
46. Hanauer, S.B. A Never Ending STORI. *Clin. Gastroenterol. Hepatol.* **2018**, *16*, 1034–1036. [CrossRef] [PubMed]
47. Cheifetz, A.; Smedley, M.; Martin, S.; Reiter, M.; Leone, G.; Mayer, L.; Plevy, S. The Incidence and Management of Infusion Reactions to Infliximab: A Large Center Experience. *Am. J. Gastroenterol.* **2003**, *98*, 1315–1324. [CrossRef]

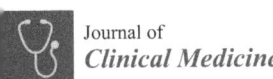

Review

Therapeutic Drug Monitoring in Perianal Fistulizing Crohn's Disease

Mir Zulqarnain [1], Parakkal Deepak [2] and Andres J. Yarur [3],*

[1] Department of Medicine, Medical College of Wisconsin, Milwaukee, WI 53226, USA; mzulqarnain@mcw.edu
[2] Division of Gastroenterology, Washington University in St. Louis School of Medicine, St. Louis, MO 63110, USA; deepak.parakkal@wustl.edu
[3] Division of Gastroenterology, Medical College of Wisconsin, Milwaukee, WI 53226, USA
* Correspondence: ajyarur@gmail.com

Abstract: Perianal fistulas are a common complication of Crohn's disease (CD) that has, historically, been challenging to manage. Despite the strong available evidence that anti-tumor necrosis factor (anti-TNF) agents are useful in the treatment of perianal fistulizing Crohn's disease (PFCD), a significant number of these patients do not respond to therapy. The use of therapeutic drug monitoring (TDM) in patients with CD receiving biologic agents has evolved and is currently positioned as an important tool to optimize and guide biologic treatment. Considering the treatment of PFCD can represent a challenge; identifying novel tools to improve the efficacy of current treatments is an important unmet need. Given its emerging role in other phenotypes of Crohn's disease, the use of TDM could also offer an opportunity to enhance the effectiveness of available therapies and improve outcomes in the subset of patients with PFCD receiving biologics. Overall, there is mounting evidence that higher anti-TNF drug levels are associated with better rates of "fistula healing". However, studies have been limited by their use of subjective outcomes and observational designs. Ultimately, further interventional, randomized controlled trials looking into the relationship between drug exposure and fistula outcomes are needed.

Keywords: Crohn's disease; therapeutic drug monitoring; anti-tumor necrosis factor; perianal fistulas; infliximab; ustekinumab; vedolizumab; adalimumab

1. Introduction

Crohn's disease (CD) is an increasingly prevalent chronic inflammatory bowel disease (IBD) characterized by the development of inflammation in the gastrointestinal tract [1,2]. Among those patients with Crohn's disease, some develop perianal fistulizing Crohn's disease (PFCD). This is a debilitating phenotype that can be seen in up to a third of patients [3–5]. Its incidence increases with distal disease and its presence is associated with an overall worse prognosis [3,6]. It can lead to significant pain, perineal disfigurement, and fecal incontinence. Furthermore, patients with severe, refractory disease may also require proctectomy and permanent ostomy [7]. A multidisciplinary approach that includes combined medical and surgical therapies guided by radiologic and endoscopic diagnostics has shown to have a higher success rate in managing this phenotype than medical therapy alone [8]. Although there are multiple medical options available for the management of PFCD, most of them are limited in their overall efficacy.

Over the last decade, anti-tumor necrosis factor (anti-TNF) agents, particularly infliximab (IFX), have demonstrated their effectiveness in this subset of patients and have become first-line medical therapy in the treatment of PFCD. However, as with luminal Crohn's disease, a significant fraction of patients do not respond to therapy. This has led into the investigation of pharmacokinetic mechanisms of non-response, such as low drug levels and anti-drug antibodies with fistula healing. Observational studies have revealed limited evidence that the use of TDM in patients with PFCD on biologics may potentially have a role in improving outcomes. In this narrative review, we sought to summarize the current evidence behind those biologic therapies utilized in PFCD while highlighting the emerging role of TDM in patients presenting with this phenotype.

2. Evidence behind the Current Biologic Therapies Utilized in the Management of Perianal Fistulizing Crohn's Disease

Although there is growing evidence supporting the role of biologics in PFCD, there is a significant gap in knowledge regarding the positioning, optimization, and use of the biologics that are now available. Within these agents, IFX is one of the most recognized options due to the availability of randomized controlled trials supporting its efficacy in this patient population. The exact role of the newer generations of biologics, such as vedolizumab (VDZ) and ustekinumab (UST), remains less clear [9,10].

The first double-blind, placebo-controlled trial which studied anti-TNFs in PFCD was published in 1999 by Present et al. [11]. The study included 94 patients who were randomized to induction therapy with IFX dosed at 5 mg/kg, 10 mg/kg, or placebo at 0, 2, and 6 weeks. The primary endpoint of the trial was defined as a reduction of 50% or more in the number of draining fistulas at two or more consecutive study visits, which were required to be 21 days apart. The resolution of a draining fistula was defined as the lack of drainage upon gentle finger compression. The authors found that 68% of those patients receiving IFX at a dose of 5 mg/kg and 56% of those receiving IFX at a dose of 10 mg/kg achieved this primary endpoint. This rate of effectiveness was significantly higher than the 26% seen in the group that received placebo. Complete response, defined as absence of drainage on two consecutive visits, was seen in 55%, 38%, and 13% of patients treated with IFX 5 mg/kg, IFX 10 mg/kg, and placebo, respectively. The response rate in this initial trial did not appear dose related, with the 5 mg/kg group having a higher rate of response than the 10 mg/kg group.

A subsequent multicenter, double-blind, randomized, placebo-controlled trial performed by Sands et al. investigated the efficacy of IFX as a maintenance therapy for PFCD [12]. In this study, patients received an open label induction regimen of IFX 5 mg/kg at weeks 0, 2, and 6. Those patients that responded to treatment were then randomized to continue IFX 5 mg/kg or placebo every 8 weeks for 54 weeks. Response to treatment was defined as a reduction of at least 50% from baseline in the number of draining fistulas at weeks 10 and 14 after the induction regimen. The primary outcome was loss of response through week 54 of treatment defined as: recurrence of draining fistulas, need for additional or alternate therapy for worsening or persistent (luminal) disease, need for surgery, or self-discontinuation of the medication by the patient due to lack of efficacy. At the end of the follow-up, those patients that received IFX therapy had a significantly lower rate of loss of response when compared to those that received placebo (more than 40 weeks vs. 14 weeks, respectively [$p < 0.001$]).

What makes these trials unique is that they are among the few randomized controlled trials investigating a biologic agent for PCFD. However, a considerable limitation is the subjective nature of the primary endpoint of "fistula closure", as it was based on the investigators' physical evaluation of the patients and did include a more objective endpoint such as cross-sectional imaging. Additionally, the endpoint of "50% reduction in fistulas from baseline" was also left to the clinician's assessment and different clinicians may have interpreted this endpoint differently. In an ideal scenario, a clinical trial should have a more objective, centrally read primary outcome. This has been recognized by investigators and a recent systematic review noted that radiologic outcomes are becoming more increasingly incorporated into the primary endpoints of trials investigating PFCD [13].

The efficacy of another anti-TNF, adalimumab (ADA), was shown in a sub-group analysis of the CHARM trial which demonstrated that at week 26 of treatment, complete fistula closure (defined as closure of all fistulas that were draining at screening visits) was achieved in 30% in the ADA-treated patients versus 13% of those receiving placebo [14]. This difference remained significant through week 56. Most notably, all the patients that achieved complete fistula closure at week 26 remained in remission at week 56. Another retrospective cohort study conducted in 15 tertiary centers in Spain showed that at 6 months of therapy, 66% of patients treated with ADA experienced an improvement in complex fistulas [15]. A particular strength of this study was the use of magnetic resonance imaging to assess PFCD activity. The authors did find a correlation between clinical and radiological disease activity ($\kappa = 0.68$). A more recent meta-analysis consisting of seven studies and 379 patients found that 36% (95% CI: 0.31–0.41) of patients receiving ADA had obtained complete fistula closure (defined as no draining fistulas on examination) at follow up periods ranging from 4 to 56 weeks [16].

Unlike IFX and ADA, the role of other biologics, such as certolizumab-pegol, VDZ, and UST, is less certain. Sub-group analysis of larger studies such as the GEMINI II trial and registry data show that a higher percentage of patients on VDZ experience fistula closure when compared to placebo [17–23]. This association is supported by the recent ENTERPRISE trial, a phase 4, randomized, double-blind, multicenter trial which evaluated the efficacy of VDZ in PFCD in patients with CD with 1-3 MRI-confirmed perianal fistulas [10]. One arm received VDZ, 300 mg IV at weeks 0, 2, 6, 14, and 22, while the other arm received the same regimen with an additional VDZ dose at week 10. At week 30, 53.6% of all subjects included in the study achieved the primary endpoint of having greater than a 50% decrease from baseline in the number of draining perianal fistulae (defined as no longer draining despite gentle finger compression). The arm randomized to receive an extra dose of VDZ at week 10 did not have better outcomes when compared to the arm that had the standard treatment regimen. However, despite the strength of being a prospective study, the generalizability of this trial was limited due to its small sample size and lack of a placebo-arm.

Regarding ustekinumab, the recent BioLAP multicenter retrospective study showed that, out of patients who had been received ustekinumab (UST) therapy for at least 3 months, 38.5% with active PFCD at initiation of treatment reached the endpoint of "clinical success" at 6 months [9]. Clinical success was defined by the absence of draining purulent material as determined by a clinician, as well as not having a need for new medical or surgical intervention. This study also showed that, among patients with a history of PFCD that was inactive at the time of ustekinumab initiation, only 22% had a recurrence of perianal disease. Despite the encouraging results, the study is limited by its poor definition of fistulas and retrospective design.

3. Therapeutic Drug Monitoring: Current Application in Inflammatory Bowel Disease

Despite the proven efficacy of biologics in IBD, up to 30% experience primary non-response, while approximately another 40% develop secondary non-response over time, requiring dose optimization or the need to switch therapy. The development of immunogenicity against the drug and/or sub-optimal drug levels can explain a significant number of therapeutic failures [24].

The advent of therapeutic drug monitoring, defined as the evaluation of serum drug concentrations and the presence/titers of anti-drug antibodies at a specific point in time has helped clinicians guide treatment by allowing them to identify those patients that may experience a benefit with dose optimization versus those where increase the dose is likely futile and should switch therapies and/or strategies. Numerous studies have demonstrated that higher serum biologic concentrations are associated with improved objective therapeutic outcomes, such as mucosal healing and normalization of inflammatory markers [25–32]. However, these studies have shown an association and not causation. Drug levels may be lower in patients with a higher disease burden and higher drug clearance. An important debate has been regarding the use of "pro-active" TDM of anti-TNFs, where drug doses are adjusted with the goal of maintaining a specific drug threshold, independently of disease activity [33,34]. The results have been conflicting, mainly due to the heterogenicity in the characteristics of patients, potential difference in target drug levels, and limitations in study design, among others.

4. Anti-Tumor Necrosis Factor Drug Levels and Outcomes in Perianal Fistulizing Crohn's Disease

Studies looking into TDM and the association of anti-TNF drug levels and drug efficacy have also been conducted in sub-group of CD disease patients with specific phenotypes (Table 1). Emerging evidence has shown a strong association between higher anti-TNF drug levels and fistula healing in PFCD. A retrospective cohort study by Davidov et al. included 36 patients with active PFCD who received IFX at a standard dose of 5 mg/kg at weeks 0, 2, and 6, followed by every 8 weeks and looked at the association of drug levels and clinical response at week 14, defined as "decreased drainage of fistulas as reported by the patient and verified by a physician" [35]. The authors found that the group of patients with "clinical response" had higher median trough IFX levels when compared to those that did not (week 2, 20 vs. 5.6 µg/mL, $p = 0.0001$; week 6, 13.3 vs. 2.55 µg/mL $p = 0.0001$; and week 14, 4.1 vs. 0.14 µg/mL, $p = 0.01$). Specifically, IFX serum levels ≥ 9.25 µg/mL at Week 2 and ≥ 7.25 µg/mL at Week 6 were noted to be best associated with response to treatment at week 14. Despite its positive findings, this study had several limitations including a small sample size, retrospective study design, lack of follow up fistula imaging on most patients and the inherent subjective nature in which the outcomes were measured.

A larger retrospective study performed by Yarur et al. included 117 PFCD patients with an active fistula and showed that, at a median of 29 weeks of IFX therapy, those with healing of perianal fistula (defined as absence of drainage after gentle compression) had higher trough IFX concentrations in comparison to those with active disease (15.8 µg/mL versus 4.4 µg/mL; $p < 0.001$) [36]. Quartile analysis of serum IFX concentrations showed that IFX levels > 10.1 µg/mL and >20.3 µg/mL were associated with three- and eight-fold chance of fistula healing, respectively. Additionally, patients with fistula healing had a lower likelihood of having serum anti-IFX antibodies (OR, 0.04; 95% CI, 0.004–0.3, $p < 0.0001$) and IFX levels ≥ 10.1 mcg/mL were significantly associated with fistula closure (OR, 2.9; 95% CI, 1.1–8.7, $p < 0.036$). Notably, a subset of included patients achieved fistula healing only at levels of ≥ 20 mcg/mL, which potentially supports the approach of optimizing drug levels to this threshold prior to abandoning therapy in patients who have not experienced fistula healing at lower trough IFX levels. The study was limited given its retrospective study design and due to its failure in distinguishing simple vs. complex fistulas. As in other TDM studies, the results only proved an association and not causation. A particular strength of the study was that it contained the largest sample size of any study investigating this topic and did include patients who had received dose optimization/escalation, opening the possibility to assess the rates of fistula healing on those patients with a high IFX exposure.

Strik et al. added to this growing body of literature with a retrospective study investigating ADA in addition to IFX in the treatment of PCFD [37]. Patients maintained on these anti-TNFs were separated into two groups based on the status of their fistulas (actively draining or non-draining). Fistula closure was defined as the absence of purulent discharge upon gentle finger compression and/or fistula closure on MRI of the pelvis. The authors found that serum trough levels were significantly higher in patients with fistula closure as compared to those with active drainage in both IFX (6.0 µg/mL vs. 2.3 µg/mL; $p < 0.001$) and ADA groups (7.4 µg/mL vs. 4.8 µg/mL; $p = 0.003$). An IFX trough level of ≥ 5 µg/mL and an ADA trough level ≥ 5.9 was significantly associated with perianal fistula closure. For IFX, higher closure rates were seen in those naïve to biologics and with combination therapy as opposed to the patients receiving monotherapy. In the ADA group, the treatment duration and combined use of a seton was associated with higher rates of fistula closure. The objectivity provided by MRI (as opposed to the subjectivity of physical exam) was a particular strength of this study.

Table 1. Studies demonstrating association between increased biologic drug levels with fistula healing in PFCD.

Author (Year)	Population	No. of Subjects	Anti-TNF	Primary Outcome	Drug Concentration in Active Fistulas (µg/mL)	Drug Concentration in Healed/Closed Fistulas (µg/mL)	Strengths	Limitations
Davidov et al. [35] (2016)	Adults	36	IFX	Decrease in drainage of fistulas	Week 2: 5.6 µg/mL Week 6: 2.55 µg/mL Week 14: 0.14 µg/mL	Week 2: 20.0 µg/mL Week 6: 13.3 µg/mL Week 14: 4.1 µg/mL	Similar demographics in both groups	small sample size, no imaging, subjective outcome
Yarur et al. [36] (2016)	Adults	117	IFX	absence of drainage	4.4 µg/mL	15.8 µg/mL	Large sample size	Retrospective, didn't distinguish simple vs. complex fistulas
Strik et al. [37] (2019)	Adults	47 IFX 19 ADA	IFX ADA	absence of discharge upon gentle finger and/or fistula closure on MRI	IFX: 2.3 µg/mL ADA: 4.8 µg/mL	IFX: 6.0 µg/mL ADA: 7.4 µg/mL	Assessment with imaging	Retrospective, didn't distinguish simple vs. complex fistulas
Plevris et al. [38] (2020)	Adults	29 IFX 35 ADA	IFX ADA	Absence of drainage	IFX: 3.2 µg/mL ADA: 2.7 µg/mL	IFX: 8.1 µg/mL ADA: 12.6 µg/mL	Secondary outcome of fistula closure	Retrospective, no imaging
Et Matary et al. [39] (2019)	Pediatric	27	IFX	Decrease in drainage of fistulas	5.4 µg/mL	12.7 ug/mL	Prospective study	Small sample size
Ruemmele et al. [40] (2018)	Pediatric	36	ADA	Closure of baseline fistulas or decrease in number by ≥50%	Week 16: 7.0 ug/mL Week 52: 6.1 ug/mL	Week 16: 7.4 ug/mL Week 52: 10.0 ug/mL	Well defined endpoints	Not powered to detect statistical difference, not randomized, not placebo controlled
Papamichael et al. [41] (2021)	Adults	Induction group n = 282 maintenance group n = 139	IFX	Fistula response: reduction of at least 50% of draining fistulas from baseline	No Response: 4.0 µg/mL	Response: 5.7 µg/mL	large sample size, the use of stringent endpoints	No imaging assessment of fistula, not randomized
De Gregario et al. [42] (2021)	Adults	117 IFX 76 ADA	IFX	Radiologic healing (inflammatory subscore ≤6 on Van Assche Index)	IFX: 3.9 µg/mL ADA: 6.2 µg/mL	IFX: 6.0 µg/mL ADA: 9.1 µg/mL	Use of radiographic parameters	Not placebo controlled, not randomized
Schwartz, D. A et al. [10] (2021)	Adults	VDZ (16) VDZ +10 (18)	VDZ	≥50% decrease from baseline in the number of draining perianal fistulae at week 30	~33 µg/mL (pooled trough conc. week 10)	~28 µg/mL (pooled trough conc. week 10)	Multicenter- RCT, use of MRI	Small sample size, no placebo arm

Plevris et al. also investigated both IFX and ADA for PFCD with a retrospective cross-sectional study including 64 patients on maintenance therapy for at least 24 weeks [38]. Drug levels were measured ±4 weeks of the clinical assessment of the fistula. IFX drug and antibody levels were measured at trough, while for ADA drug and antibody levels were measured at any time between doses. The primary outcome was perianal fistula healing (defined as the absence of drainage) and the secondary outcome was perianal fistula closure (defined as no external skin opening in the peri-anal area). Patients with fistula healing had higher levels of anti-TNF trough levels vs. those without fistula healing (ADA: 12.6 vs. 2.7 µg/mL, $p < 0.01$; IFX: 8.1 vs. 3.2 µg/mL, $p < 0.01$). Patients with fistula closure also had significantly higher anti-TNF trough levels vs. those without fistula closure (ADA: 14.8 vs. 5.7 µg/mL, $p < 0.01$; IFX: 8.2 vs. 3.2 µg/mL, $p < 0.01$). Receiver operating characteristic analysis revealed a cutoff of ≥ 6.8 µg/mL for fistula healing and ≥ 9.8 µg/mL for fistula closure in patients receiving ADA and an optimum trough of ≥ 7.1 µg/mL for both fistula healing and closure for IFX. Again, the retrospective design of the study and lack of objective evaluation of the fistulas with imaging were limitations of this study.

El-Matary et al. performed a multicenter prospective cohort study including 27 pediatric patients (<17 years) with PCFD who were treated with IFX and who had serum trough drug titers measured before the fourth dose [39]. The median IFX pre-fourth dose level in the responders (defined as a decrease in drainage of fistulas) was 12.7 ug/mL, compared with 5.4 ug/mL in the group with no response ($p = 0.02$). A particular strength of this study was its prospective study design; however, the small sample size, lack of long term follow up, and the subjective primary outcome were notable limitations.

In a post-hoc analysis, Ruemmele et al. performed a sub-analysis of the data from the IMAgINE 1 and IMAgINE 2 trials [40]. These trials cumulatively followed pediatric patients for 292 weeks and demonstrated the efficacy of ADA in fistula closure and fistula improvement (as defined as closure of all baseline fistulas or decrease in number by ≥ 50%, respectively, for at least two consecutive visits). The patients were randomly assigned to receive either high dose ADA (defined as 20 mg every other week [EOW] or 40 mg EOW if >40 kg) or standard doses (defined as 10 mg every other week [EOW] or 20 mg EOW if >40 kg). Although the concentration of ADA in patients with fistula closure trended slightly higher than those not achieving fistula closure at weeks 16 (7.4 µg/mL vs. 7.0 µg/mL) and 52 (10 µg/mL vs. 6.1 µg/mL), there was no statistically significant difference between the two groups. While this contradicted the adult studies and findings of El Matary et al., the limited study was not powered to detect statistical differences between treatment groups, did not have a placebo-arm, and lacked objective assessment of fistula closure with pelvic MRI.

The most recent evidence supporting optimizing post-induction IFX levels arises from a post hoc analysis of the ACCENT-II trial by Papamichael et al., which evaluated patients with fistulizing CD receiving induction and maintenance infliximab therapy [41]. Measured outcomes included fistula response (defined as a reduction of at least 50% of draining fistulas from baseline), complete fistula remission (defined as absence of draining fistulas), CRP normalization (defined as a CRP level ≤ 5 mg/L), and, finally, a composite outcome of both complete fistula remission combined with CRP normalization at week 14 and week 54. Higher week 14 IFX concentrations were independently associated with week 14 fistula response (odds ratio [OR]: 1.16; 95% confidence interval [CI]: 1.02–1.32; $p = 0.019$), and composite remission (OR: 2.32; 95% CI: 1.55–3.49; $p < 0.001$). Higher week 14 IFX concentrations were also independently associated with week 54 composite remission (OR: 2.05; 95% CI: 1.10–3.82; $p = 0.023$). ROC curve analysis identified an IFX concentration of ≥ 9.6 µg/mL at week 6 to be associated with complete fistula response at week 54. Most notably, the analysis revealed that IFX concentrations of ≥ 26.1 µg/mL at week 6 and ≥ 8.7 µg/mL at week 14 were associated with the highest rates of early composite remission (36% and 48%, respectively). Furthermore, IFX concentrations ≥ 11.3 µg/mL at week 14 were associated with the highest rate of long-term composite remission. These findings are interesting and open the debate on whether proactively increasing infliximab doses early on therapy may improve short- and long-term outcomes. Randomized controlled trials are warranted to support this hypothesis.

A cross-sectional retrospective study by De Gregario et al. added a more objective viewpoint to existing evidence by documenting the association of anti-TNF levels and radiologic fistula outcomes [42]. This study included 193 patients with PFCD on maintenance IFX or ADA who had drug levels checked within 6 months of a pelvic MRI. Radiologic disease activity was scored using the Van Assche Index (VAI) with an inflammatory subscore calculated using multiple indices: T2-weighted imaging hyperintensity, collections > 3 mm diameter, and rectal wall involvement. The primary endpoint was radiologic healing (inflammatory subscore ≤ 6). The secondary endpoint was radiologic remission (inflammatory subscore = 0). Patients with radiologic healing had higher median drug levels compared with those with active disease (IFX 6.0 vs. 3.9 µg/mL; ADA 9.1 vs. 6.2 µg/mL; $p < 0.05$ for both). Patients with radiologic remission also had higher median drug levels compared with those with active disease (IFX 7.4 vs. 3.9 µg/mL; $p < 0.05$; ADA 9.8 vs. 6.2 µg/mL; $p = 0.07$). This study is unique because most of the other retrospective trials had a largely subjective definition of fistula healing and lacked the objectivity provided by imaging studies. Despite this distinguishing attribute, the study does have multiple limitations. The VAI is not a validated scoring index and since the imaging was not centrally reviewed, there was inherent risk of variability and bias from the different radiologists interpreting the images.

Prospective randomized studies looking into the association of fistula healing and VDZ and UST serum levels are scarce. Data from the ENTERPRISE study did show that, in the group that received VDZ with an extra dose at week 10, patients with fistula healing had a higher pooled VDZ trough concentration between weeks 6 and 22 of the study. However, since more patients terminated treatment early in this group, and given the overall small sample size, the authors were unable to draw a definitive conclusion regarding the relationship between VDZ drug exposure and treatment response [10].

5. Discussion

The management of PFCD typically combines a medical and surgical approach. Biologics, especially anti-TNF agents, have demonstrated an important role in the treatment of PFCD. The current evidence supports an association between higher IFX and ADA serum drug levels with higher rates of fistula healing. Considering these findings, it would be tempting for many clinicians to assume that increasing drug doses could improve outcomes. However, randomized controlled trials are needed to prove this hypothesis. The lower drug levels seen in those patients that do not achieve fistula healing could potentially be explained by a higher inflammatory burden and higher drug clearance. The current literature is also significantly limited by deficits in study design, low sample sizes, variability in patient selection, failure to stratify different types of fistulas, and lack of objective endpoints.

One ongoing interventional randomized controlled study by Gu et al. may offer a better insight on how TDM could effectively be used in PFCD [43]. The PROACTIVE trial (Prospective randomized controlled trial of adults with perianal fistulizing Crohn's disease and optimized therapeutic IFX levels) is enrolling patients with active PFCD randomized to either a proactive TDM group or standard dosing group with a 54 week follow up period. The proactive TDM group will have IFX dosing optimized to target higher trough concentrations at various time points (≥ 25 µg/mL at week 2, ≥ 20 µg/mL at week 6 and ≥ 10 µg/mL during maintenance therapy). The standard arm will be treated with the standard 5 mg/Kg dose of IFX at weeks 0, 2, and 6 weeks followed by every 8 weeks. The primary outcome of the study will be fistula healing at week 32 and secondary outcomes include fistula closure, fistula healing, radiological fistula healing, economic costs, and patient-reported outcomes. The addition of a radiologic outcome will serve to support the more subjective, clinical primary outcome. This is helpful as many of the studies reviewed lack this level of objectivity.

This randomized trial may also help prove causation and not just correlation when it comes to increased drug levels and improved fistula healing. Currently there is a strong association between the two, but the decreased serum levels in non-healing fistulas may be due to other factors, such as increased drug clearance and a higher inflammatory burden. This concern is supported by the ATLAS study which showed that there are also localized tissue factors that play a role in variations of local and systemic drug levels [44]. This study was unique in that it not only reported an accurate measurement of tissue levels of anti-TNF drug in luminal Crohn's disease, but also found that these levels correlated well with the serum drug levels. The key finding of the study suggested that areas of severe luminal inflammation act as a 'sink' for the drug and resulted in diminished localized tissue drug levels. This drop in specific tissue drug levels may, thereby, be reducing its concentration and, therefore, efficacy in another area of inflammation, thus, leading to a mismatch in serum and tissue drug levels in these patients. The authors proposed this as an explanation for why patients with "normal" serum drug levels may still have uncontrolled disease and suggested that increasing these levels may result in improved outcomes. More recently, the same authors observed that increased serum infliximab levels were also associated with improved fistula healing in PFCD as compared to those with luminal disease. This leads to the question of possibly insufficient drug concentrations within the perianal tissues as a possible mechanistic explanation in treatment failure.

This question was recently explored by a pilot study assessing the fistula tissue levels of anti-TNF agents (infliximab and adalimumab) by use of ultraperformance liquid chromatography-mass spectrometry [45]. The authors obtained tissue samples from the fistula tracts of seven patients with Crohn's perianal disease (five patients on adalimumab and two patients on infliximab) on maintenance treatment and compared tissue drug activity to negatives controls and spiked positive controls. They observed a lack of drug activity in all fistula samples taken from Crohn's on maintenance therapy despite activity in positive controls. This raises the question on how tissue and serum pharmacokinetics are related and what role that the administration of higher doses may have on outcomes.

Higher dosing sub-groups do not always have better outcomes, as seen in the study cited above by Present et al. [11]. Although increasing dose and shortening intervals between doses has been shown to increase drug levels and clinical response in luminal disease there is significant pharmacologic variation between individuals. Patient characteristics such as high body weight, low albumin, and presence of ATI have been documented factors in increasing clearance of serum anti-TNF and leading to decreased serum levels [46]. There is also evidence that suggests shortening dose intervals may be a better way in increasing serum drug concentrations as opposed to simply increasing the medication dosage, especially in patients with low serum albumin levels. The development of an optimal, individualized dosing strategy for PFCD must consider all of these factors.

Another major question that warrants further investigation is the role that non-anti-TNF biologics can play in the treatment algorithm of PFCD and how the use of TDM for those drugs may help to optimize therapy in this patient population. Aside from observational evidence showing a possible dose-related response, there are limited randomized controlled data to guide the incorporation of these agents into the management of PFCD.

A recent multicenter randomized, controlled trial (ENTERPRISE) supported the use of VDZ in the treatment algorithm of PFCD by demonstrating a 53.6% pooled success rate in achieving the primary endpoint of having greater than a 50% decrease from baseline in the number of draining perianal fistulae [10]. This study also boasted a 71.4% fistula closure rate during the 30 week follow up period. Additionally, patients that responded to treatment trended towards a higher VDZ trough concentration between weeks 6 and 22 in the study arm that administered an extra dose of VDZ at week 10. However, despite these significant findings, the study was substantially limited by its lack of placebo-arm, small sample size ($n = 38$) and inability to support the findings with radiographic data.

No randomized controlled trials have assessed the efficacy of UST in PFCD; however, the recently published BioLAP multicenter, retrospective study showed that, out of patients who had been received UST therapy for at least 3 months, 38.5% with active PFCD at initiation of treatment reached the endpoint of "clinical success" at 6 months [9]. The interpretation of these data is limited by the subjective definition of the main outcome as it relied on a physician's interpretation of fistula drainage and not a more objective outcome such as radiographic healing. Additionally, due to the retrospective nature of this study, the authors were not able to assess the relationship between serum UST levels and fistula response. They did find, however, that the lack of optimization of UST was associated with improved outcomes, but this was attributed to the refractory nature of disease in those that required aggressive drug optimization. Given this potential confounder and lack of drug level comparison between responders and non-responders in this study, the role of TDM with UST and PFCD remains unclear. Although this study shows a definite correlation between UST use and fistula healing, the exact role of UST in the treatment of PFCD remains uncertain and further prospective, randomized studies are needed.

Lastly, although this review focuses on the optimization of medical therapy with TDM, it is important to remember the crucial role of surgery in the management of PFCD. A combined medical and surgical approach in managing PFCD has shown to have better outcomes than medical therapy alone [47–49]. Irrespective of the prescribed medical therapies, individualized interventions, such as abscess drainage, seton placement, fistulectomy, fistulotomy, ligation, and advancement flaps, may be needed and, therefore, surgical consultation should be obtained to further guide these decisions.

6. Conclusions

PFCD is a challenging and debilitating phenotype of CD that has been historically difficult to manage. Anti-TNF agents, especially IFX, have emerged as the cornerstone of medical management in these patients. High quality evidence supporting the efficacy of most biologics and the potential role of TDM in PFCD is limited. Overall, the evidence supports that higher anti-TNF drug levels correlate with higher efficacy; however, no high quality, interventional data are available. This is partly because performing high quality clinical trials in PFCD can be challenging and costly. Moreover, conducting, and interpreting TDM studies impose their own challenges. Drug level concentrations may vary between laboratories and assays, which limits the extrapolation and comparison of results. Moreover, endpoints may vary across studies and patient demographics and selection may also complicate the interpretation of the data. Despite these challenges, further investigations in TDM are undergoing and may lead to a future of individualized and optimized management in patients not only with PFCD, but with IBD in general.

Author Contributions: M.Z. was responsible for drafting all sections of the paper, including first draft, and correcting subsequent revisions. P.D. was responsible for editing and review of subsequent drafts. A.J.Y. was responsible for editing and review of each draft preparation, as well as taking on the role of senior, supervisory author. All authors have read and agreed to the published version of the manuscript.

Funding: This research received no external funding.

Institutional Review Board Statement: Not applicable.

Informed Consent Statement: Not applicable.

Data Availability Statement: Not applicable.

Conflicts of Interest: M.Z., no disclosures. P.D. participated in consulting or advisory board, for Janssen, Pfizer, Prometheus Biosciences, Boehringer Ingelheim, Arena Pharmaceuticals, Scipher Medicine, and CorEvitas, LLC, as well as receiving funding under a sponsored research agreement unrelated to the data in the paper from Takeda Pharmaceutical, Arena Pharmaceuticals, Bristol Myers Squibb-Celgene, and Boehringer Ingelheim. A.J.Y., Consultant Takeda, Arena pharmaceuticals, Prometheus Labs and Bristol Myers Squibb. Speaker bureau, Bristol Myers Squibb.

References

1. Abraham, C.; Cho, J.H. Inflammatory Bowel Disease. *N. Engl. J. Med.* **2009**, *361*, 2066–2078. [CrossRef] [PubMed]
2. Molodecky, N.A.; Soon, I.S.; Rabi, D.M.; Ghali, W.A.; Ferris, M.; Chernoff, G.; Benchimol, E.I.; Panaccione, R.; Ghosh, S.; Barkema, H.W.; et al. Increasing Incidence and Prevalence of the Inflammatory Bowel Diseases with Time, Based on Systematic Review. *Gastroenterology* **2012**, *142*, 46–54.e42. [CrossRef] [PubMed]
3. Hellers, G.; Bergstrand, O.; Ewerth, S.; Holmström, B. Occurrence and outcome after primary treatment of anal fistulae in Crohn's disease. *Gut* **1980**, *21*, 525–527. [CrossRef]
4. Schwartz, D.A.; Loftus, E.V., Jr.; Tremaine, W.J.; Panaccione, R.; Harmsen, W.S.; Zinsmeister, A.R.; Sandborn, W.J. The natural history of fistulizing Crohn's disease in Olmsted County, Minnesota. *Gastroenterology* **2002**, *122*, 875–880. [CrossRef]
5. Ardizzone, S.; Porro, G.B. Perianal Crohn's disease: Overview. *Dig. Liver Dis.* **2007**, *39*, 957–958. [CrossRef] [PubMed]
6. Beaugerie, L.; Seksik, P.; Nion–Larmurier, I.; Gendre, J.; Cosnes, J. Predictors of Crohn's Disease. *Gastroenterology* **2006**, *130*, 650–656. [CrossRef]
7. Bell, S.J.; Williams, A.B.; Wiesel, P.; Wilkinson, K.; Cohen, R.C.G.; Kamm, M.A. The clinical course of fistulating Crohn's disease. *Aliment. Pharmacol. Ther.* **2003**, *17*, 1145–1151. [CrossRef]
8. Yassin, N.A.; Askari, A.; Warusavitarne, J.; Faiz, O.D.; Athanasiou, T.; Phillips, R.K.S.; Hart, A.L. Systematic review: The combined surgical and medical treatment of fistulising perianal Crohn's disease. *Aliment. Pharmacol. Ther.* **2014**, *40*, 741–749. [CrossRef]
9. Chapuis-Biron, C.; Kirchgesner, J.; Pariente, B.; Bouhnik, Y.; Amiot, A.; Viennot, S.; Serrero, M.; Fumery, M.; Allez, M.; Siproudhis, L.; et al. Ustekinumab for Perianal Crohn's Disease: The BioLAP Multicenter Study From the GETAID. *Am. J. Gastroenterol.* **2020**, *115*, 1812–1820. [CrossRef]
10. Schwartz, D.A.; Peyrin-Biroulet, L.; Lasch, K.; Adsul, S.; Danese, S. Efficacy and Safety of 2 Vedolizumab Intravenous Regimens for Perianal Fistulizing Crohn's Disease: ENTERPRISE Study. *Clin. Gastroenterol. Hepatol. Off. Clin. Pract. J. Am. Gastroenterol. Assoc.* **2021**, in press. [CrossRef]
11. Present, D.H.; Rutgeerts, P.; Targan, S.; Hanauer, S.B.; Mayer, L.; Van Hogezand, R.A.; Podolsky, D.K.; Sands, B.E.; Braakman, T.; DeWoody, K.L.; et al. Infliximab for the Treatment of Fistulas in Patients with Crohn's Disease. *N. Engl. J. Med.* **1999**, *340*, 1398–1405. [CrossRef] [PubMed]
12. Sands, B.E.; Anderson, F.H.; Bernstein, C.N.; Chey, W.Y.; Feagan, B.G.; Fedorak, R.; Kamm, M.A.; Korzenik, J.R.; Lashner, B.A.; Onken, J.E.; et al. Infliximab Maintenance Therapy for Fistulizing Crohn's Disease. *N. Engl. J. Med.* **2004**, *350*, 876–885. [CrossRef] [PubMed]
13. Caron, B.; D'Amico, F.; Danese, S.; Peyrin-Biroulet, L. Endpoints for Perianal Crohn's Disease Trials: Past, Present and Future. *J. Crohn's Colitis* **2021**, *15*, 1387–1398. [CrossRef] [PubMed]
14. Colombel, J.; Sandborn, W.J.; Rutgeerts, P.; Enns, R.; Hanauer, S.B.; Panaccione, R.; Schreiber, S.; Byczkowski, D.; Li, J.; Kent, J.D.; et al. Adalimumab for Maintenance of Clinical Response and Remission in Patients with Crohn's Disease: The CHARM Trial. *Gastroenterology* **2007**, *132*, 52–65. [CrossRef]
15. Castaño-Milla, C.; Chaparro, M.; Saro, C.; Acosta, M.B.-D.; García-Albert, A.M.; Bujanda, L.; Martín-Arranz, M.D.; Carpio, D.; Muñoz, F.; Manceñido, N.; et al. Effectiveness of Adalimumab in Perianal Fistulas in Crohn's Disease Patients Naive to Anti-TNF Therapy. *J. Clin. Gastroenterol.* **2015**, *49*, 34–40. [CrossRef]
16. Fu, Y.-M.; Chen, M.; Liao, A.-J. A Meta-Analysis of Adalimumab for Fistula in Crohn's Disease. *Gastroenterol. Res. Pract.* **2017**, *2017*, 1745692. [CrossRef]
17. Chapuis-Biron, C.; Bourrier, A.; Nachury, M.; Nancey, S.; Bouhnik, Y.; Serrero, M.; Armengol-Debeir, L.; Buisson, A.; Tran-Minh, M.-L.; Zallot, C.; et al. Vedolizumab for perianal Crohn's disease: A multicentre cohort study in 151 patients. *Aliment. Pharmacol. Ther.* **2020**, *51*, 719–727. [CrossRef]
18. Feagan, B.G.; Schwartz, D.; Danese, S.; Rubin, D.T.; Lissoos, T.W.; Xu, J.; Lasch, K. Efficacy of Vedolizumab in Fistulising Crohn's Disease: Exploratory Analyses of Data from GEMINI 2. *J. Crohn's Colitis* **2018**, *12*, 621–626. [CrossRef]
19. Biemans, V.B.C.; Jong, A.E.V.D.M.-D.; Van Der Woude, C.J.; Löwenberg, M.; Dijkstra, G.; Oldenburg, B.; de Boer, N.; Van Der Marel, S.; Bodelier, A.G.L.; Jansen, J.M.; et al. Ustekinumab for Crohn's Disease: Results of the ICC Registry, a Nationwide Prospective Observational Cohort Study. *J. Crohn's Colitis* **2020**, *14*, 33–45. [CrossRef]
20. Attauabi, M.; Burisch, J.; Seidelin, J.B. Efficacy of ustekinumab for active perianal fistulizing Crohn's disease: A systematic review and meta-analysis of the current literature. *Scand. J. Gastroenterol.* **2021**, *56*, 53–58. [CrossRef]
21. Sandborn, W.W.; Feagan, B.G.; Stoinov, S.; Honiball, P.J.; Rutgeerts, P.; Mason, D.; Bloomfield, R.; Schreiber, S.; PRECISE 1 Study Investigators. Certolizumab Pegol for the Treatment of Crohn's Disease. *N. Engl. J. Med.* **2007**, *357*, 228–238. [CrossRef] [PubMed]
22. Schreiber, S.; Khaliq-Kareemi, M.; Lawrance, I.C.; Thomsen, O.Ø.; Hanauer, S.B.; McColm, J.; Bloomfield, R.; Sandborn, W.J.; PRECISE 2 Study Investigators. Maintenance Therapy with Certolizumab Pegol for Crohn's Disease. *N. Engl. J. Med.* **2007**, *357*, 239–250. [CrossRef] [PubMed]
23. Schreiber, S.; Lawrance, I.C.; Thomsen, O.Ø.; Hanauer, S.B.; Bloomfield, R.; Sandborn, W.J. Randomised clinical trial: Certolizumab pegol for fistulas in Crohn's disease-subgroup results from a placebo-controlled study. *Aliment. Pharmacol. Ther.* **2010**, *33*, 185–193. [CrossRef] [PubMed]
24. Papamichael, K.; Gils, A.; Rutgeerts, P.; Levesque, B.G.; Vermeire, S.; Sandborn, W.J.; Casteele, N.V. Role for Therapeutic Drug Monitoring During Induction Therapy with TNF Antagonists in IBD: Evolution in the definition and management of primary nonresponse. *Inflamm. Bowel Dis.* **2015**, *21*, 182–197. [CrossRef]

25. Papamichael, K.; Cheifetz, A.S. Use of anti-TNF drug levels to optimise patient management. *Front. Gastroenterol.* **2016**, *7*, 289–300. [CrossRef]
26. Vande Casteele, N.; Khanna, R.; Levesque, B.G.; Stitt, L.; Zou, G.Y.; Singh, S.; Lockton, S.; Hauenstein, S.; Ohrmund, L.; Greenberg, G.R.; et al. The relationship between infliximab concentrations, antibodies to infliximab and disease activity in Crohn's disease. *Gut* **2015**, *64*, 1539–1545. [CrossRef]
27. Casteele, N.V.; Ferrante, M.; Van Assche, G.; Ballet, V.; Compernolle, G.; Van Steen, K.; Simoens, S.; Rutgeerts, P.; Gils, A.; Vermeire, S. Trough Concentrations of Infliximab Guide Dosing for Patients with Inflammatory Bowel Disease. *Gastroenterology* **2015**, *148*, 1320–1329.e3. [CrossRef]
28. Papamichael, K.; Van Stappen, T.; Vande Casteele, N.; Gils, A.; Billiet, T.; Tops, S.; Claes, K.; Van Assche, G.; Rutgeerts, P.; Vermeire, S.; et al. Infliximab Concentration Thresholds During Induction Therapy Are Associated with Short-term Mucosal Healing in Patients with Ulcerative Colitis. *Clin. Gastroenterol. Hepatol.* **2016**, *14*, 543–549. [CrossRef]
29. Rosario, M.; French, J.L.; Dirks, N.L.; Sankoh, S.; Parikh, A.; Yang, H.; Danese, S.; Colombel, J.-F.; Smyth, M.; Sandborn, W.J.; et al. Exposure–efficacy Relationships for Vedolizumab Induction Therapy in Patients with Ulcerative Colitis or Crohn's Disease. *J. Crohn's Colitis* **2017**, *11*, 921–929. [CrossRef]
30. Pouillon, L.; Vermeire, S.; Bossuyt, P. Vedolizumab trough level monitoring in inflammatory bowel disease: A state-of-the-art overview. *BMC Med.* **2019**, *17*, 89. [CrossRef]
31. Battat, R.; Kopylov, U.; Bessissow, T.; Bitton, A.; Cohen, A.; Jain, A.; Martel, M.; Seidman, E.; Afif, W. Association between Ustekinumab Trough Concentrations and Clinical, Biomarker, and Endoscopic Outcomes in Patients with Crohn's Disease. *Clin. Gastroenterol. Hepatol.* **2017**, *15*, 1427–1434.e2. [CrossRef] [PubMed]
32. Ungar, B.; Levy, I.; Yavne, Y.; Yavzori, M.; Picard, O.; Fudim, E.; Loebstein, R.; Chowers, Y.; Eliakim, R.; Kopylov, U.; et al. Optimizing Anti-TNF-α Therapy: Serum Levels of Infliximab and Adalimumab Are Associated with Mucosal Healing in Patients with Inflammatory Bowel Diseases. *Clin. Gastroenterol. Hepatol.* **2016**, *14*, 550–557.e2. [CrossRef] [PubMed]
33. D'Haens, G.; Vermeire, S.; Lambrecht, G.; Baert, F.; Bossuyt, P.; Pariente, B.; Buisson, A.; Bouhnik, Y.; Filippi, J.; Woude, J.V.; et al. Increasing Infliximab Dose Based on Symptoms, Biomarkers, and Serum Drug Concentrations Does Not Increase Clinical, Endoscopic, and Corticosteroid-Free Remission in Patients with Active Luminal Crohn's Disease. *Gastroenterology* **2018**, *154*, 1343–1351.e1. [CrossRef] [PubMed]
34. Assa, A.; Matar, M.; Turner, D.; Broide, E.; Weiss, B.; Ledder, O.; Guz-Mark, A.; Rinawi, F.; Cohen, S.; Topf-Olivestone, C.; et al. Proactive Monitoring of Adalimumab Trough Concentration Associated with Increased Clinical Remission in Children with Crohn's Disease Compared with Reactive Monitoring. *Gastroenterology* **2019**, *157*, 985–996.e2. [CrossRef] [PubMed]
35. Davidov, Y.; Ungar, B.; Bar-Yoseph, H.; Carter, D.; Haj-Natour, O.; Yavzori, M.; Chowers, Y.; Eliakim, R.; Ben-Horin, S.; Kopylov, U. Association of Induction Infliximab Levels with Clinical Response in Perianal Crohn's Disease. *J. Crohn's Colitis* **2016**, *11*, 549–555. [CrossRef] [PubMed]
36. Yarur, A.J.; Kanagala, V.; Stein, D.J.; Czul, F.; Quintero, M.A.; Agrawal, D.; Patel, A.; Best, K.; Fox, C.; Idstein, K.; et al. Higher infliximab trough levels are associated with perianal fistula healing in patients with Crohn's disease. *Aliment. Pharmacol. Ther.* **2017**, *45*, 933–940. [CrossRef] [PubMed]
37. Strik, A.S.; Löwenberg, M.; Buskens, C.J.; Gecse, K.B.; Ponsioen, C.I.; Bemelman, W.A.; D'Haens, G.R. Higher anti-TNF serum levels are associated with perianal fistula closure in Crohn's disease patients. *Scand. J. Gastroenterol.* **2019**, *54*, 453–458. [CrossRef]
38. Plevris, N.; Jenkinson, P.W.; Arnott, I.D.; Jones, G.R.; Lees, C. Higher anti-tumor necrosis factor levels are associated with perianal fistula healing and fistula closure in Crohn's disease. *Eur. J. Gastroenterol. Hepatol.* **2020**, *32*, 32–37. [CrossRef]
39. El-Matary, W.; Walters, T.D.; Huynh, H.Q.; Debruyn, J.; Mack, D.R.; Jacobson, K.; Sherlock, M.E.; Church, P.; Wine, E.; Carroll, M.W.; et al. Higher Postinduction Infliximab Serum Trough Levels Are Associated with Healing of Fistulizing Perianal Crohn's Disease in Children. *Inflamm. Bowel Dis.* **2019**, *25*, 150–155. [CrossRef]
40. Ruemmele, F.M.; Rosh, J.; Faubion, W.A.; Dubinsky, M.C.; Turner, D.; Lazar, A.; Eichner, S.; Maa, J.-F.; Alperovich, G.; Robinson, A.M.; et al. Efficacy of Adalimumab for Treatment of Perianal Fistula in Children with Moderately to Severely Active Crohn's Disease: Results from IMAgINE 1 and IMAgINE 2. *J. Crohn's Colitis* **2018**, *12*, 1249–1254. [CrossRef]
41. Papamichael, K.; Casteele, N.V.; Jeyarajah, J.; Jairath, V.; Osterman, M.T.; Cheifetz, A.S. Higher Postinduction Infliximab Concentrations Are Associated with Improved Clinical Outcomes in Fistulizing Crohn's Disease: An ACCENT-II Post Hoc Analysis. *Am. J. Gastroenterol.* **2021**, *116*, 1007–1014. [CrossRef] [PubMed]
42. De Gregorio, M.; Lee, T.; Krishnaprasad, K.; Amos, G.; An, Y.K.; Bastian-Jordan, M.; Begun, J.; Borok, N.; Brown, D.; Cheung, W.; et al. Higher Anti-tumor Necrosis Factor-α Levels Correlate With Improved Radiologic Outcomes in Crohn's Perianal Fistulas. *Clin. Gastroenterol. Hepatol. Off. Clin. Pract. J. Am. Gastroenterol. Assoc.* **2021**, *in press*. [CrossRef] [PubMed]
43. Gu, B.; De Gregorio, M.; Pipicella, J.L.; Casteele, N.V.; Andrews, J.M.; Begun, J.; Connell, W.; D'Souza, B.; Gholamrezaei, A.; Hart, A.; et al. Prospective randomised controlled trial of adults with perianal fistulising Crohn's disease and optimised therapeutic infliximab levels: PROACTIVE trial study protocol. *BMJ Open* **2021**, *11*, e043921. [CrossRef]
44. Yarur, A.J.; Jain, A.; Sussman, D.A.; Barkin, J.S.; Quintero, M.A.; Princen, F.; Kirkland, R.; Deshpande, A.R.; Singh, S.; Abreu, M.T. The association of tissue anti-TNF drug levels with serological and endoscopic disease activity in inflammatory bowel disease: The ATLAS study. *Gut* **2016**, *65*, 249–255. [CrossRef]

45. Adegbola, S.O.; Sarafian, M.; Sahnan, K.; Pechlivanis, A.; Phillips, R.K.; Warusavitarne, J.; Faiz, O.; Haddow, J.; Knowles, C.; Tozer, P.; et al. Lack of anti-TNF drugs levels in fistula tissue—A reason for nonresponse in Crohn's perianal fistulating disease? *Eur. J. Gastroenterol. Hepatol.* **2021**, *34*, 18–26. [CrossRef] [PubMed]
46. Dotan, I.; Ron, Y.; Yanai, H.; Becker, S.; Fishman, S.; Yahav, L.; Ben Yehoyada, M.; Mould, D.R. Patient Factors That Increase Infliximab Clearance and Shorten Half-life in Inflammatory Bowel Disease: A population pharmacokinetic study. *Inflamm. Bowel Dis.* **2014**, *20*, 2247–2259. [CrossRef]
47. Marzo, M.; Felice, C.; Pugliese, D.; Andrisani, G.; Mocci, G.; Armuzzi, A.; Guidi, L. Management of perianal fistulas in Crohn's disease: An up-to-date review. *World J. Gastroenterol.* **2015**, *21*, 1394–1403. [CrossRef]
48. van Praag, E.M.M.; Buskens, C.J.; Hompes, R.; Bemelman, W.A. Surgical management of Crohn's disease: A state of the art review. *Int. J. Colorectal Dis.* **2021**, *36*, 1133–1145. [CrossRef]
49. Miranda, E.F.; Nones, R.B.; Kotze, P.G. Correlation of serum levels of anti-tumor necrosis factor agents with perianal fistula healing in Crohn's disease: A narrative review. *Intest. Res.* **2021**, *19*, 255–264. [CrossRef]

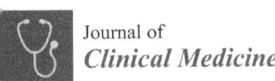

Review

Therapeutic Drug Monitoring of Biologics in IBD: Essentials for the Surgical Patient

Rodrigo Bremer Nones [1], Phillip R. Fleshner [2], Natalia Sousa Freitas Queiroz [3], Adam S. Cheifetz [4], Antonino Spinelli [5,6], Silvio Danese [6,7], Laurent Peyrin-Biroulet [8], Konstantinos Papamichael [4,†] and Paulo Gustavo Kotze [1,9,*,†]

1. Health Sciences Postgraduate Program, School of Medicine, Pontifical Catholic University of Paraná (PUCPR), Curitiba 80215-901, Brazil; robremernones@gmail.com
2. Division of Colon and Rectal Surgery, Cedars-Sinai Medical Center, Los Angeles, CA 90048, USA; pfleshner@aol.com
3. Department of Gastroenterology, University of São Paulo School of Medicine, Sao Paulo 05403-000, Brazil; nataliasfqueiroz@gmail.com
4. Department of Medicine and Division of Gastroenterology, Beth Israel Deaconess Medical Center, Harvard Medical School, Boston, MA 02215, USA; acheifet@bidmc.harvard.edu (A.S.C.); kpapamic@bidmc.harvard.edu (K.P.)
5. Division of Colon and Rectal Surgery, IRCCS Humanitas Research Hospital, Via Manzoni 56, 20089 Milan, Italy; antoninospinelli@gmail.com
6. Department of Biomedical Sciences, Humanitas University, Via Rita Levi Montalcini 4, 20090 Milan, Italy; sdanese@hotmail.com
7. IBD Centre, Humanitas Research Hospital, 20089 Milan, Italy
8. Department of Gastroenterology, University Hospital of Nancy, 54500 Nancy, France; peyrinbiroulet@gmail.com
9. IBD Outpatient Clinics, Pontifical Catholic University of Paraná (PUCPR), Curitiba 80215-901, Brazil
* Correspondence: pgkotze@hotmail.com
† These authors share last co-authorship.

Abstract: Despite significant development in the pharmacological treatment of inflammatory bowel diseases (IBD) along with the evolution of therapeutic targets and treatment strategies, a significant subset of patients still requires surgery during the course of the disease. As IBD patients are frequently exposed to biologics at the time of abdominal and perianal surgery, it is crucial to identify any potential impact of biological agents in the perioperative period. Even though detectable serum concentrations of biologics do not seem to increase postoperative complications after abdominal procedures in IBD, there is increasing evidence on the role of therapeutic drug monitoring (TDM) in the perioperative setting. This review aims to provide a comprehensive summary of published studies reporting the association of drug concentrations and postoperative outcomes, postoperative recurrence (POR) after an ileocolonic resection for Crohn's disease (CD), colectomy rates in ulcerative colitis (UC), and perianal fistulizing CD outcomes in patients treated with biologics. Current data suggest that serum concentrations of biologics are not associated with an increased risk in postoperative complications following abdominal procedures in IBD. Moreover, higher concentrations of anti-TNF agents are associated with a reduction in colectomy rates in UC. Finally, higher serum drug concentrations are associated with reduced rates of POR after ileocolonic resections and increased rates of perianal fistula healing in CD. TDM is being increasingly used to guide clinical decision making with favorable outcomes in many clinical scenarios. However, given the lack of high quality data deriving mostly from retrospective studies, the evidence supporting the systematic application of TDM in the perioperative setting is still inconclusive.

Keywords: therapeutic drug monitoring; inflammatory bowel disease; surgery; Crohn's disease; ulcerative colitis; anti-TNF therapy; vedolizumab; ustekinumab

1. Introduction

Inflammatory bowel disease (IBD) is characterized by a course of chronic and recurrent bowel inflammation and eventually cumulative and irreversible bowel damage [1,2]. In cases where moderate to severe disease activity is present, biological therapy is the cornerstone treatment as it can prevent disease progression [3]. There are several biological agents approved globally to treat both Crohn's disease (CD) and ulcerative colitis (UC), with different mechanisms of action: tumor-necrosis factor (TNF) inhibitors, anti-integrins, and anti-interleukins [4,5].

One of the most challenging decisions in the treatment of patients with IBD is the choice of the biological agent. Although each of the different biologics has the potential to induce remission, one cannot predict individual response. Approximately one-third of patients may have a primary nonresponse to an initial agent. Secondary loss of response, after initial improvement, is also frequent in the management of CD and UC [6,7]. Data on genetic and microbiological signatures and new biomarkers are needed in order to guide this appropriate medication choice [8]. This is a critical aspect for precision medicine in IBD [9].

Another feature of precision medicine in IBD is founded on the pharmacokinetic study of currently approved drugs, also known as therapeutic drug monitoring (TDM). This strategy, based on measurement of serum concentrations and antibodies to a specific agent, assumes that there are specific thresholds for concentration of biologics above which there is increased chance of induction and maintenance of remission [10]. TDM can be used reactively on evidence of therapy failure or proactively with the goal of anticipating and preventing therapeutic failure [11,12]. There are still many controversies regarding TDM in regard to when it should be performed and which range of drug concentrations should be considered adequate for each agent and clinical scenario.

Currently, the management of IBD is based in a multidisciplinary approach, including medical and surgical options for different disease phenotypes. Despite the approval of new biologics and small molecules, and newer strategies such as earlier treatment and treat-to-target, surgery is still required in a substantial portion of CD and UC patients [13–15]. Patients who are refractory to optimal medical therapy and those with disease complications (e.g., dysplasia, perforation, and strictures) comprise the most common indication for surgery in IBD [16–18]. Most patients who undergo surgery have been previously exposed to biologic therapy. Thus, it is essential for the surgeon to understand the relationship between biologic agents and surgery, including situations where serum drug concentrations can influence perioperative outcomes [19,20]. The aim of this review is to summarize essential concepts of TDM for IBD surgeons, by discussing the common clinical situations where it can influence pre-, peri-, and postoperative scenarios in CD and UC, specifically examining TDM in postoperative morbidity, CD recurrence, need for colectomy in UC and perianal fistula treatment.

2. Tdm and Postoperative Complications in IBD

2.1. Anti-TNF Agents

Currently, there is still controversy whether the preoperative use of biologics impacts postoperative outcomes in IBD. Data regarding serum concentrations of biologics in the perioperative period are based on one large multicenter prospective trial (The Postoperative Infection in Inflammatory Bowel Disease—PUCCINI) and few prospective single-center studies [21–23].

A large retrospective study from Waterman et al. [24] including 473 CD-related surgical procedures (195 in patients previously treated with anti-TNFs and 278 in matched controls) was the first to evaluate the association between serum biologic drug concentrations and postoperative complications. It found that detectable infliximab concentrations did not increase the rates of postoperative wound infection ($p = 0.21$). However, only 16 UC patients had preoperative levels measured.

A study from Lau et al. was the first prospective study in patients undergoing surgery for IBD with preoperative evaluation of serum concentrations of infliximab [22]. In this study, 123 patients with CD underwent abdominal surgery. Infliximab concentration higher than 3 µg/mL was related to an increased rate of overall complications (Odds ratio (OR) 2.5; $p = 0.03$) and infectious complications (OR 3.0; $p = 0.03$). Overall complications and readmissions rates were significantly higher in patients with drug concentrations higher than 8 µg/mL. In the UC cohort (n = 94), patients with infliximab concentrations > 3 µg/mL compared to those with drug concentrations $\leq$ 3 µg/mL had similar rates of adverse postoperative outcomes when stratified according to the specific type of surgery. Postoperative morbidity was seen in 31/77 (40%) patients with undetectable concentrations and in 8/17 (41%) patients with detectable infliximab concentrations ($p = 0.61$).

The large multicenter PUCCINI trial [21], prospectively assessed the risk of surgery and biologics, including IBD patients who underwent abdominal operations. Among 955 procedures (ileocolonic resections (n = 410), small bowel or colonic segmental resections (n = 185), and subtotal colectomy with ileostomy (n = 168)), 382 with use of anti-TNFs up to 12 weeks before surgery, the rates of overall infectious complications were similar between patients previously treated with anti-TNFs and controls (20% vs. 19.4%, $p = 0.801$) or detectable anti-TNF drug concentrations (19.7% vs. 19.6%, $p = 0.985$). In the same vein, similar rates of surgical site infections were found in patients with prior anti-TNF therapy exposure (12.4% vs. 11.5%, $p = 0.692$) or detectable drug concentrations (10.3% vs. 12.1%, $p = 0.513$). Both prior anti-TNF exposure and detectable drug concentrations were not significantly associated with the risk of overall infectious complications or surgical site infections. Data regarding serum concentrations of vedolizumab and ustekinumab and their relationship with postoperative outcomes from the same study are eagerly awaited.

A French study also prospectively analyzed the possible influence of serum concentrations of anti-TNFs on postoperative outcomes after ileocolic resection in patients with CD [23]. From the 209 patients initially included, 76 had serum concentrations of infliximab or adalimumab available prior to surgery. Trough concentrations > 1 ug/mL (OR = 0.69, 95% (confidence interval) CI 0.21–2.22) and > 3 ug/mL (OR = 0.95, 95% CI 0.28–2.96) were not related to an increased rate of postoperative complications.

2.2. Anti-Integrins and Anti-Interleukins

Regarding vedolizumab, only one study has assessed the impact of preoperative vedolizumab drug concentrations on postoperative outcomes in patients undergoing major abdominal surgery for IBD [25]. Of the 72 patients with preoperative exposure, 38 (53%) patients had detectable (>1.6 µg/mL), and 34 (47%) had undetectable vedolizumab concentrations. In the UC cohort (n = 42), 48% had undetectable vedolizumab concentration in contrast to 52% who had a detectable one. Postoperative morbidity was comparable between these groups. The CD cohort included 27 patients, of which 48% had undetectable vedolizumab concentrations. Similar to UC, in the CD cohort (n = 27) there were no statistically significant differences in overall complications between patients with (48%) or without (52%) undetectable vedolizumab concentrations. Interestingly, there was a significantly lower incidence of postoperative ileus in CD patients with detectable vedolizumab concentrations compared to patients with undetectable concentrations ($p < 0.04$). Although the association between vedolizumab and postoperative ileus needs to be validated, it may reflect the ability of this specific agent to bind to the integrin α4β7 receptor present on mast cells [26,27].

Similar to vedolizumab, there are limited data on the effect of preoperative ustekinumab concentrations on postoperative surgical outcomes in IBD. The only report, presented at DDW 2021, included 36 patients with IBD. Ustekinumab concentrations were detectable (≥ 0.9 µg/mL) in 25 (69%) and undetectable in 11 (31%) patients [28]. Among the patients with detectable drug concentrations, the median ustekinumab concentration was 6.4 µg/mL (range 0.9–25). Overall postoperative morbidity (27% vs. 28%, $p = 0.72$),

30-day readmission rate (18% vs. 8%, $p = 0.57$), postoperative ileus (18% vs. 8%, $p = 0.57$), and wound infection (9% vs. 4%, $p = 0.52$) were comparable between the two groups.

It is clear that our knowledge gap in the evaluation of serum drug concentrations and postoperative outcomes for non-TNF agents is significant. As previously stated, we eagerly await data from the PUCCINI trial, where serum concentrations of both vedolizumab and ustekinumab and their relationship with postoperative outcomes will be analyzed [21]. Table 1 summarizes available data with anti-TNF agents, vedolizumab, and ustekinumab regarding influence of serum drug concentrations on postoperative outcomes.

Table 1. Therapeutic drug monitoring and perioperative outcome.

Author	Journal (Year)	Type of Study	Number of Patients	Biologic	Outcome Studied	Results
Lau et al. [22]	Ann Surg (2015)	Single-center prospective	123 CD 94 UC	IFX	Overall and infectious postoperative complications with serum concentrations	In CD, IFX concentrations > 3 µg/mL associated with increased overall and infectious complications. IFX concentrations > 8 µg/mL associated with overall complications and readmissions. No relation in UC patients
Fumery et al. [23]	Am J Gastroenterol (2017)	Multicenter prospective	76 CD	IFX/ADA	Overall early (30 day) postoperative complications with serum concentrations	Trough concentrations > 1µg/mL (OR = 0.69, 95%CI: 0.21–2.22) and >3 µg/mL (OR = 0.95, 95%CI: 0.28-2.96) were not associated to increased rates of postoperative complications
Cohen et al. [21]	Gastroenterology (2019) [abstract only]	Multicenter prospective	573 IBD	Anti-TNF agents	Infectious complications and surgical site infections with serum concentrations	No relation between detectable serum drug concentrations or previous exposure to anti-TNF agents with increased infectious postoperative complications or surgical site infections
Parrish AB et al. [25]	Dis Colon Rectum (2021)	Single-center prospective	72 IBD	VDZ	Overall and infectious postoperative complications with serum concentrations	No significant differences in overall postoperative morbidity between detectable (>1.6 µg/ml) and undetectable concentration groups. In CD, there was a significantly lower incidence of postoperative ileus with detectable VDZ concentrations compared to patients with an undetectable VDZ concentration ($p < 0.04$).
Kumar et al. [28]	Gastroenterology (2021) [abstract only]	Single-center prospective	36 IBD	UST	Overall and infectious postoperative complications with serum concentrations	There were no significant differences between the undetectable vs. detectable concentration ($\geq$0.9 µg/ml) groups in regards to overall postoperative morbidity

Legend: CD- Crohn's disease, UC- ulcerative colitis, IBD- inflammatory bowel disease, IFX- infliximab, ADM- adalimumab, VDZ- vedolizumab, UST- ustekinumab, OR- odds ratio, CI- confidence intervals; TNF- tumor necrosis factor.

3. Tdm and Postoperative Recurrence in CD

Even though there is appropriate evidence on the role of anti-TNFs in the prevention of endoscopic recurrence after ileocolonic resection, the effect of drug concentrations on recurrence rates has not been adequately explored and available data is scarce. A recent systematic review identified only four studies which assessed infliximab concentrations and endoscopic postoperative recurrence (POR) in CD, with higher concentrations mostly associated with lower POR rates [29].

The PREVENT (Prospective, Multicenter, Randomized, Double-Blind, Placebo-Controlled Trial Comparing Infliximab and Placebo in the Prevention of Recurrence in Crohn's Disease Patients Undergoing Surgical Resection Who Are at an Increased Risk of Recurrence) trial [30] evaluating 297 patients who had an ileocolonic resection for CD and received either infliximab or placebo showed that among patients who had endoscopic POR, 52.4% had a week 72 undetectable drug concentration; 31.3% had infliximab concentrations 0.1 to 1.85 µg/mL; 18.8%, 1.85 to 4.44 µg/mL; 26.7%, 4.44 to 7.77 µg/mL and 13.3% had drug concentrations higher than 7.77 µg/mL. Patients with positive, negative, or inconclusive antibodies to infliximab (ATI), had an endoscopic POR rate of 64.7% (11/17), 46.7% (7/15), and 30.1% (22/73), respectively.

A study from Israel showed that lower infliximab trough concentrations and ATI were associated with endoscopic POR [31]. Significantly higher median infliximab concentrations were found in patients with a Rutgeerts' score of i0 (3.1 [interquartile range (IQR) 0.1–4.1] µg/mL) as compared to those with a score of i4 (0.1 [IQR 0.1–3] µg/mL; $p = 0.037$). When limited to patients naïve to anti-TNF prior to surgery the difference in infliximab concentrations (2.3 [IQR 0.3–3.8] vs. 1.1 [IQR 0.1–3.3] µg/mL, $p = 0.048$) and ATI (7.7% vs. 60%, $p = 0.044$) remained significant. In the same study, the same association was not observed for 41 adalimumab patients.

In a post hoc analysis of a small randomized controlled trial (RCT), Bodini et al. described the correlation between adalimumab concentrations and POR in six patients treated with monotherapy [32]. Serum concentrations were evaluated every 8 weeks for 2 years. Patients with clinical or endoscopic POR compared to those with clinical or endoscopic remission had lower adalimumab concentrations (median (IQR) [7.5 (4.4–9.8) µg/mL vs. 13.9 (8.9–23.6) µg/mL, $p < 0.01$).

Boivineau et al. [33], presenting results of 19 CD patients on adalimumab after ileocolic resections showed that serum adalimumab concentrations measured 3 months after surgery were higherin patients with normal mucosa (Rutgeerts' score $\leq$ i1) versus those with endoscopic POR (Rutgeerts' score $\geq$ i2) (7.95 µg/mL vs. 3.25 µg/mL, respectively, $p = 0.0485$). The same study found an inverse correlation between adalimumab concentrations Rutgeerts' score ($p = 0.004$), and 86% of patients with concentrations less than 4.2 µg/mL had endoscopic POR compared to 15% of patients with concentrations $\geq$ 4.2 µg/mL ($p = 0.025$).

A sub-analysis from the POCER (Postoperative Crohn's Endoscopic Recurrence) trial demonstrated opposite results. In this study, there were 52 patients with serum concentrations of adalimumab measured after ileocolic resection [34]. When combining endoscopic outcomes from 6 and 18 months, patients in endoscopic remission compared to those with POR (Rutgeerts $\geq$ i2) had similar adalimumab concentrations (9.98 µg/mL vs. 8.43 µg/mL, respectively, $p = 0.387$). There were also no statistically significant differences ($p = 0.495$) when adalimumab concentrations were compared between each different Rutgeerts' score category (i0 to i4).

Table 2 summarizes data on the application of TDM in POR in CD. Low serum concentrations of anti-TNF agents and immunogenicity seem to be associated with a higher risk of endoscopic POR in patients undergoing an ileocolonic resection for CD. The role of TDM to better optimize not only anti-TNF therapy, but also biologics with a different mechanism of action for preventing and treating POR, should be evaluated in large prospective studies and RCTs.

Table 2. Therapeutic drug monitoring of anti-TNF therapy and postoperative recurrence after ileocolonic resection for CD.

Author	Journal (Year)	Type of Study	Number of Patients	Anti-TNF Agent	Outcome Studied	Results
Regueiro et al. (PREVENT trial) [30]	Gastroenterology (2016)	Multicenter prospective (RCT)	147	IFX	POR rates with serum concentrations (secondary outcome)	Inverse correlation between serum IFX concentrations and POR rates (the higher the concentration, the lower the rates of POR)
Fay et al. [31]	Inflamm Bowel Dis (2017)	Multicenter retrospective	73	IFX/ADA	POR rates with serum concentrations	Lower IFX trough concentrations (median, 1.1 µg/mL versus 2.4 µg/mL; $p = 0.008$) and ATI (5.6% vs. 71.4%, $p = 0.0001$) were significantly associated with endoscopic POR. Same association not observed in ADA patients
Boivineau et al. [33]	J Crohn's Colitis (2020)	Multicenter prospective	19	ADA	POR rates with serum concentrations	Median serum ADA concentration was 7.95 µg/mL in patients with normal mucosa (Rutgeerts' score $\leq$ i1) and 3.25 µg/mL in patients with endoscopic POR (Rutgeerts' score $\geq$ i2), respectively ($p = 0.0485$). Serum ADA concentration was inversely correlated to the Rutgeerts' score ($p = 0.004$)

Legend: IFX—infliximab, ADA—adalimumab, ATI—antibodies toward infliximab, POR—post-operative recurrence, RCT- randomized controlled trial., TNF-tumor necrosis factor.

4. Tdm and Colectomy Rates in UC

Recent data demonstrated a possible relation between low serum concentrations of infliximab and the need for colectomy in UC patients. Papamichael et al. assessed the long-term follow-up of 99 UC patients with primary non-response to infliximab [35]. Lower week 2 and week 6 infliximab concentrations at were found in patients who required colectomy (n = 55) as compared to patients with no need for surgery. An infliximab concentration $\leq$ 16.5 µg/mL at week 2 week 6 was an independent predictor of colectomy. When stratification of infliximab concentrations was performed in quartiles, patients with concentrations in the lower quartiles (<10 µg/mL) had higher rates of colectomy at weeks 2 (70%) and 6 (89%).

Similar data from the Leuven group described the outcome of 285 UC patients with refractory disease on infliximab [36]. Overall, 57/285 (20%) patients needed colectomy during the disease course. Week 14 infliximab concentrations were available in a subset of patients (n = 112). A serum week 14 infliximab concentration greater than 2.5 ug/mL was predictive both for relapse-free survival ($p < 0.001$) and colectomy-free survival ($p = 0.034$).

Acute severe ulcerative colitis (ASUC), refractory to intravenous corticosteroids (CS), is a challenging condition to treat, and colectomy rates remain high regardless of the efficacy of salvage therapies such as cyclosporine and infliximab [37,38]. A substantial portion of patients do not respond to infliximab, possibly due to low drug exposure as a result of increased disease inflammatory burden and high drug clearance and drug fecal loss [39–42].

The relation of colectomy rates in ASUC and the clearance of infliximab was also recently studied. Battat et al. demonstrated that, in 39 patients with ASUC, those with colectomy at 6 months had higher median baseline calculated infliximab clearance compared to those without (0.733 vs. 0.569 L/day, respectively, $p = 0.005$) [41]. A clearance threshold of infliximab of 0.627 L/day identified patients who underwent colectomy with a sensitivity (SN) and specificity (SP) of 80% and 82.8%, respectively (AUC 0.80). These data described that with higher clearance of the drug, consequent lower serum concentrations are associated with greater chance of colectomy [41]. A study from Kevans et al. including 36 patients with steroid-refractory ASUC showed that longer induction infliximab half-life and lower drug clearance were associated with week 14 clinical response and week 54 at CS-free remission [42].

Based on the currently available data, emphasis should be given to studying the role of TDM in ASUC and choosing the optimal infliximab dosing. Table 3 describes the main studies regarding this topic in detail. Due to paucity of data from prospective studies and RCTs, the American Gastroenterological Association makes no recommendation on routine use of intensive versus standard infliximab dosing in hospitalized adult patients with ASUC being treated with infliximab [43]. The prospective multi-center PROTOS (Pharmacokinetics of IFX and TNF Concentrations in Serum, Stool, and Colonic Mucosa in Acute Severe Ulcerative Colitis) study is currently underway aiming to define infliximab pharmacokinetics and guide infliximab dosing strategies in patients with ASUC.

Table 3. Therapeutic drug monitoring of infliximab and colectomy rates in UC.

Author	Journal (Year)	Type of Study	Number of Patients	Anti-TNF Agent	Outcome Studied	Results
Arias et al. [36]	Clin Gastroenterol Hepatol (2014)	Single-center retrospective	112 UC	IFX	Colectomy-free survival with serum concentrations at week 14	A serum IFX concentration > 2.5 µg/mL at week 14 was predictive not only of relapse-free survival ($p < 0.001$), but also of colectomy-free survival ($p < 0.034$).
Papamichael et al. [35]	J Crohn's Colitis (2016)	Multicenter retrospective	99 UC	IFX	Colectomy rates with serum concentrations at weeks 2 and 6	A ROC analysis identified IFX concentration thresholds of 16.5 and 5.3 µg/mL at weeks 2 and 6, respectively, associated with colectomy. Patients with concentrations on the lower quartile (<10 µg/mL) had higher rates of colectomy at weeks 2 (70%) and 6 (89%), respectively
Battat et al. [41]	Clin Gastroenterol Hepatol (2020)	Single-center retrospective	39 ASUC	IFX	Clearance of IFX with colectomy rates in ASUC	Median baseline calculated clearance of IFX was higher in patients with colectomy at 6 months than in patients without (0.733 vs. 0.569 L/day; $p = 0.005$). A clearance threshold of IFX of 0.627 L/day identified patients who required colectomy (AUC, SN: 80.0%; SP: 82.8%). A higher proportion of patients with IFX clearance of 0.627 L/day or more needed colectomy within 6 months (61.5%) than patients with lower clearance values (7.7%) ($p = 0.001$). Multivariable analysis identified that the baseline IFX clearance value was the only factor associated with colectomy

Legend: IFX—infliximab, UC—ulcerative colitis, ASUC—acute severe ulcerative colitis, ROC—receiver operation curve, TNF-tumor necrosis factor.

5. TDM and Perianal Fistulizing CD

Current data on the use of TDM and perianal fistulizing CD are limited to anti-TNF agents. Data from adult populations are based on cross-sectional studies or retrospective observational cohorts (Table 4). Most studies demonstrate that there is a positive correlation between infliximab and adalimumab concentrations and fistula closure

A post hoc analysis of ACCENT-II RCT (282 patients after induction therapy and 139 patients on maintenance therapy) recently published by Papamichael et al. [48] demonstrated that higher concentrations of IFX at week 14 were independently associated with composite remission defined as complete fistula closure and CRP normalization at week 14 (OR: 2.32; 95% CI: 1.55–3.49; $p < 0.001$) and week 54 (OR: 2.05; 95% CI: 1.10–3.82; $p = 0.023$). IFX concentrations predictive of composite remission were ≥ 20.2 µg/mL, ≥ 15 µg/mL and ≥ 7.2 µg/mL at weeks 2, 6, and 14, respectively. These correlations comprise the only evidence derived from a prospective trial, despite it being a post hoc analysis.

On the pediatric population, two prospective studies were conducted. El-Matary et al. followed 27 patients prospectively and found that an IFX concentration higher than 12.7 µg/mL at week 14 was associated with fistula healing at week 24 (SN 0.62, SP: 0.65) [50]. In addition to this study, Ruemmele et al. randomly assigned 36 patients to receive standard or high doses of ADA. No statistical difference in fistula closure was demonstrated between the different dosing regimens, and ADA levels at weeks 16 and 52 did not correlate with fistula closure in this underpowered study [51].

The studies of TDM and perianal fistulizing CD are associated with some important limitations, mainly related to how the response to treatment was evaluated (with MRI outcomes), as well as for not clearly defining fistula classification (simple versus complex). Prospective data on TDM for perianal fistulizing CD are awaited. The results of the PROACTIVE (Prospective Randomised Controlled Trial of Adults with Perianal Fistulising Crohn's Disease and Optimised Therapeutic Infliximab Levels) RCT regarding adults with perianal fistulizing CD and proactively optimized infliximab concentrations) [52] is expected to shed more light regarding the role of proactive TDM in this situation.

Table 4. Therapeutic drug monitoring of anti-TNF therapy and perianal fistulizing CD.

Author	Journal (Year)	Number of Patients	Timing of TDM	Anti-TNF Agent	Median (IQR) Drug Concentration in Healed Fistulas, µg/mL	Median (IQR) Drug Concentration in Active Fistulas, µg/mL	Observations
Yarur et al. [44]	Alimentary Pharmacol Ther (2016)	117	Maintenance	IFX	15.8 (9.9–27)	4.4 (0–9.8)	Single-center, cross-sectional retrospective study.
Strik et al. [45]	Scand J Gastroenterol (2019)	IFX = 47 ADA = 19	Maintenance	IFX ADA	6.0 (5.4–6.9) 7.4 (6.5–10.8)	2.3 (1.1–4.0) 4.8 (1.7–6.2)	Single center, cross-sectional retrospective study.
Davidov et al. [46]	J Crohn's Colitis (2017)	36	Week 2 Week 6 Week 14	IFX	20.0 (16.2–26.3) 13.3 (7.6–19) 4.1 (0.7–5.7)	5.6 (2.8–9.2) 2.6 (0.4–7.0) 0.1 (0.01–2.3)	2-center, retrospective cohort study. Proactive TDM.
Plevris et al. [47]	Eur J Gastroenterol Hepatol (2019)	IFX = 29 ADA = 35	Maintenace	IFX	8.1 12.6	3.2 2.7	Single center, cross-sectional retrospective study.
Papamichael et al. [48]	Am J Gastroenterol (2021)	Induction: 282 Maintenance: 139	Week 14	IFX	9.3 (4.9–16.2)	3.2 (1.1–7.0)	Post hoc analysis of ACCENT II trial. Composite remission (defined as a combined complete fistula response and CRP normalization) data.
Zhu et al. [49]	Dig Dis Sci (2021)	157	6 infusions 12 infusions 18 infusions	IFX	3.5 (0.9–8.7) 2.8 (0.5–6.2) 2.8 (0.4–4.1)	1.9 (0.6–5.2) 1.6 (0.4–3.9) 0.7 (0–2.8)	Retrospective single-center study. Radiological remission data.

Legend: IFX—infliximab, ADA—adalimumab, CRP—C reactive protein, TDM—therapeutic drug monitoring, TNF–tumor necrosis factor, IQR: interquartile range.

6. Discussion

This review provides a comprehensive assessment of the data on the role of TDM and surgical outcomes in patients with IBD (Figure 1). Although there are limited studies supporting the widespread use of the TDM in the perioperative setting, there is growing evidence demonstrating its potential benefits.

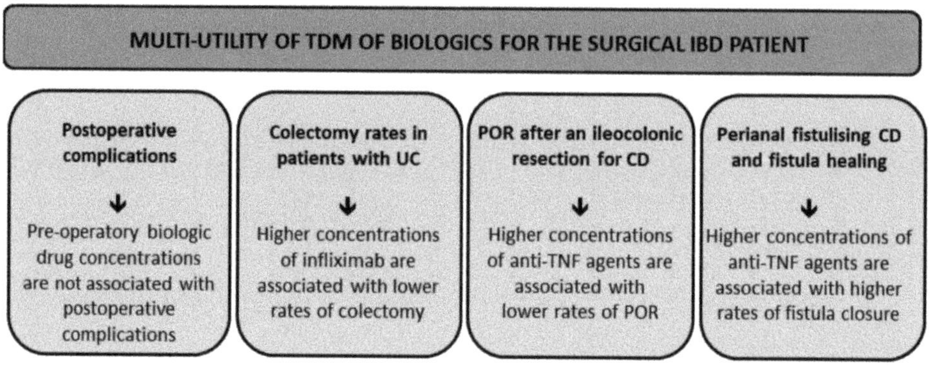

MULTI-UTILITY OF TDM OF BIOLOGICS FOR THE SURGICAL IBD PATIENT

Postoperative complications	Colectomy rates in patients with UC	POR after an ileocolonic resection for CD	Perianal fistulising CD and fistula healing
↓	↓	↓	↓
Pre-operatory biologic drug concentrations are not associated with postoperative complications	Higher concentrations of infliximab are associated with lower rates of colectomy	Higher concentrations of anti-TNF agents are associated with lower rates of POR	Higher concentrations of anti-TNF agents are associated with higher rates of fistula closure

Figure 1. Multi-utility of TDM of biologics for the surgical IBD patient. Legend: UC—ulcerative colitis, POR—post-operative recurrence, CD—Crohn's disease.

Abdominal and perianal surgery in IBD patients demands high expertise and a multidisciplinary approach. IBD patients are frequently malnourished, with a high inflammatory burden, often have a past history of previous surgeries, and are frequently exposed to biologics, corticosteroids, and immunomodulators [53]. Consequently, the surgical complications are expected to be higher among these patients than among patients undergoing abdominal surgery for other reasons [54,55]. Thus, early studies identifying the potential relation between postoperative complications and preoperative exposure to biologics should be considered carefully, as numerous confounding factors might influence surgical outcomes in this population. Prospective studies with precise biomarkers, such as quantification of tissue penetration of the drugs in surgical specimens are encouraged to better describe the effect of preoperative biologics on postoperative complications.

Although a positive exposure–response relationship between higher drug concentrations and favorable therapeutic outcomes has been consistently demonstrated [10], this association seems less clear in the context of postoperative recurrence of CD. In the study by Fay et al. [31], despite the significant difference between groups with or without POR, low IFX concentrations (2.4 [0.45–4.1] µg/mL) were still observed in patients with no POR supporting the hypothesis that the actual threshold in the postoperative scenario can be somewhat different than in luminal CD, without a prior surgery. Moreover, it should be emphasized that disease recurrence could be significantly influenced by the higher biologic clearance as a consequence of more severe disease at baseline along with the amount of residual inflamed bowel, a confounding factor poorly explored in the available literature.

There is growing data suggesting the use of proactive TDM during induction for UC and likely for ASUC. Post hoc analyses of the ACT-1 and ACT-2 RCTs demonstrate a positive correlation between infliximab concentrations and favorable outcomes, such as clinical response and remission as well as mucosal healing. Higher infliximab concentrations were also associated with higher rates of week 8 mucosal healing in patients with UC [56]. However, trials evaluating accelerated IFX induction regimen in the setting of ASUC are controversial. A recent meta-analysis of seven studies did not show any difference in in-hospital colectomy rates between accelerated infliximab induction therapy and standard induction therapy [57]. However, there were likely significant confounding factors in these studies. Given that ASUC constitutes a life-threatening condition with reported mortality rates reaching 1% in a recent systematic review and meta-analysis from population-based studies [58], RCT accounting for disease severity and IFX pharmacokinetics are warranted to define the best IFX dosing strategy.

Perianal fistulas are a disabling complication of CD and can have a significant impact on patients' quality of life [59]. Unfortunately, closure of fistula tracts and radiologic healing are considered ambitious outcomes with low remission rates with any therapy, even anti-TNF. Recent studies regarding anti-TNF therapy have shown that higher than previously reported drug concentrations might be needed to attain complete healing of fistulae [44,45]. It has been suggested that increasing the dose of anti-TNFs with the aim of achieving higher drug concentrations could be helpful in this setting [18]. However, whether this is related to improved mucosal healing rather than a direct action of the drug on fistula tracks remains unclear. Notably, a recent pilot study investigating the role of tissue drug concentrations in fistula tracts of CD patients on anti-TNF therapy found an absence of drug detection in fistula tissue [60]. These observations increase uncertainties surrounding the potential role of tissue penetrance of anti-TNF agents of in response to treatment.

7. Conclusions

The use of TDM is becoming more available globally. Application of serum concentrations and antibody measurement with anti-TNF agents is most commonly used. As indications for surgery in CD and UC persist, despite important advances in medical management of IBD, it is important to define the possible impact of biological agents in the perioperative period. Thus, surgeons should be aware of the possible practical application of the use of TDM in the treatment of IBD and in the peri-surgical period.

Detectable serum concentrations of biologics do not appear to increase postoperative complications after abdominal procedures in IBD. Higher concentrations of anti-TNF agents are associated with a reduction in colectomy rates in UC and may have a role in those admitted with ASUC. Mirroring luminal disease, higher concentrations of anti-TNF agents seem to be associated with reduced rates of postoperative recurrence after ileocolonic resections and higher rates of perianal fistula healing in CD.

Precision medicine is a natural consequence of the development of diagnostic methods and therapeutic agents in IBD. Application of TDM in surgical patients may be an important piece of the "right therapy to the right patient at the right time" aphorism. More prospective data analyzing the relation of serum concentrations of biologics in the perioperative period are awaited.

Author Contributions: Conceptualization, K.P. and P.G.K.; writing—original draft preparation, all authors; writing—review and editing, all authors. All authors have read and agreed to the published version of the manuscript.

Funding: This research received no external funding.

Conflicts of Interest: RBN has no conflict of interest. PRF is a consultant for Takeda NSFQ has served as a speaker and advisory board member of Janssen, Takeda, and Abbvie. ASC reports consultancy fees from Janssen, Abbvie, Artugen, Procise, Prometheus, Arena, Grifols, Bacainn, and Bristol Myers Squibb. AS is a consultant for Takeda. SD has served as a speaker, consultant, and advisory board member for Schering-Plough, AbbVie, Actelion, Alphawasserman, AstraZeneca, Cellerix, Cosmo Pharmaceuticals, Ferring, Genentech, Grunenthal, Johnson and Johnson, Millenium Takeda, MSD, Nikkiso Europe GmbH, Novo Nordisk, Nycomed, Pfizer, Pharmacosmos, UCB Pharma, and Vifor. LPB has served as a speaker, consultant, and advisory board member for Merck, Abbvie, Janssen, Genentech, Mitsubishi, Ferring, Norgine, Tillots, Vifor, Hospira/Pfizer, Celltrion, Takeda, Biogaran, Boerhinger-Ingelheim, Lilly, HAC- Pharma, Index Pharmaceuticals, Amgen, Sandoz, Forward Pharma GmbH, Celgene, Biogen, Lycera, Samsung Bioepis, and Theravance. KP reports lecture fees from Mitsubishi Tanabe Pharma and Physicians Education Resource LLC; consultancy fee from Prometheus Laboratories Inc; and scientific advisory board fees from ProciseDx Inc. and

Scipher Medicine Corporation. PGK is a speaker and consultant for Abbvie, Janssen, Pfizer, and Takeda. He also does clinical research for Lilly, Takeda, and Pfizer.

References

1. Roda, G.; Chien Ng, S.; Kotze, P.G.; Argollo, M.; Panaccione, R.; Spinelli, A.; Kaser, A.; Peyrin-Biroulet, L.; Danese, S. Crohn's disease. *Nat. Rev. Dis. Primers* **2020**, *6*, 22. [CrossRef] [PubMed]
2. Ungaro, R.; Mehandru, S.; Allen, P.B.; Peyrin-Biroulet, L.; Colombel, J.F. Ulcerative colitis. *Lancet* **2017**, *389*, 1756–1770. [CrossRef]
3. Van Assche, G.; Vermeire, S.; Rutgeerts, P. The potential for disease modification in Crohn's disease. *Nat. Rev. Gastroenterol. Hepatol.* **2010**, *7*, 79–85. [CrossRef] [PubMed]
4. Torres, J.; Bonovas, S.; Doherty, G.; Kucharzik, T.; Gisbert, J.P.; Raine, T.; Adamina, M.; Armuzzi, A.; Bachmann, O.; Bager, P.; et al. ECCO Guidelines on Therapeutics in Crohn's Disease: Medical Treatment. *J. Crohns Colitis* **2020**, *14*, 4–22. [CrossRef] [PubMed]
5. Rubin, D.T.; Ananthakrishnan, A.N.; Siegel, C.A.; Sauer, B.G.; Long, M.D. ACG Clinical Guideline: Ulcerative Colitis in Adults. *Am. J. Gastroenterol.* **2019**, *114*, 384–413. [CrossRef] [PubMed]
6. Lima, C.C.G.; Queiroz, N.S.F.; Sobrado, C.W.; Silva, G.L.R.; Nahas, S.C. Critical Analysis Of Anti-TNF Use In The Era Of New Biological Agents In Inflammatory Bowel Disease. *Arq. Gastroenterol.* **2020**, *57*, 323–332. [CrossRef] [PubMed]
7. Roda, G.; Jharap, B.; Narula, N.; Colombel, J.F. Loss of Response to Anti-TNFs: Definition, Epidemiology, and Management. *Clin. Transl. Gastroenterol.* **2016**, *7*, e135. [CrossRef]
8. Fiocchi, C.; Iliopoulos, D. What's new in IBD therapy: An "omics network" approach. *Pharmacol. Res.* **2020**, *159*, 104886. [CrossRef]
9. Fiocchi, C.; Dragoni, G.; Iliopoulos, D.; Katsanos, K.; Hernandez Ramirez, V.; Suzuki, K.; Scientific Workshop Steering Committee. Results of the Seventh Scientific Workshop of ECCO: Precision medicine in—What, why, and how. *J. Crohns Colitis* **2021**, *15*, 1410–1430. [CrossRef] [PubMed]
10. Papamichael, K.; Cheifetz, A.S.; Melmed, G.Y.; Irving, P.M.; Casteele, N.V.; Kozuch, P.L.; Raffals, L.E.; Baidoo, L.; Bressler, B.; Devlin, S.M.; et al. Appropriate Therapeutic Drug Monitoring of Biologic Agents for Patients With Inflammatory Bowel Diseases. *Clin. Gastroenterol. Hepatol.* **2019**, *17*, 1655-1668.e3. [CrossRef] [PubMed]
11. De Martins, C.A.; Moss, A.C.; Sobrado, C.W.; Queiroz, N.S.F. Practical Aspects of Proactive TDM for Anti-TNF Agents in IBD: Defining Time Points and Thresholds to Target. *Crohn's Colitis 360* **2019**, *1*, otz049. [CrossRef]
12. Papamichael, K.; Cheifetz, A.S. Therapeutic drug monitoring in inflammatory bowel disease. *Curr. Opin. Gastroenterol.* **2019**, *35*, 302–310. [CrossRef] [PubMed]
13. Cosnes, J.; Gower-Rousseau, C.; Seksik, P.; Cortot, A. Epidemiology and natural history of inflammatory bowel diseases. *Gastroenterology* **2011**, *140*, 1785–1794. [CrossRef] [PubMed]
14. Bernell, O.; Lapidus, A.; Hellers, G. Risk Factors for Surgery and Postoperative Recurrence in Crohn's Disease. *Ann. Surg.* **2000**, *231*, 38. [CrossRef]
15. El Ouali, S.; Click, B.; Holubar, S.D.; Rieder, F. Natural history, diagnosis and treatment approach to fibrostenosing Crohn's disease. *United Eur. Gastroenterol. J.* **2020**, *8*, 263–270. [CrossRef]
16. Frolkis, A.D.; Dykeman, J.; Negrón, M.E.; Debruyn, J.; Jette, N.; Fiest, K.M.; Frolkis, T.; Barkema, H.; Rioux, K.P.; Panaccione, R.; et al. Risk of surgery for inflammatory bowel diseases has decreased over time: A systematic review and meta-analysis of population-based studies. *Gastroenterology* **2013**, *145*, 996–1006. [CrossRef]
17. Fumery, M.; Singh, S.; Dulai, P.S.; Gower-Rousseau, C.; Peyrin-Biroulet, L.; Sandborn, W.J. Natural History of Adult Ulcerative Colitis in Population-based Cohorts: A Systematic Review. *Clin. Gastroenterol. Hepatol.* **2018**, *16*, 343-356.e3. [CrossRef] [PubMed]
18. Kotze, P.G.; Shen, B.; Lightner, A.; Yamamoto, T.; Spinelli, A.; Ghosh, S.; Panaccione, R. Modern management of perianal fistulas in Crohn's disease: Future directions. *Gut* **2018**, *67*, 1181–1194. [CrossRef] [PubMed]
19. Kulaylat, A.N.; Kulaylat, A.S.; Schaefer, E.W.; Mirkin, K.; Tinsley, A.; Williams, E.; Koltun, W.A.; Hollenbeak, C.S.; Messaris, E. The Impact of Preoperative Anti-TNFα Therapy on Postoperative Outcomes Following Ileocolectomy in Crohn's Disease. *J. Gastrointest. Surg.* **2020**, *25*, 467–474. [CrossRef] [PubMed]
20. Perin, R.L.; Queiroz, N.S.F.; Kotze, P.G. Preoperative Anti-TNF Agents and Morbidity After Ileocolonic Resections in Crohn's Disease: Are Biologics the Only Ones to Blame? *J. Gastrointest. Surg.* **2021**, *25*, 1352–1353. [CrossRef] [PubMed]
21. Cohen, B.; Fleshner, P.; Kane, S. Anti-tumor necrosis factor is not associated with postoperative infections: Results from prospective cohort of ulcerative colitis and Crohn's disease patients undergoing surgery to identify risk factors for postoperative infections (PUCCINI). *Gastroenterology* **2019**, *156*, S-80. [CrossRef]
22. Lau, C.; Dubinsky, M.; Melmed, G.; Vasiliauskas, E.; Berel, D.; McGovern, D.; Ippoliti, A.; Shih, D.; Targan, S.; Fleshner, P. The impact of preoperative serum anti-TNFα therapy levels on early postoperative outcomes in inflammatory bowel disease surgery. *Ann. Surg.* **2015**, *261*, 487–496. [CrossRef] [PubMed]
23. Fumery, M.; Seksik, P.; Auzolle, C.; Munoz-Bongrand, N.; Gornet, J.M.; Boschetti, G.; Cotte, E.; Buisson, A.; Dubois, A.; Pariente, B.; et al. Postoperative Complications after Ileocecal Resection in Crohn's Disease: A Prospective Study from the REMIND Group. *Am. J. Gastroenterol.* **2017**, *112*, 337–345. [CrossRef] [PubMed]
24. Waterman, M.; Xu, W.; Dinani, A.; Steinhart, A.H.; Croitoru, K.; Nguyen, G.C.; McLeod, R.S.; Greenberg, G.R.; Cohen, Z.; Silverberg, M.S. Preoperative biological therapy and short-term outcomes of abdominal surgery in patients with inflammatory bowel disease. *Gut* **2013**, *62*, 387–394. [CrossRef]

25. Parrish, A.B.; Lopez, N.E.; Truong, A.; Zaghiyan, K.; Melmed, G.Y.; McGovern, D.P.B.; Ha, C.; Syal, G.; Bonthala, N.; Jain, A.; et al. Preoperative Serum Vedolizumab Levels Do Not Impact Postoperative Outcomes in Inflammatory Bowel Disease. *Dis. Colon Rectum* **2021**, *64*, 1259–1266. [CrossRef] [PubMed]
26. The, F.; Bennink, R.J.; Ankum, W.M.; Buist, M.R.; Busch, O.R.C.; Gouma, D.J.; van der Heide, S.; Wijngaard, R.M.V.D.; de Jonge, W.J.; E Boeckxstaens, G. Intestinal handling-induced mast cell activation and inflammation in human postoperative ileus. *Gut* **2008**, *57*, 33–40. [CrossRef] [PubMed]
27. Schleier, L.; Wiendl, M.; Heidbreder, K.; Binder, M.-T.; Atreya, R.; Rath, T.; Becker, E.; Schulz-Kuhnt, A.; Stahl, A.; Schulze, L.L.; et al. Non-classical monocyte homing to the gut via α4β7 integrin mediates macrophage-dependent intestinal wound healing. *Gut* **2020**, *69*, 252–263. [CrossRef]
28. Kumar, R.; Syal, G.; Ha, C.; Melmed, G.; Vasilauskas, E.; Feldman, E.J.; Landers, C.; Jain, A.; Targan, R.S.; Zaghiyan, K.; et al. Su457 Does Preoperative Serum Ustekinumab Concentration Predict Thirty-Day Postoperative Outcomes In Patients With Inflammatory Bowel Disease Undergoing Abdominal Surgery? *Gastroenterology* **2021**, *160*, S-699–S-700. [CrossRef]
29. Baraúna, F.S.B.; Kotze, P.G. Correlation between trough levels of infliximab and postoperative endoscopic recurrence in crohn's disease patients submitted to ileocolonic resections: A systematic review. *Arq. Gastroenterol.* **2021**, *58*, 107–113. [CrossRef] [PubMed]
30. Regueiro, M.; Feagan, B.G.; Zou, B.; Johanns, J.; Blank, M.A.; Chevrier, M.; Plevy, S.; Popp, J.; Cornillie, J.F.; Lukas, M.; et al. Infliximab Reduces Endoscopic, but Not Clinical, Recurrence of Crohn's Disease after Ileocolonic Resection. *Gastroenterology* **2016**, *150*, 1568–1578. [CrossRef] [PubMed]
31. Fay, S.; Ungar, B.; Paul, S.; Levartovsky, A.; Yavzori, M.; Fudim, E.; Picard, O.; Eliakim, R.; Ben-Horin, S.; Roblin, X.; et al. The Association between Drug Levels and Endoscopic Recurrence in Postoperative Patients with Crohn's Disease Treated with Tumor Necrosis Factor Inhibitors. *Inflamm. Bowel Dis.* **2017**, *23*, 1924–1929. [CrossRef]
32. Bodini, G.; Savarino, V.; Peyrin-Biroulet, L.; de Cassan, C.; Dulbecco, P.; Baldissarro, I.; Fazio, V.; Giambruno, E.; Savarino, E. Low serum trough levels are associated with post-surgical recurrence in Crohn's disease patients undergoing prophylaxis with adalimumab. *Dig. Liver Dis.* **2014**, *46*, 1043–1046. [CrossRef] [PubMed]
33. Boivineau, L.; Guillon, F.; Altweg, R. Serum Adalimumab Concentration After Surgery Is Correlated With Postoperative Endoscopic Recurrence in Crohn's Disease Patients: One Step Before Proactive Therapeutic Drug Monitoring. *J. Crohns Colitis* **2020**, *14*, 1500–1501. [CrossRef]
34. Wright, E.K.; Kamm, M.A.; De Cruz, P.; Hamilton, A.L.; Selvaraj, F.; Princen, F.; Gorelik, A.; Liew, D.; Prideaux, L.; Lawrance, I.C.; et al. Anti-TNF Therapeutic Drug Monitoring in Postoperative Crohn's Disease. *J. Crohns Colitis* **2018**, *12*, 653–661. [CrossRef]
35. Papamichael, K.; Rivals-Lerebours, O.; Billiet, T.; Vande Casteele, N. Long-Term Outcome of Patients With Ulcerative Colitis and Primary Non-response to Infliximab. *J. Crohns Colitis* **2016**, *10*, 1015–1023. [CrossRef] [PubMed]
36. Arias, M.T.; Vande Casteele, N.; Vermeire, S.; de Buck van Overstraeten, A.; Billiet, T.; Baert, F.; Wolthuis, A.; Van Assche, G.; Noman, M.; Hoffman, I.; et al. A panel to predict long-term outcome of infliximab therapy for patients with ulcerative colitis. *Clin. Gastroenterol. Hepatol.* **2015**, *13*, 531–538. [CrossRef] [PubMed]
37. Mak, W.Y.; Zhao, M.; Ng, S.C.; Burisch, J. The epidemiology of inflammatory bowel disease: East meets west. *J. Gastroenterol. Hepatol.* **2020**, *35*, 380–389. [CrossRef] [PubMed]
38. Holvoet, T.; Lobaton, T.; Hindryckx, P. Optimal Management of Acute Severe Ulcerative Colitis (ASUC): Challenges and Solutions. *Clin. Exp. Gastroenterol.* **2021**, *14*, 71–81. [CrossRef] [PubMed]
39. Ungar, B.; Mazor, Y.; Weisshof, R.; Yanai, H.; Ron, Y.; Goren, I.; Waizbard, A.; Yavzori, M.; Fudim, E.; Picard, O.; et al. Induction infliximab levels among patients with acute severe ulcerative colitis compared with patients with moderately severe ulcerative colitis. *Aliment. Pharmacol. Ther.* **2016**, *43*, 1293–1299. [CrossRef] [PubMed]
40. Brandse, J.F.; van den Brink, G.R.; Wildenberg, M.E.; van der Kleij, D.; Rispens, T.; Jansen, J.M.; Mathôt, R.A.; Ponsioen, C.Y.; Löwenberg, M.; D'Haens, G.R. Loss of Infliximab Into Feces Is Associated With Lack of Response to Therapy in Patients With Severe Ulcerative Colitis. *Gastroenterology* **2015**, *149*, 350-355.e2. [CrossRef] [PubMed]
41. Battat, R.; Hemperly, A.; Truong, S.; Whitmire, N.; Boland, B.S.; Dulai, P.S.; Holmer, A.K.; Nguyen, N.H.; Singh, S.; Casteele, N.V.; et al. Baseline Clearance of Infliximab is Associated with Requirement for Colectomy in Patients with Acute Severe Ulcerative Colitis. *Clin. Gastroenterol. Hepatol.* **2021**, *19*, 511-518.e6. [CrossRef] [PubMed]
42. Kevans, D.; Murthy, S.; Mould, D.R.; Silverberg, M.S. Accelerated Clearance of Infliximab is Associated With Treatment Failure in Patients With Corticosteroid-Refractory Acute Ulcerative Colitis. *J. Crohns Colitis* **2018**, *12*, 662–669. [CrossRef] [PubMed]
43. Feuerstein, J.D.; Isaacs, K.L.; Schneider, Y.; Siddique, S.M.; Falck-Ytter, Y.; Singh, S. AGA Clinical Practice Guidelines on the Management of Moderate to Severe Ulcerative Colitis. *Gastroenterology* **2020**, *158*, 1450–1461. [CrossRef]
44. Yarur, A.J.; Kanagala, V.; Stein, D.J.; Czul, F.; Quintero, M.A.; Agrawal, D.; Patel, A.; Best, K.; Fox, C.; Idstein, K.; et al. Higher infliximab trough levels are associated with perianal fistula healing in patients with Crohn's disease. *Aliment. Pharmacol. Ther.* **2017**, *45*, 933–940. [CrossRef] [PubMed]
45. Strik, A.S.; Löwenberg, M.; Buskens, C.J.; Gecse, K.B.; Ponsioen, I.C.; Bemelman, W.A.; D'Haens, R.G. Higher anti-TNF serum levels are associated with perianal fistula closure in Crohn's disease patients. *Scand. J. Gastroenterol.* **2019**, *54*, 453–458. [CrossRef] [PubMed]

46. Davidov, Y.; Ungar, B.; Bar-Yoseph, H.; Carter, D.; Haj-Natour, O.; Yavzori, M.; Chowers, Y.; Eliakim, R.; Ben-Horin, S.; Kopylov, U. Association of Induction Infliximab Levels with Clinical Response in Perianal Crohn's Disease. *J. Crohns Colitis* **2017**, *11*, 549–555. [CrossRef]
47. Plevris, N.; Jenkinson, P.W.; Arnott, I.D.; Jones, G.R.; Lees, C.W. Higher anti-tumor necrosis factor levels are associated with perianal fistula healing and fistula closure in Crohn's disease. *Eur. J. Gastroenterol. Hepatol.* **2020**, *32*, 32–37. [CrossRef]
48. Papamichael, K.; Vande Casteele, N.; Jeyarajah, J.; Jairath, V.; Osterman, M.T.; Cheifetz, A.S. Higher Postinduction Infliximab Concentrations Are Associated With Improved Clinical Outcomes in Fistulizing Crohn's Disease: An ACCENT-II Post Hoc Analysis. *Am. J. Gastroenterol.* **2021**, *116*, 1007–1014. [CrossRef] [PubMed]
49. Zhu, M.; Xu, X.; Feng, Q.; Cui, Z.; Wang, T.; Yan, Y.; Ran, Z. Effectiveness of Infliximab on Deep Radiological Remission in Chinese Patients with Perianal Fistulizing Crohn's Disease. *Dig. Dis. Sci.* **2021**, *66*, 1658–1668. [CrossRef]
50. El-Matary, W.; Walters, T.D.; Huynh, H.Q.; de Bruyn, J.; Mack, D.R.; Jacobson, K.; Sherlock, M.E.; Church, P.; Wine, E.; Carroll, M.W.; et al. Higher Postinduction Infliximab Serum Trough Levels Are Associated With Healing of Fistulizing Perianal Crohn's Disease in Children. *Inflamm. Bowel Dis.* **2019**, *25*, 150–155. [CrossRef] [PubMed]
51. Ruemmele, F.M.; Rosh, J.; Faubion, W.A.; Dubinsky, M.C.; Turner, D.; Lazar, A.; Eichner, S.; Maa, J.-F.; Alperovich, G.; Robinson, A.M.; et al. Efficacy of Adalimumab for Treatment of Perianal Fistula in Children with Moderately to Severely Active Crohn's Disease: Results from IMAgINE 1 and IMAgINE 2. *J. Crohns Colitis* **2018**, *12*, 1249–1254. [CrossRef] [PubMed]
52. Gu, B.; De Gregorio, M.; Pipicella, J.L.; Vande Casteele, N.; Andrews, J.M.; Begun, J.; Connell, W.; D'Souza, B.; Gholamrezaei, A.; Hart, A.; et al. Prospective randomised controlled trial of adults with perianal fistulising Crohn's disease and optimised therapeutic infliximab levels: PROACTIVE trial study protocol. *BMJ Open* **2021**, *11*, e043921. [CrossRef] [PubMed]
53. Ahmed Ali, U.; Martin, S.T.; Rao, A.D.; Kiran, R.P. Impact of preoperative immunosuppressive agents on postoperative outcomes in Crohn's disease. *Dis. Colon Rectum* **2014**, *57*, 663–674. [PubMed]
54. Kirchhoff, P.; Clavien, P.-A.; Hahnloser, D. Complications in colorectal surgery: Risk factors and preventive strategies. *Patient Saf. Surg.* **2010**, *4*, 5. [CrossRef]
55. Bellolio, F.; Cohen, Z.; Macrae, H.M.; O'Connor, B.I.; Huang, H.; Victor, J.C.; McLeod, R.S. Outcomes following surgery for perforating Crohn's disease. *J. Br. Surg.* **2013**, *100*, 1344–1348. [CrossRef] [PubMed]
56. Adedokun, O.J.; Sandborn, W.J.; Feagan, B.G.; Rutgeerts, P.; Xu, Z.; Marano, C.W.; Johanns, J.; Zhou, H.; Davis, H.M.; Cornillie, F.; et al. Association between serum concentration of infliximab and efficacy in adult patients with ulcerative colitis. *Gastroenterology* **2014**, *147*, 1296-1307.e5. [CrossRef] [PubMed]
57. Nalagatla, N.; Falloon, K.; Tran, G.; Borren, N.Z.; Avalos, D.; Luther, J.; Colizzo, F.; Garber, J.; Khalili, H.; Melia, J.; et al. Effect of Accelerated Infliximab Induction on Short- and Long-term Outcomes of Acute Severe Ulcerative Colitis: A Retrospective Multicenter Study and Meta-analysis. *Clin. Gastroenterol. Hepatol.* **2019**, *17*, 502-509.e1. [CrossRef] [PubMed]
58. Dong, C.; Metzger, M.; Holsbø, E.; Perduca, V.; Carbonnel, F. Systematic review with meta-analysis: Mortality in acute severe ulcerative colitis. *Aliment. Pharmacol. Ther.* **2020**, *51*, 8–33. [CrossRef]
59. Panés, J.; Rimola, J. Perianal fistulizing Crohn's disease: Pathogenesis, diagnosis and therapy. *Nat. Rev. Gastroenterol. Hepatol.* **2017**, *14*, 652–664. [CrossRef]
60. Adegbola, S.O.; Sarafian, M.; Sahnan, K.; Pechlivanis, A.; Phillips, R.K.S.; Warusavitarne, J.; Faiz, O.; Haddow, J.; Knowles, C.; Tozer, P.; et al. Lack of anti-TNF drugs levels in fistula tissue—A reason for nonresponse in Crohn's perianal fistulating disease? *Eur. J. Gastroenterol. Hepatol.* **2021**, *34*, 18–26. [CrossRef]

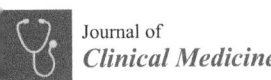

Review

Therapeutic Drug Monitoring of Infliximab in Acute Severe Ulcerative Colitis

Benjamin L. Gordon [1] and Robert Battat [2],*

[1] Division of Gastroenterology and Hepatology, New York-Presbyterian/Weill Cornell Medical Center, New York, NY 10065, USA; beg2013@nyp.org
[2] Center for Clinical and Translational Research in Inflammatory Bowel Diseases, Centre Hospitalier de l'Université de Montréal, Montreal, QC H2X 0A9, Canada
* Correspondence: robert.battat@umontreal.ca

Abstract: Therapeutic drug monitoring (TDM) is a useful strategy in ulcerative colitis (UC). Nearly a quarter of UC patients will experience acute severe UC (ASUC) in their lifetime, including 30% who will fail first-line corticosteroid therapy. Steroid-refractory ASUC patients require salvage therapy with infliximab, cyclosporine, or colectomy. Fewer data are available for the use of TDM of infliximab in ASUC. The pharmacokinetics of ASUC make TDM in this population more complex. High inflammatory burden is associated with increased infliximab clearance, which is associated with lower infliximab drug concentrations. Observational data support the association between increased serum infliximab concentrations, lower clearance, and favorable clinical and endoscopic outcomes, as well as decreased rates of colectomy. Data regarding the benefit of accelerated or intensified dosing strategies of infliximab—as well as target drug concentration thresholds—in ASUC patients remain more equivocal, though limited by their observational nature. Studies are underway to further evaluate optimal dosing and TDM targets in this population. This review examines the evidence for TDM in patients with ASUC, with a focus on infliximab.

Keywords: acute severe ulcerative colitis; therapeutic drug monitoring; infliximab; pharmacokinetics; dose optimization; inflammatory bowel disease; ulcerative colitis

Citation: Gordon, B.L.; Battat, R. Therapeutic Drug Monitoring of Infliximab in Acute Severe Ulcerative Colitis. *J. Clin. Med.* **2023**, *12*, 3378. https://doi.org/10.3390/jcm12103378

Academic Editor: Konstantinos Papamichael

Received: 15 April 2023
Revised: 1 May 2023
Accepted: 5 May 2023
Published: 10 May 2023

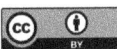

Copyright: © 2023 by the authors. Licensee MDPI, Basel, Switzerland. This article is an open access article distributed under the terms and conditions of the Creative Commons Attribution (CC BY) license (https://creativecommons.org/licenses/by/4.0/).

1. Introduction

Ulcerative colitis (UC) is one of two major chronic inflammatory bowel diseases (IBD). Up to 25% of UC patients will experience an episode of acute severe ulcerative colitis (ASUC) that requires hospitalization [1,2]. Delayed management of ASUC is associated with significant morbidity and mortality, including toxic megacolon, fulminant colitis, bowel perforation, refractory bleeding, venous thromboembolism, and bacterial infection [3,4]. Colectomy rates for hospitalized patients with ASUC range from 25% to 30%, including 20% of patients requiring colectomy during their first hospital admission [1,2,5,6]. Despite the advent of biologic therapy and advances in the management of ASUC, there is still measurable mortality associated with it [6].

First-line medical therapy in patients with ASUC remains intravenous corticosteroids. However, 30% of ASUC patients will fail steroid therapy, of whom up to 50% will require colectomy [3,7–9]. Patients who do not demonstrate improvement within 3–5 days of initiation of corticosteroids are unlikely to respond to steroids and require either rescue therapy or colectomy [10].

Rescue therapy for ASUC includes infliximab (IFX) and intravenous cyclosporine. Multiple trials have shown that infliximab is beneficial in steroid-refractory ASUC patients, including one randomized controlled trial (RCT) which demonstrated that infliximab decreased short-term colectomy rates compared to placebo (29% vs. 67%) [11–13]. Cyclosporine has similarly been proven to be superior to placebo in these patients [14,15]. In multiple head-to-head RCTs of infliximab and cyclosporine in ASUC, there have been no differences in short- or long-term rates of clinical response, colectomy, or mortality [16,17]. A recent meta-analysis of trials compared rescue IFX to cyclosporine therapy in steroid-refractory ASUC [1]. In RCTs of severe UC patients receiving infliximab, pooled rates of therapeutic response, 3-month colectomy, and 12-month colectomy were 43.8%, 26.6%, and 34.4%, respectively. Similar results were observed with cyclosporine (41.7%, 26.4%, and 40.8%, respectively). In nonrandomized studies, rates were considerably higher for both infliximab (74.8%, 24.1%, and 20.7%, respectively) and cyclosporine (55.4%, 42.5%, and 36.8%, respectively) [1].

Infliximab is generally preferred over cyclosporine in ASUC patients for ease of use. Initial responders to infliximab remain on maintenance infliximab therapy. Cyclosporine requires frequent dose adjustments due to a narrow therapeutic window. In addition, responders to cyclosporine must be converted to alternate therapies, and the most robust data exist for subsequent thiopurines, which is no longer preferred as a first-line UC therapy.

For cyclosporine, data do not support intensive dosing. In a RCT of high-dose intravenous cyclosporine (4 mg/kg) versus standard dose intravenous cyclosporine (2 mg/kg), there was no significant difference in short-term colectomy rates, despite the high-dose group having significantly increased mean cyclosporine blood levels [18]. However, data regarding dose optimization and therapeutic drug monitoring (TDM) in infliximab are still being elucidated. For this reason, in this review, we will discuss TDM in ASUC, with a focus on infliximab.

2. Pharmacokinetics of Infliximab in ASUC

It is well understood that the clearance of anti-TNF (tumor necrosis factor) agents in ASUC is propagated by numerous mechanisms related broadly to increased inflammatory burden. The pharmacokinetics of infliximab in ASUC are impacted by increased levels of TNF-α, anti-TNF neutralization, heightened proteolytic degradation of immune complexes, and reduced tissue penetration, all of which leads to low serum concentrations of infliximab, which may subsequently augment immunogenicity [8,19–25]. Moreover, many ASUC patients suffer from malnutrition in the acute setting, and thus drug levels of infliximab may be negatively affected by both decreased protein intake as well as increased intestinal protein loss, resulting in hypoalbuminemia and increased infliximab clearance, as infliximab is albumin-bound [8,10,26,27].

Fecal drug loss can occur in the setting of a severely impaired mucosal barrier in patients with ASUC. Not only does this lead to lower drug levels, but it also results in effectively decreased episodic doses of infliximab, which promotes immunogenicity and antibody formation against infliximab [9]. The formation of antibodies to infliximab has ramifications on dose optimization of infliximab, and it impacts treatment decisions. In one large study using an IBD database, in infliximab-treated patients (n = 63,176) with antibodies to infliximab (ATI), dose escalation was associated with adequate infliximab levels (>5 µg/mL) at the subsequent assessment [28]. Dose escalation was also associated with a greater increase in drug concentration (5.9 vs. 0.2 µg/mL) and ATI reductions (1.9 vs. 4.3 U/mL) compared to patients with no escalation [28].

Little is known about the relationship between efficacy and serum, colonic mucosa, and stool concentrations of drugs. Mucosal 5-acetylsalicylic acid (5-ASA) concentrations are associated with endoscopic outcomes [29] but there is a paucity of data on the relationship of infliximab concentrations between tissue, serum, and fecal compartments. A recent study on TNF antagonist concentrations in colonic tissue provides minimal information on infliximab in UC. Only six patients with UC were included, of which an unspecified number received infliximab or adalimumab. Furthermore, a majority of samples analyzed in the study were from uninflamed tissue and neither clinical outcomes nor objective endoscopic scores were assessed [23]. The study demonstrated a positive correlation between serum and tissue TNF antagonist concentration in uninflamed tissue but not in inflamed tissue. Serum TNF antagonist concentrations only correlated with the degree of endoscopic inflammation in uninflamed tissue. Patients with active mucosal disease had high rates of discordant serum to tissue drug concentrations [23].

Data in ASUC are consistent with observations that infliximab concentrations are lower with higher inflammatory burden. In an observational retrospective study, Ungar et al. demonstrated that mean infliximab trough levels at day 14 were significantly lower in patients with ASUC compared to patients with moderately severe UC (7.1 vs. 14.4 µg/mL) [30] (Table 1). As ASUC impacts the pharmacokinetics of infliximab and decreases drug levels, there may be benefit to TDM in this population.

Table 1. Summary of Pharmacokinetic Studies of Infliximab in ASUC.

Author (Year)	Study Design	Population	Number of Subjects	Measurement of IFX Pharmacokinetics	Outcomes
Yarur (2016) [23]	Prospective Cross-Sectional	IBD patients on maintenance IFX or adalimumab	30 (including 6 UC)	Anti-TNF serum concentration and anti-TNF tissue concentration (from colonic and ileal biopsies)	Anti-TNF tissue concentrations correlated with anti-TNF serum concentrations, except in inflamed tissue. Ratio of anti-TNF to TNF in tissue was highest in uninflamed tissue and lowest in severely inflamed tissue
Dotan (2014) [25]	Prospective Observational	IBD patients receiving IFX	54 patients (25 UC, 25 Crohn's disease, and 4 indeterminate) with 169 IFX concentrations	IFX trough concentrations and antibodies against IFX prior to IFX infusion	Low albumin, high body weight, and presence of antibodies against IFX were associated with higher IFX clearance
Fasanmade (2009) [26]	Post-hoc analysis of 2 RCTs (ACT 1 and 2)	Moderate-to-severe UC randomized to IFX 5 mg/kg or 10 mg/kg or placebo	482	IFX serum concentrations immediately before and after IFX doses and antibodies against IFX	IFX clearance was higher in patients with antibodies to IFX. IFX clearance was inversely correlated with serum albumin
Brandse (2016) [20]	Prospective Cohort	Anti-TNF naïve moderate–severe UC patients receiving IFX induction therapy	19	Serial IFX serum concentrations and antibodies against IFX	IFX nonresponders were more likely to have antibodies against IFX (odds ratio 30.0, 95% CI 2.2–406). Patients with CRP > 50 mg/L at baseline had lower serum IFX concentrations at week 6 compared to patients with lower CRP
Brandse (2015) [21]	Prospective Cohort	Anti-TNF naïve patients with moderately to severely active UC, initiated on IFX	30 (26 with severe endoscopic disease)	IFX serum concentration at week 2 and IFX fecal concentration at day 1 from induction	Clinical nonresponders at week 2 had significantly increased fecal IFX levels at day 1 from induction compared to responders (5.01 vs. 0.54 µg/mL)
Ungar (2016) [30]	Retrospective	Hospitalized steroid-refractory ASUC patients compared to moderately severe UC initiated on IFX	32 total (including 16 ASUC)	IFX trough concentrations and antibodies to IFX at day 14 from induction	IFX trough concentrations were significantly lower in ASUC patients compared to moderately severe UC patients (7.2 vs. 14.4 µg/mL)

3. Outcomes Associated with Infliximab Pharmacokinetics in ASUC

The potential utility of TDM in ASUC initially came out of the established benefit of dose optimization in patients with moderate-to-severe UC. In a post-hoc analysis of 728 patients with moderate-to-severe UC in the ACT-1 and ACT-2 (Active Ulcerative Colitis Trials 1 and 2) trials, patients with clinical response, mucosal healing, and/or clinical remission had higher median serum concentrations of infliximab at weeks 8, 30, and 54 compared to patients without clinical or endoscopic response [31]. In a separate study of 155 patients with IBD, in patients with subtherapeutic infliximab concentrations, dose escalation led to complete or partial clinical response in 86% of patients [32]. Lastly, Brandse et al. published two separate prospective, observational studies evaluating infliximab concentrations in serum and stool in patients with moderate-to-severe UC. Primary infliximab nonresponders were found to have lower serum infliximab concentrations, increased fecal infliximab concentrations, and higher rates of antibody formation to infliximab, suggesting that higher infliximab clearance and drug wasting in the stool are associated with worse clinical outcomes [20,21].

In ASUC patients, supportive data exist showing that serum infliximab concentrations have predictive value for clinical response, clinical remission, and need for colectomy. In a prospective observational study of 115 patients with steroid-refractory acute UC (including 42 with ASUC), Seow et al. demonstrated that patients with detectable serum infliximab trough concentrations—during both induction and maintenance—had higher rates of clinical remission (69% vs. 15%) and lower rates of colectomy (7% vs. 55%) compared to patients with undetectable trough concentrations [22]. In another prospective observational study of 285 patients with refractory UC (including 39 patients with ASUC), serum levels of infliximab > 2.5 µg/mL at week 14 were associated with higher rates of relapse-free survival as well as colectomy-free survival [33]. In a retrospective study of 99 patients with UC (including 23 patients with ASUC), Papamichael et al. showed that infliximab concentration < 16.5 µg/mL at week 2 after induction was an independent predictor of colectomy [34]. Furthermore, in a study of 24 ASUC patients, elevated fecal infliximab concentrations were associated with both decreased remission rates and higher risk of colectomy [35] (Table 2).

Table 2. Summary of Outcomes Associated with Infliximab Pharmacokinetics in ASUC.

Author (Year)	Study Design	Population	Number of Subjects	Measurement of IFX Pharmacokinetics	Outcomes Associated with IFX Pharmacokinetics
Seow (2010) [22]	Prospective Observational	Steroid-refractory acute moderate-to-severe UC patients initiated on IFX	115 total (including 42 ASUC)	Detectable serum IFX trough concentration during induction and maintenance periods (found in 39% of subjects)	Higher rates of clinical remission (69% vs. 15%), lower rates of colectomy (7 vs. 55%), and higher rates of endoscopic improvement (76% vs. 28%) were found in patients with detectable troughs compared to those with undetectable troughs
Arias (2015) [33]	Prospective Observational	UC patients refractory to cyclosporine or immunomodulators, initiated on IFX	285 total (including 39 ASUC)	Serum IFX level at week 14 of treatment	Serum IFX level > 2.5 µg/mL at week 14 was associated with increased rates of relapse-free survival and colectomy-free survival
Papamichael (2016) [34]	Retrospective Observational Multicenter	Anti-TNF naïve UC patients with primary nonresponse to IFX induction therapy	99 total (including 23 ASUC)	Serum IFX levels at weeks 2 and 6 of treatment	Serum IFX level < 16.5 µg/mL at week 2 (hazard ratio 5.6, 95% CI 1.1–27.8) was independently associated with colectomy
Beswick (2018) [35]	Prospective Observational Pilot	Hospitalized steroid-refractory ASUC patients, initiated on IFX	24 total (all 24 with ASUC)	Fecal IFX concentration at day 1 post-first dose of IFX	Fecal IFX level > 1 mg/mL at day 1 was associated with lower rates of clinical remission at week 6 (odds ratio 0.04, 95% CI 0.02–0.9) and higher rates of colectomy (odds ratio 176, 95% CI 2.1–14,452)

Table 2. Cont.

Author (Year)	Study Design	Population	Number of Subjects	Measurement of IFX Pharmacokinetics	Outcomes Associated with IFX Pharmacokinetics
Paul (2013) [36]	Prospective Observational	IBD patients receiving IFX who required IFX dose optimization for active disease	52 total (18 UC, including 10 ASUC)	IFX trough concentrations prior to IFX optimization and at week 8 after optimization; differences in trough concentrations were calculated (called delta IFX)	Delta IFX > 0.5 µg/mL was associated with mucosal healing (sensitivity 0.88, specificity 0.77)
Papamichael (2016) [37]	Retrospective	UC patients receiving IFX induction	101 total (including 16 ASUC)	Serum IFX levels at weeks 2, 6, and 14 after induction	Early mucosal healing was associated with increased serum IFX levels at weeks 2 (22.9 vs. 19.3 µg/mL), 6 (17.6 vs. 10.3 µg/mL), and 14 (7.4 vs. 1.5 µg/mL) compared to those without healing
Battat (2021) [27]	Retrospective	Hospitalized ASUC patients, initiated on IFX	39 total (all 39 with ASUC)	Baseline calculated IFX clearance using existing formula (that included sex, presence of antibodies to IFX, and serum albumin)	IFX clearance > 0.627 L/day was associated with higher rates of colectomy within 6 months compared to those with lower clearance (61.5% vs. 7.7%)
Kevans (2018) [38]	Retrospective	Steroid-refractory ASUC patients, initiated on IFX	36 total (all 36 with ASUC)	IFX clearance using pharmacokinetic modeling (that included serum IFX levels, antibodies to IFX, weight, and serum albumin)	Lower IFX clearance was associated with higher rates of clinical response at week 14 and steroid-free remission at week 54

Serum infliximab concentrations have also been associated with favorable endoscopic outcomes. For example, in Seow's study of 115 acute UC patients (including 42 with ASUC), a detectable serum infliximab trough concentration was associated with higher rates of endoscopic improvement (decrease in endoscopic Mayo score of at least one point) compared to patients with undetectable trough concentrations (76% vs. 28%) [22]. In a prospective observational study of 52 patients with active IBD on maintenance infliximab requiring dose optimization (including 18 UC patients, 10 with severe endoscopic activity), an increase in infliximab trough level was associated with mucosal healing, and 50% of IBD patients achieved mucosal healing after dose intensification [36]. In a retrospective study of 101 UC patients (including 16 with ASUC), Papamichael et al. showed that patients with early mucosal healing (at weeks 10–14 from initiation of therapy) had higher serum infliximab concentrations at weeks 2, 6, and 14 after treatment initiation than those without healing [37]. This study also demonstrated that the presence of ASUC was associated with being in the lowest quartile of infliximab concentration among all UC patients in the study (11 of 16 ASUC patients were in the lowest quartile)—the authors of this study thus suggested that accelerated dosing be used in ASUC patients. A number of the studies outlined present their data in aggregate, including all moderate and severe UC patients, without subgroup analysis of ASUC patients. This may limit the application of these data to ASUC patients.

Clearance of infliximab is also an important determinant of pharmacokinetics and outcomes in ASUC. Higher infliximab clearance has been associated with colectomy and treatment failure. In a retrospective study of 39 patients with ASUC, elevated (>0.627 L/day) baseline calculated infliximab clearance (using sex, presence of antibodies to infliximab, and serum albumin) prior to induction was associated with higher rates of colectomy compared to patients with lower clearance values (61.5% vs. 7.7%) [27]. In another retrospective study of 36 ASUC patients, Kevans et al. demonstrated that lower clearance of infliximab (utilizing pharmacokinetic modeling of a number of parameters, including serum infliximab concentrations, antibodies to infliximab, weight, and serum albumin) was associated with week 14 clinical response and week 54 steroid-free remission [38] (Table 2).

4. Intensive Infliximab Dosing Strategies in ASUC

Despite evidence suggesting that increased serum infliximab concentrations and decreased infliximab clearance are associated with improved clinical and endoscopic outcomes, data regarding intensified and accelerated infliximab dosing strategies in this population are conflicting. Initial literature on intensive dosing strategies were first investigated in moderate-to-severe UC, providing the rationale for its use in ASUC. For instance, in subgroup analyses of the ACT-1 and 2 trials, a 10 mg/kg dosing strategy of infliximab significantly reduced the risk of colectomy at 54 weeks compared to placebo (8% vs. 17%), but a 5 mg/kg dosing strategy did not (12%) [39].

However, data comparing different dosing strategies of infliximab in ASUC are contradictory. Some observational data suggest a benefit to intensive infliximab induction dosing strategies in ASUC with either multiple early doses or higher doses at standard intervals. In a retrospective study of 50 ASUC patients comparing standard induction of infliximab (5 mg/kg at weeks 0, 2, and 6) to accelerated induction (3 doses of 5 mg/kg within a median period of 24 days), Gibson et al. showed that an accelerated dosing strategy was associated with lower rates of early colectomy (7% vs. 40%) [40].

Other data have not shown a benefit to intensified dosing in this cohort. In a systematic review of seven retrospective studies (181 patients receiving accelerated infliximab dosing and 436 receiving standard infliximab dosing), there were similar rates of in-hospital colectomy among the accelerated dosing group and standard dosing group (9% vs. 8%); furthermore, similar proportions required colectomy at 3, 6, 12, and 24 months [41]. In a separate meta-analysis of five observational studies, Feuerstein et al. found that there was no significant difference in short-term colectomy risk between ASUC patients given intensive infliximab dosing (shortened interval dosing during induction or higher-dose during induction) compared to standard infliximab dosing (relative risk (RR) 1.61, 95% confidence interval (CI, 0.74–3.52) [10]. Other smaller retrospective studies have similarly found no difference in short-term colectomy risk in ASUC patients receiving higher-dose induction or accelerated dosing compared to those receiving standard induction dosing [42–44] (Table 3). While limited data exist on different intensive dosing strategies, a meta-analysis of two observational studies found that upfront higher dose infliximab (10 mg/kg) was associated with lower rates of colectomy than accelerated dosing with 5 mg/kg (RR 0.24, 95% CI, 0.08–0.68) [10].

Table 3. Summary of Intensive Dosing Strategy Studies in ASUC.

Author (Year)	Study Design	Population	Number of Subjects	Intensive Dosing Strategy	Primary Outcome	Results
Gibson (2015) [40]	Retrospective Cohort	Hospitalized patients receiving IFX for steroid-refractory ASUC	50 total (n = 35 standard dosing; n = 15 accelerated dosing	Three induction doses of IFX 5 mg/kg in median 24 days	Colectomy during IFX induction	Significantly decreased rates of early colectomy in the accelerated arm (7% vs. 40%)
Shah (2018) [42]	Retrospective Cohort with Propensity Score Matching	Hospitalized, IFX-naïve, acute UC patients receiving induction IFX	146 total (n = 120 standard dose; n = 26 high dose)	10 mg/kg induction dose of IFX	30-day colectomy	No significant difference in 30-day colectomy rates between high dose and standard dose groups in the unmatched cohort (15.4% vs. 17.5%) and matched cohort (9.5% vs. 9.5%)

Table 3. Cont.

Author (Year)	Study Design	Population	Number of Subjects	Intensive Dosing Strategy	Primary Outcome	Results
Chao (2019) [43]	Retrospective Cohort	Hospitalized ASUC patients receiving IFX	72 total (n = 37 standard dose induction; 35 high dose induction)	10 mg/kg induction dosing of IFX	Three-month colectomy	No significant difference in three-month colectomy rates between high dose and standard dose groups (14.3% vs. 5.4%)
Govani (2020) [44]	Retrospective Cohort	Hospitalized ASUC patients receiving IFX	66 total (n = 33 standard dosing; 33 accelerated dosing)	Two doses of IFX prior to day 14	90-day colectomy	No significant difference in 90-day colectomy rates between accelerated dosing and standard dosing groups (30.3% vs. 24.2%)
Nalagatla (2019) [41]	Retrospective Cohort and Meta-analysis of 7 Retrospective Studies (3 full text, 4 abstract)	Hospitalized patients receiving IFX for steroid-refractory ASUC	Retrospective Cohort: 213 total (n = 132 standard dosing; n = 81 accelerated dosing) Meta-analysis: 617 total (n = 436 standard dosing; n = 181 accelerated dosing)	10 mg/kg induction dosing of IFX or 5 mg/kg dosing at intervals shorter than weeks 0, 2, and 6	Retrospective Cohort: in-hospital colectomy Meta-analysis: in-hospital colectomy or one-month colectomy	No significant difference in in-hospital colectomy between accelerated dosing and standard dosing groups (9% vs. 8%) No significant difference in early colectomy between accelerated dosing and standard dosing in the meta-analysis (odds ratio 0.76, 95% CI 0.36–1.61)
Feuerstein (2020) [10]	Meta-analysis of 5 Observational Studies	Hospitalized patients receiving IFX for steroid-refractory ASUC	Total subjects not given	Shortened interval between IFX dosing (<2 weeks, dose stacking) or 10 mg/kg induction dosing	Short-term risk of colectomy	No significant difference in short-term risk of colectomy between intensive and standard dosing groups (relative risk 1.61, 95% CI 0.74–3.52)

Interpreting observational data of intensive dosing in ASUC patients is complex. Selection bias may exist in groups with accelerated or intensified dosing for patients with higher probability to have inadequate response to standard induction therapy [10]. In addition, there may be subgroups of individuals that required personalized selective dosing that are not captured by broadly comparing two treatment strategies. Further studies comparing clearance-based dosing to standard dosing in ASUC are needed.

5. Specific Threshold Target Concentrations for Infliximab

Observational data have shown higher infliximab drug concentrations to be associated with clinical remission, endoscopic remission, and lower rates of colectomy [22,33–37]. However, the use of specific infliximab concentrations to guide therapy is complicated by several factors: ASUC patients exhibit particularly unfavorable pharmacokinetics, specific infliximab drug concentrations targets are unknown in this context, and multiple measurement timepoints and assays exist.

Despite this, indirect data for specific infliximab thresholds from moderate-to-severe UC may inform the ASUC setting. In a post-hoc analysis of ACT-1 and ACT-2 (n = 728), serum infliximab levels of 41 µg/mL at week 8 of induction were associated with clinical response (sensitivity 63%, specificity 62%, positive predictive value 80%) [31]. In a separate literature review, Chiefetz et al. identified two studies with week 2 infliximab thresholds of >11.5–15.3 µg/mL for clinical response and remission, and week 14 infliximab thresholds of >5.1–6.7 µg/mL for mucosal healing [45–47].

Multiple infliximab thresholds have also been evaluated in ASUC. A retrospective study of 101 UC patients (including 16 with ASUC) found that infliximab concentrations of 28.3, 15.0, and 2.1 µg/mL at weeks 2, 6, and 14, respectively, were associated with short-term mucosal healing [37]. Moreover, in a prospective observational study of 285 patients with refractory UC (including 39 patients with ASUC), Arias et al. showed that serum levels of infliximab > 2.5 µg/mL at week 14 were associated with an absence of clinical relapse (sensitivity 81%, specificity 75%) and higher rates of relapse-free survival as well as colectomy-free survival [33]. However, a smaller retrospective study of 76 patients with IBD (including 18 with UC, number of ASUC unspecified) found no significant difference in mean infliximab troughs between patients who had clinical response to intensification of infliximab compared to those who did not (3.3 µg/mL vs. 2.3 µg/mL) [48].

Expert consensus statements for TDM in IBD recommend targeting infliximab concentrations of at least 20–25 µg/mL at week 2, 15–20 µg/mL at week 6, and 7–10 µg/mL at week 14 [45]. The caveat to these recommendations is that target thresholds should be tailored to disease severity and desired therapeutic outcome, as higher drug concentrations may be needed for ASUC [45].

6. Maintenance Monitoring following Infliximab Salvage Therapy for ASUC

Infliximab TDM strategies post-induction are variable, and few data exist on TDM during maintenance infliximab therapy after infliximab rescue therapy for ASUC. In a small retrospective study of 41 ASUC patients, including 20 patients who were maintained on infliximab after discharge (and who had follow-up data for one year), only 4 of 20 patients (20%) had a serum infliximab level checked after discharge [49]. As a comparison, thiopurine metabolites were monitored in 15 of 27 (56%) patients [49].

To our knowledge, in adult ASUC patients, no other data exist on TDM for maintenance therapy after salvage therapy, although this has been studied prospectively in the pediatric population [50]. In this pediatric study of 38 ASUC patients receiving infliximab, higher infliximab clearance (calculated by serum albumin, ATI, and white blood cell count) was associated with lack of remission at 26 weeks from induction; furthermore, patients with clinical remission at 26 weeks had numerically—albeit not significantly—higher infliximab trough concentrations (19.5 vs. 14.2 µg/mL) [50]. The PROTOS study, "Pharmacokinetics of IFX and TNF Concentrations in Serum, Stool, and Colonic Mucosa in Acute Severe Ulcerative Colitis", is an ongoing open-label, prospective, observational study to better assess the pharmacokinetics of infliximab in adult ASUC patients in the acute and maintenance setting [51]—studies such as this will potentially provide better data regarding timing of TDM and drug concentration thresholds of this cohort during the induction and maintenance period.

7. Cost-Effectiveness of TDM of Infliximab in ASUC

The use of TDM of infliximab has not only proven to be a useful strategy in IBD, but it has also been shown to be cost-effective. In one prospective observational multicenter study of 96 IBD patients with loss of response to infliximab managed according to a TDM algorithm compared to 56 historical controls treated empirically with dose intensification, there were similar rates of clinical response at 12 weeks. However, patients managed with TDM were less likely to have infliximab dose escalations and by cost analysis there was an estimated 15% savings with the TDM algorithm [52]. A separate systematic review identifying two RCTs (including 247 Crohn's disease patients and 85 UC patients) found that the cost savings from TDM dosing strategies ranged from 28% to 34% [53]. However, while the use of infliximab in ASUC has been demonstrated to be cost-effective compared to both cyclosporine and surgery [54], to our knowledge, there have been no studies of cost-effectiveness of TDM of infliximab in ASUC patients. This remains an area for future research.

8. Conclusions and Future Directions

The pharmacokinetics of infliximab are altered in the severely inflamed state of ASUC, leading to lower drug concentrations and higher clearance. Observational data show that lower infliximab levels and higher clearance are associated with worse symptoms, more colonic inflammation, and higher rates of colectomy. However, observational studies on the use of intensive dosing strategies to overcome lower infliximab concentrations in ASUC are equivocal.

Based on the reported pharmacokinetics of infliximab in ASUC, very high doses of infliximab are likely to be required to induce clinical and endoscopic responses. In addition, there are inter-individual differences in infliximab clearance between ASUC patients. Thus, some ASUC patients may benefit from intensive dosing strategies, while others only require standard dosing. Determining the optimal dosing strategy for each patient in a personalized manner would likely lead to improved outcomes. However, to date there are no trials comparing clearance-based dosing strategies to standard dosing.

Besides robust data supporting TDM strategies in ASUC, another potential obstacle to the broader adoption of TDM is cost and time lag between sample collection and results. In a survey of 403 gastroenterologists and their attitudes towards TDM of anti-TNF agents in IBD, the largest barriers to widespread TDM implementation were perceived to be insurance coverage (78%), out-of-pocket costs (76%), and lag time between sample collection and result (39%) [55]. Point-of-care assays for TDM exist [56] and should be further explored in ASUC to address time lag concerns. In addition, further cost-effectiveness studies may further impact payor decisions to support TDM in ASUC.

Two ongoing clinical trials will hopefully provide answers to some of these unmet questions. PREDICT UC or "Optimising Infliximab Induction Therapy for Acute Severe Ulcerative Colitis" is a multicenter RCT investigating whether accelerated dose infliximab (5 mg/kg at weeks 0, 1, and 3) or higher-dose infliximab (10 mg/kg at weeks 0 and week 1) is superior to standard dose infliximab (5 mg/kg at weeks 0, 2, and 6) in improving clinical response and decreasing short-term colectomy rates [57]. The study was completed in September 2022, and data should become available soon. Additionally, TITRATE, or inducTIon for acuTe ulceRATivE Colitis, is a multicenter RCT evaluating whether proactive individualized intensified infliximab dosing in ASUC patients—using a pharmacokinetics-driven dashboard system—can lead to better clinical and endoscopic responses at week 6 compared to standard dosing [58]. This study is planned to be completed in December 2024. Further studies will clarify the use of TDM in ASUC patients and potentially improve outcomes in this population.

Author Contributions: B.L.G. and R.B. performed the literature review and wrote the paper. All authors have read and agreed to the published version of the manuscript.

Funding: This research received no external funding.

Institutional Review Board Statement: Not applicable.

Informed Consent Statement: Not applicable.

Data Availability Statement: No new data were created or analyzed in this study. Data sharing is not applicable to this article.

Conflicts of Interest: B.L.G.: None to report; R.B.: Speaker/moderator: Bristol Myers Squibb, Janssen, AbbVie, Takeda; Advisory boards: AbbVie, Pfizer, Lilly, Janssen, Bristol Myers Squibb.

References

1. Narula, N.; Marshall, J.K.; Colombel, J.F.; Leontiadis, G.I.; Williams, J.G.; Muqtadir, Z.; Reinisch, W. Systematic review and meta-analysis: Infliximab or cyclosporine as rescue therapy in patients with severe ulcerative colitis refractory to steroids. *Am. J. Gastroenterol.* **2016**, *111*, 477–491. [CrossRef]
2. Dinesen, L.C.; Walsh, A.J.; Protic, M.N.; Heap, G.; Cummings, F.; Warren, B.F.; George, B.; Mortensen, N.J.; Travis, S.P. The pattern and outcome of acute severe colitis. *J. Crohn's Colitis* **2010**, *4*, 431–437. [CrossRef]
3. Turner, D.; Walsh, C.M.; Steinhart, A.H.; Griffiths, A.M. Response to Corticosteroids in Severe Ulcerative Colitis: A Systematic Review of the Literature and a Meta-Regression. *Clin. Gastroenterol. Hepatol.* **2007**, *5*, 103–110. [CrossRef]
4. Carvello, M.; Watfah, J.; Włodarczyk, M.; Spinelli, A. The Management of the Hospitalized Ulcerative Colitis Patient: The Medical-Surgical Conundrum. *Curr. Gastroenterol. Rep.* **2020**, *22*, 11. [CrossRef]
5. Aratari, A.; Papi, C.; Clemente, V.; Moretti, A.; Luchetti, R.; Koch, M.; Capurso, L.; Caprilli, R. Colectomy rate in acute severe ulcerative colitis in the infliximab era. *Dig. Liver Dis.* **2008**, *40*, 821–826. [CrossRef]

6. Lynch, R.W.; Lowe, D.; Protheroe, A.; Driscoll, R.; Rhodes, J.M.; Arnott, I.D.R. Outcomes of rescue therapy in acute severe ulcerative colitis: Data from the United Kingdom inflammatory bowel disease audit. *Aliment. Pharmacol. Ther.* **2013**. [CrossRef]
7. Rubin, D.T.; Ananthakrishnan, A.N.; Siegel, C.A.; Sauer, B.G.; Long, M.D. ACG Clinical Guideline: Ulcerative Colitis in Adults. *Am. J. Gastroenterol.* **2019**, *114*, 384–413. [CrossRef]
8. Hindryckx, P.; Novak, G.; Vande Casteele, N.; Laukens, D.; Parker, C.; Shackelton, L.M.; Narula, N.; Khanna, R.; Dulai, P.; Levesque, B.G.; et al. Review article: Dose optimisation of infliximab for acute severe ulcerative colitis. *Aliment. Pharmacol. Ther.* **2017**, *45*, 617–630. [CrossRef]
9. Seah, D.; De Cruz, P. Review article: The practical management of acute severe ulcerative colitis. *Aliment. Pharmacol. Ther.* **2016**, *43*, 482–513. [CrossRef]
10. Feuerstein, J.D.; Isaacs, K.L.; Schneider, Y.; Siddique, S.M.; Falck-Ytter, Y.; Singh, S.; AGA Institute Clinical Guidelines Committee. AGA Clinical Practice Guidelines on the Management of Moderate to Severe Ulcerative Colitis. *Gastroenterology* **2020**, *158*, 1450–1461. [CrossRef]
11. Jarnerot, G.; Hertervig, E.; Friis-Liby, I.; Blomquist, L.; Karlén, P.; Grännö, C.; Vilien, M.; Ström, M.; Danielsson, Å.; Verbaan, H.; et al. Infliximab as Rescue Therapy in Severe to Moderately Severe Ulcerative Colitis: A Randomized, Placebo-controlled Study. *Gastroenterology* **2005**, *128*, 1805–1811. [CrossRef]
12. Sands, B.E.; Miehsler, W.; Tremain, W.J.; Rutgeerts, P.J.; Hanauer, S.B.; Mayer, L.; Targan, S.R.; Podolsky, D.K. Infliximab in the treatment of severe, steroid-refractory ulcerative colitis: A pilot study. *Inflamm. Bowel Dis.* **2001**, *7*, 83–88. [CrossRef]
13. Sjoberg, M.; Magnuson, A.; Bjork, J.; Benoni, C.; Almer, S.; Friis-Liby, I.; Hertervig, E.; Olsson, M.; Karlén, P.; Eriksson, A.; et al. Infliximab as rescue therapy in hospitalised patients with steroid-refractory acute ulcerative colitis: A long-term follow-up of 211 Swedish patients. *Aliment. Pharmacol. Ther.* **2013**, *38*, 377–387. [CrossRef]
14. Lichtiger, S.; Present, D.H.; Kornbluth, A.; Gelernt, I.; Bauer, J.; Galler, G.; Michelassi, F.; Hanauer, S. Cyclosporine in severe ulcerative colitis refractory to steroid therapy. *N. Engl. J. Med.* **1994**, *330*, 1841–1845. [CrossRef]
15. Campbell, S.; Travis, S.; Jewell, D. Ciclosporin use in acute ulcerative colitis: A long-term experience. *Eur. J. Gastroenterol. Hepatol.* **2005**, *17*, 79–84. [CrossRef]
16. Laharie, D.; Bourreille, A.; Branche, J.; Allez, M.; Bouhnik, Y.; Filippi, J.; Zerbib, F.; Savoye, G.; Nachury, M.; Moreau, J.; et al. Ciclosporin versus infliximab in patients with severe ulcerative colitis refractory to intravenous steroids: A parallel, open-label randomised controlled trial. *Lancet* **2012**, *380*, 1909–1915. [CrossRef]
17. Williams, J.G.; Alam, M.F.; Alrubaiy, L.; Arnott, I.; Clement, C.; Cohen, D.; Gordon, J.N.; Hawthorne, A.B.; Hilton, M.; Hutchings, H.A.; et al. Infliximab versus ciclosporin for steroid-resistant acute severe ulcerative colitis (CONSTRUCT): A mixed methods, open-label, pragmatic randomised trial. *Lancet Gastroenterol. Hepatol.* **2016**, *1*, 15–24. [CrossRef]
18. Van Assche, G.; D'Haens, G.; Noman, M.; Vermeire, S.; Hiele, M.; Asnong, K.; Arts, J.; D'Hoore, A.; Penninckx, F.; Rutgeerts, P. Randomized, double-blind comparison of 4 mg/kg versus 2 mg/kg intravenous cyclosporine in severe ulcerative colitis. *Gastroenterology* **2003**, *125*, 1025–1031. [CrossRef]
19. Irving, P.M.; Gecse, K.B. Optimizing Therapies Using Therapeutic Drug Monitoring: Current Strategies and Future Perspectives. *Gastroenterology* **2022**, *162*, 1512–1524. [CrossRef]
20. Brandse, J.F.; Mathôt, R.A.; van der Kleij, D.; Rispens, T.; Ashruf, Y.; Jansen, J.M.; Rietdijk, S.; Löwenberg, M.; Ponsioen, C.Y.; Singh, S.; et al. Pharmacokinetic Features and Presence of Antidrug Antibodies Associate with Response to Infliximab Induction Therapy in Patients with Moderate to Severe Ulcerative Colitis. *Clin. Gastroenterol. Hepatol.* **2016**, *14*, 251–258.e1-2. [CrossRef]
21. Brandse, J.F.; van den Brink, G.R.; Wildenberg, M.E.; van der Kleij, D.; Rispens, T.; Jansen, J.M.; Mathôt, R.A.; Ponsioen, C.Y.; Löwenberg, M.; D'Haens, G.R. Loss of Infliximab into Feces Is Associated with Lack of Response to Therapy in Patients with Severe Ulcerative Colitis. *Gastroenterology* **2015**, *149*, 350–355.e2. [CrossRef]
22. Seow, C.H.; Newman, A.; Irwin, S.P.; Steinhart, A.H.; Silverberg, M.S.; Greenberg, G.R. Trough serum infliximab: A predictive factor of clinical outcome for infliximab treatment in acute ulcerative colitis. *Gut* **2010**, *59*, 49–54. [CrossRef]
23. Yarur, A.J.; Jain, A.; Sussman, D.A.; Barkin, J.S.; Quintero, M.A.; Princen, F.; Kirkland, R.; Deshpande, A.R.; Singh, S.; Abreu, M.T. The association of tissue anti-TNF drug levels with serological and endoscopic disease activity in inflammatory bowel disease: The ATLAS study. *Gut* **2016**, *65*, 249–255. [CrossRef]
24. Rosen, M.J.; Minar, P.; Vinks, A.A. Review article: Applying pharmacokinetics to optimise dosing of anti-TNF biologics in acute severe ulcerative colitis. *Aliment. Pharmacol. Ther.* **2015**, *41*, 1094–1103. [CrossRef]
25. Dotan, I.; Ron, Y.; Yanai, H.; Becker, S.; Fishman, S.; Yahav, L.; Ben Yehoyada, M.; Mould, D.R. Patient factors that increase infliximab clearance and shorten half-life in inflammatory bowel disease: A population pharmacokinetic study. *Inflamm. Bowel Dis.* **2014**, *20*, 2247–2259. [CrossRef]
26. Fasanmade, A.A.; Adedokun, O.J.; Ford, J.; Hernandez, D.; Johanns, J.; Hu, C.; Davis, H.M.; Zhou, H. Population pharmacokinetic analysis of infliximab in patients with ulcerative colitis. *Eur. J. Clin. Pharmacol.* **2009**, *65*, 1211–1228. [CrossRef]
27. Battat, R.; Hemperly, A.; Truong, S.; Whitmire, N.; Boland, B.S.; Dulai, P.S.; Holmer, A.K.; Nguyen, N.H.; Singh, S.; Vande Casteele, N.; et al. Baseline Clearance of Infliximab Is Associated with Requirement for Colectomy in Patients With Acute Severe Ulcerative Colitis. *Clin. Gastroenterol. Hepatol.* **2021**, *19*, 511–518.e6. [CrossRef]
28. Battat, R.; Lukin, D.; Scherl, E.J.; Pola, S.; Kumar, A.; Okada, L.; Yang, L.; Jain, A.; Siegel, C.A. Immunogenicity of Tumor Necrosis Factor Antagonists and Effect of Dose Escalation on Anti-Drug Antibodies and Serum Drug Concentrations in Inflammatory Bowel Disease. *Inflamm. Bowel Dis.* **2021**, *27*, 1443–1451. [CrossRef]

29. Frieri, G.; Giacomelli, R.; Pimpo, M.; Palumbo, G.; Passacantando, A.; Pantaleoni, G.; Caprilli, R. Mucosal 5-aminosalicylic acid concentration inversely correlates with severity of colonic inflammation in patients with ulcerative colitis. *Gut* **2000**, *47*, 410–414. [CrossRef]
30. Ungar, B.; Mazor, Y.; Weisshof, R.; Yanai, H.; Ron, Y.; Goren, I.; Waizbard, A.; Yavzori, M.; Fudim, E.; Picard, O.; et al. Induction infliximab levels among patients with acute severe ulcerative colitis compared with patients with moderately severe ulcerative colitis. *Aliment. Pharmacol. Ther.* **2016**, *43*, 1293–1299. [CrossRef]
31. Adedokun, O.J.; Sandborn, W.J.; Feagan, B.G.; Rutgeerts, P.; Xu, Z.; Marano, C.W.; Johanns, J.; Zhou, H.; Davis, H.M.; Cornillie, F.; et al. Association between serum concentration of infliximab and efficacy in adult patients with ulcerative colitis. *Gastroenterology* **2014**, *147*, 1296–1307.e5. [CrossRef] [PubMed]
32. Afif, W.; Loftus, E.V., Jr.; Faubion, W.A.; Kane, S.V.; Bruining, D.H.; Hanson, K.A.; Sandborn, W.J. Clinical utility of measuring infliximab and human anti-chimeric antibody concentrations in patients with inflammatory bowel disease. *Am. J. Gastroenterol.* **2010**, *105*, 1133–1139. [CrossRef] [PubMed]
33. Arias, M.T.; Vande Casteele, N.; Vermeire, S.; de Buck van Overstraeten, A.; Billiet, T.; Baert, F.; Wolthuis, A.; Van Assche, G.; Noman, M.; Hoffman, I.; et al. A panel to predict long-term outcome of infliximab therapy for patients with ulcerative colitis. *Clin. Gastroenterol. Hepatol.* **2015**, *13*, 531–538. [CrossRef] [PubMed]
34. Papamichael, K.; Rivals-Lerebours, O.; Billiet, T.; Vande Casteele, N.; Gils, A.; Ferrante, M.; Van Assche, G.; Rutgeerts, P.J.; Mantzaris, G.J.; Peyrin-Biroulet, L.; et al. Long-Term Outcome of Patients with Ulcerative Colitis and Primary Non-response to Infliximab. *J. Crohn's Colitis* **2016**, *10*, 1015–1023. [CrossRef]
35. Beswick, L.; Rosella, O.; Rosella, G.; Headon, B.; Sparrow, M.P.; Gibson, P.R.; van Langenberg, D.R. Exploration of Predictive Biomarkers of Early Infliximab Response in Acute Severe Colitis: A Prospective Pilot Study. *J. Crohn's Colitis* **2018**, *12*, 289–297. [CrossRef]
36. Paul, S.; Del Tedesco, E.; Marotte, H.; Clavel, L.; Phelip, J.M.; Peyrin-Biroulet, L.; Roblin, X. Therapeutic drug monitoring of infliximab and mucosal healing in inflammatory bowel disease: A prospective study. *Inflamm. Bowel Dis* **2013**, *19*, 2568–2576. [CrossRef]
37. Papamichael, K.; Van Stappen, T.; Vande Casteele, N.; Gils, A.; Billiet, T.; Tops, S.; Claes, K.; Van Assche, G.; Rutgeerts, P.; Vermeire, S.; et al. Infliximab Concentration Thresholds During Induction Therapy Are Associated with Short-term Mucosal Healing in Patients with Ulcerative Colitis. *Clin. Gastroenterol. Hepatol.* **2016**, *14*, 543–549. [CrossRef]
38. Kevans, D.; Murthy, S.; Mould, D.R.; Silverberg, M.S. Accelerated Clearance of Infliximab is Associated with Treatment Failure in Patients with Corticosteroid-Refractory Acute Ulcerative Colitis. *J. Crohn's Colitis* **2018**, *12*, 662–669. [CrossRef]
39. Sandborn, W.J.; Rutgeerts, P.; Feagan, B.G.; Reinisch, W.; Olson, A.; Johanns, J.; Lu, J.; Horgan, K.; Rachmilewitz, D.; Hanauer, S.B.; et al. Colectomy rate comparison after treatment of ulcerative colitis with placebo or infliximab. *Gastroenterology* **2009**, *137*, 1250–1260. [CrossRef]
40. Gibson, D.J.; Heetun, Z.S.; Redmond, C.E.; Nanda, K.S.; Keegan, D.; Byrne, K.; Mulcahy, H.E.; Cullen, G.; Doherty, G.A. An accelerated infliximab induction regimen reduces the need for early colectomy in patients with acute severe ulcerative colitis. *Clin. Gastroenterol. Hepatol.* **2015**, *13*, 330–335. [CrossRef]
41. Nalagatla, N.; Falloon, K.; Tran, G.; Borren, N.; Avalos, D.; Luther, J.; Colizzo, F.; Garber, J.; Khalili, H.; Melia, J.; et al. Effect of Accelerated Infliximab Induction on Short- and Long-term Outcomes of Acute Severe Ulcerative Colitis: A Retrospective Multicenter Study and Meta-analysis. *Clin. Gastroenterol. Hepatol.* **2019**, *17*, 502–509.e1. [CrossRef] [PubMed]
42. Shah, S.C.; Naymagon, S.; Panchal, H.J.; Sands, B.E.; Cohen, B.L.; Dubinsky, M.C. Accelerated infliximab dosing increases 30-day colectomy in hospitalized ulcerative colitis patients: A propensity score analysis. *Inflamm. Bowel Dis.* **2018**, *24*, 651–659. [CrossRef] [PubMed]
43. Chao, C.Y.; Al Khoury, A.; Aruljothy, A.; Restellini, S.; Wyse, J.; Afif, W.; Bitton, A.; Lakatos, P.L.; Bessissow, T. High-dose infliximab rescue therapy for hospitalized acute severe ulcerative colitis does not improve colectomy-free survival. *Dig. Dis. Sci.* **2019**, *64*, 518–523. [CrossRef] [PubMed]
44. Govani, S.M.; Berinstein, J.A.; Waljee, A.K.; Stidham, R.W.; Higgins, P.D.R.; Hardiman, K.M. Use of Accelerated Induction Strategy of Infliximab for Ulcerative Colitis in Hospitalized Patients at a Tertiary Care Center. *Dig. Dis. Sci.* **2020**, *65*, 1800–1805. [CrossRef]
45. Cheifetz, A.S.; Abreu, M.T.; Afif, W.; Cross, R.K.; Dubinsky, M.C.; Loftus, E.V., Jr.; Osterman, M.T.; Saroufim, A.; Siegel, C.A.; Yarur, A.J.; et al. A Comprehensive Literature Review Expert Consensus Statement on Therapeutic Drug Monitoring of Biologics in Inflammatory Bowel Disease. *Am. J. Gastroenterol.* **2021**, *116*, 2014–2025. [CrossRef]
46. Gonczi, L.; Vegh, Z.; Golovics, P.A.; Rutka, M.; Gecse, K.B.; Bor, R.; Farkas, K.; Szamosi, T.; Bene, L.; Gasztonyi, B.; et al. Prediction of short- and medium-term efficacy of biosimilar infliximab therapy. Do trough levels and antidrug antibody levels or clinical and biochemical markers play the more important role? *J. Crohn's Colitis* **2017**, *11*, 697–705. [CrossRef]
47. Vande Casteele, N.; Jeyarajah, J.; Jairath, V.; Feagan, B.G.; Sandborn, W.J. Infliximab exposure-response relationship and thresholds associated with endoscopic healing in patients with ulcerative colitis. *Clin. Gastroenterol. Hepatol.* **2019**, *17*, 1814–1821. [CrossRef]
48. Pariente, B.; Pineton de Chambrun, G.; Krzysiek, R.; Desroches, M.; Louis, G.; De Cassan, C.; Baudry, C.; Gornet, J.-M.; Desreumaux, P.; Emilie, D.; et al. Trough levels and antibodies to infliximab may not predict response to intensification of infliximab therapy in patients with inflammatory bowel disease. *Inflamm. Bowel Dis.* **2012**, *18*, 1199–1206. [CrossRef]

49. Seah, D.; Choy, M.C.; Gorelik, A.; Connell, W.R.; Sparrow, M.P.; Van Langenberg, D.; Hebbard, G.; Moore, G.; De Cruz, P. Examining maintenance care following infliximab salvage therapy for acute severe ulcerative colitis. *J. Gastroenterol. Hepatol.* **2018**, *33*, 226–231. [CrossRef]
50. Whaley, K.G.; Xiong, Y.; Karns, R.; Hyams, J.S.; Kugathasan, S.; Boyle, B.M.; Walters, T.D.; Kelsen, J.; LeLeiko, N.; Shapiro, J.; et al. Multicenter Cohort Study of Infliximab Pharmacokinetics and Therapy Response in Pediatric Acute Severe Ulcerative Colitis. *Clin. Gastroenterol. Hepatol.* **2022**, *27*, S1542–S3565. [CrossRef]
51. Vande Casteele, N. Pharmacokinetics of Infliximab and Tumor Necrosis Factor Concentrations in Serum, Stool, and Colonic Mucosa in Acute Severe Ulcerative Colitis (PROTOS). In *ClinicalTrials.gov*; UCSD: San Diego, CA, USA, ClinicalTrials.gov. Identifier: NCT03765450. Available online: https://clinicaltrials.gov/ct2/show/study/NCT03765450 (accessed on 12 December 2022).
52. Guidi, L.; Pugliese, D.; Panici Tonucci, T.; Berrino, A.; Tolusso, B.; Basile, M.; Cantoro, L.; Balestrieri, P.; Civitelli, F.; Bertani, L.; et al. Therapeutic Drug Monitoring is More Cost-Effective than a Clinically Based Approach in the Management of Loss of Response to Infliximab in Inflammatory Bowel Disease: An Observational Multicentre Study. *J. Crohn's Colitis* **2018**, *12*, 1079–1088. [CrossRef] [PubMed]
53. Martelli, L.; Olivera, P.; Roblin, X.; Attar, A.; Peyrin-Biroulet, L. Cost-effectiveness of drug monitoring of anti-TNF therapy in inflammatory bowel disease and rheumatoid arthritis: A systematic review. *J. Gastroenterol.* **2017**, *52*, 19–25. [CrossRef] [PubMed]
54. Chaudhary, M.A.; Fan, T. Cost-Effectiveness of Infliximab for the Treatment of Acute Exacerbations of Ulcerative Colitis in the Netherlands. *Biol. Ther.* **2013**, *3*, 45–60. [CrossRef]
55. Grossberg, L.B.; Papamichael, K.; Feuerstein, J.D.; Siegel, C.A.; Ullman, T.A.; Cheifetz, A.S. A Survey Study of Gastroenterologists' Attitudes and Barriers Toward Therapeutic Drug Monitoring of Anti-TNF Therapy in Inflammatory Bowel Disease. *Inflamm. Bowel Dis.* **2017**, *24*, 191–197. [CrossRef] [PubMed]
56. Rentsch, C.A.; Ward, M.G.; Luber, R.P.; Taylor, K.M.; Gibson, D.J.; Headon, B.; Rosella, O.; Su, H.Y.; Friedman, A.B.; Dooley, M.; et al. Pharmacist-Driven Therapeutic Infliximab Monitoring at the Point of Care Using Rapidly Assessed Drug Levels in Patients with Inflammatory Bowel Disease. *Ther. Drug Monit.* **2023**. [CrossRef]
57. De Cruz, P. Optimising Infliximab Induction Therapy for Acute Severe Ulcerative Colitis (PREDICT-UC). In *ClinicalTrials.gov*; Austin Health: Melbourne, VIC, Australia, ClinicalTrials.gov. Identifier: NCT02770040. Available online: https://clinicaltrials.gov/ct2/show/NCT02770040 (accessed on 12 December 2022).
58. D'Haens, G. Induction for Acute Ulcerative Colitis (TITRATE). In *ClinicalTrials.gov*; Academisch Medisch Centrum-Universiteit van Amsterdam (AMC-UvA): Amsterdam, The Netherlands, ClinicalTrials.gov. Identifier: NCT03937609. Available online: https://clinicaltrials.gov/ct2/show/record/NCT03937609 (accessed on 12 December 2022).

Disclaimer/Publisher's Note: The statements, opinions and data contained in all publications are solely those of the individual author(s) and contributor(s) and not of MDPI and/or the editor(s). MDPI and/or the editor(s) disclaim responsibility for any injury to people or property resulting from any ideas, methods, instructions or products referred to in the content.

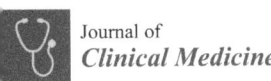

Review

What Should We Know about Drug Levels and Therapeutic Drug Monitoring during Pregnancy and Breastfeeding in Inflammatory Bowel Disease under Biologic Therapy?

Mathilde Barrau [1,†], Xavier Roblin [1,*,†], Leslie Andromaque [2], Aurore Rozieres [2], Mathias Faure [2], Stéphane Paul [3] and Stéphane Nancey [2,4]

1 Department of Gastroenterology, University Hospital of Saint-Etienne, 42000 Saint-Etienne, France; mathilde.barrau@chu-st-etienne.fr
2 CIRI—Centre International de Recherche en Infectiologie, University Lyon, Inserm U1111, University Claude Bernard Lyon 1, CNRS, UMR5308, ENS de Lyon, 69007 Lyon, France; leslie.andromaque@chu-lyon.fr (L.A.); aurore.rozieres@chu-lyon.fr (A.R.); mathias.faure@chu-lyon.fr (M.F.); stepahne.nancey@chu-lyon.fr (S.N.)
3 Department of Immunology, CIC1408, GIMAP EA3064, University Hospital of Saint-Etienne, 42055 Saint-Etienne, France
4 Department of Gastroenterology, Lyon Sud Hospital, Hospices Civils de Lyon, University Claude Bernard Lyon 1, 69003 Lyon, France
* Correspondence: xavier.roblin@chu-st-etienne.fr
† These authors contributed equally to this work.

Abstract: Data on the real long-term influences of in utero drug exposure in pregnant women on childhood development are scarce and remain not well determined and depend on the duration of in utero drug exposure and maternal drug levels. Therapeutic drug monitoring (TDM) during pregnancy may help limit fetal drug exposure while maintaining an effective dose for the treatment of the underlying inflammatory bowel disease (IBD) in women. Most antibody therapies used in patients with IBD are IgG molecules which are actively transported across the placenta, especially during the third trimester of the pregnancy. Here, we propose an up-to-date clinical review to summarize the available findings of serum drug levels in maternal blood during pregnancy, in the cord blood, infants at delivery and in breast milk of patients with IBD treated with biologics. Conversely, in comparison to adalimumab (ADA) levels, which are relatively stable during pregnancy, infliximab (IFX) drug clearance decreased significantly during the last two trimesters of the pregnancy, leading to increasing drug concentrations in the blood of the pregnant women. As most guidelines recommend using live vaccines in infants at the age of one or earlier in case of negative serum drug levels in newborns, statistical models could help clinicians in making a decision to adjust the last dose of the biologic during pregnancy and to determine the optimal date to vaccinate. Altogether, data from the literature offers strong reassurance in terms of safety for anti-TNFα therapies during pregnancy not only for IBD patients who intend to conceive, but also for pregnant women and for the physicians taking care of these patients. ADA and IFX levels in breast milk are detectable, but at very low levels, and therefore, it is recommended to pursue breast feeding under anti-TNFα therapy. Our knowledge on ustekinumab or vedolizumab levels in pregnant women remains unclear and scarce. These drugs are currently not recommended for patients with IBD in clinical practice. Therefore, TDM and proactive dose adjustment are not necessary during pregnancy since its impact on making a clinical decision have not yet been clearly demonstrated in routine practice. Overall, drug concentrations in the cord blood, an infant at birth and postpartum serum concentrations in infants, due to active placental drug transfer, may have a greater impact than the limited drug transfer in breast milk during lactation on the risk of infection and developmental outcomes. Ustekinumab and vedolizumab exposure during pregnancy and lactation are both considered low risk by the recent ECCO guidelines despite the limited data that are currently available.

Keywords: therapeutic drug monitoring; pregnancy; breastfeeding; inflammatory bowel disease

Citation: Barrau, M.; Roblin, X.; Andromaque, L.; Rozieres, A.; Faure, M.; Paul, S.; Nancey, S. What Should We Know about Drug Levels and Therapeutic Drug Monitoring during Pregnancy and Breastfeeding in Inflammatory Bowel Disease under Biologic Therapy? *J. Clin. Med.* **2023**, *12*, 7495. https://doi.org/10.3390/jcm12237495

Academic Editor: Matteo Neri

Received: 1 October 2023
Revised: 27 November 2023
Accepted: 30 November 2023
Published: 4 December 2023

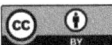

Copyright: © 2023 by the authors. Licensee MDPI, Basel, Switzerland. This article is an open access article distributed under the terms and conditions of the Creative Commons Attribution (CC BY) license (https://creativecommons.org/licenses/by/4.0/).

1. Introduction

Therapeutic drug monitoring (TDM) measures specific drug levels to guide treatment changes and helps clinicians in making decisions to adjust optimal drug frequency or dose administration, subsequently improving disease outcomes. The real long-term influences of in utero drug exposure on childhood development are yet to be investigated effectively and depend on the duration of in utero drug exposure and maternal drug levels. TDM during pregnancy may theoretically help limit fetal exposure while maintaining optimal drug levels in maternal blood. However, the consequences of drug exposure in utero on immune development and maturation in childhood are critical issues and are uncertain, and the present reassuring data have reported the absence of causal relationships between adverse events (including severe infection) in neonates and maternal drug exposure with biologics. Most antibody therapies used in patients with IBD are IgG molecules known to be transported across the placenta by an active mechanism, especially during the last trimester of the pregnancy. This review proposes here a clinical review to summarize the available findings of drug levels in infants, cord and maternal during pregnancy, as well as during breastfeeding in IBD patients treated with biologics. Additionally, the usefulness of TDM in these patients during pregnancy is also be examined. In contrast with anti-TNFα agents, it is unsurprising that little data about pharmacokinetics (PK) of recently approved monoclonal antibodies (vedolizumad, ustekinumab) are available in relation to pregnancy and breastfeeding. A better understanding of biological drug pharmacokinetics during pregnancy and breastfeeding is of primary interest for gastroenterologists. This could improve dose adjustments of biological therapies in order to minimize risks of fetal exposure and to achieve an optimal maternal disease control.

1.1. Search Strategy

We performed a systematic review of the literature in accordance with the PRISMA guidelines of 2023. We used PubMed on 20 August 2023 to systematically search and retrieve studies on the PK of IBD-related drugs throughout the trimesters of pregnancy or in women at time of delivery and the offspring. Research was also conducted for analyzing PK in breastmilk. English articles or oral presentations during DDW, ECCO or UEGW were also analyzed. The following five main keywords including "pharmacokinetics", "IBD related drugs", "pregnant women", "offspring" and "lactation" represented the search strategy. Studies including non-IBD participants were excluded. Studies which failed to meet the research aim and inclusion criteria were excluded. The search strategy and study selection were conducted by two investigators (MB and SN) independently. The results of the study selection were then discussed, and in the case of disagreement, an additional author (XR) was solicited.

1.2. Data Extraction

Once the relevant studies meeting the aim and inclusion criteria of this research were narrowed down, the data were extracted in a Microsoft Excel sheet. The study characteristics of interest were its design, the type of IBD, the sample size of pregnant women population enrolled in the study, the type, dosage and dosing interval of medication, the time-point of analysis (prior pregnancy (T0), first trimester (T1), second (T2), third (T3), at delivery (T4) and/or postpartum (T5)), age and bodyweight at inclusion. We also added the methods used to measure drug concentration. The timeframes for the trimesters were the following: T1 between 0–13 weeks, T2 between 14–26 weeks and T3 between 27–40 weeks. The PK parameters per study were also obtained as drug concentrations based on time between injection or infusion and drug measurements. We have no reported area under curve in the literature. Furthermore, it was also studied whether adapted dosages were advised by these studies on basis of a potential change in PK during pregnancy. The same study characteristics were analyzed in relation to lactation. For newborns, PK data were extracted according to the time of study, the type of IBD the mother is diagnosed with, the treatment and the analytical method used for measurements.

1.3. Mechanisms of Drug Transport for Antibody Therapies across the Human Placenta

Most drugs cross the placenta by simple diffusion of the molecules driven by concentration and electrical gradients. However, beyond simple diffusion, various other mechanisms of drug exchanges between maternal and fetal blood are involved, such as transcellular transfer (via channels, facilitated diffusion or carrier-mediated active transport, endocytosis and exocytosis) [1]. In contrast with small molecules, monoclonal antibody therapies, most of them being IgG1, are high molecular weight drugs and therefore cannot cross the placenta by simple diffusion (insignificant concentrations are detected in early pregnancy). In contrast, the maternal transfer of IgG through the placenta is mediated by active transporters using a specific receptor-mediated binding Fcγ portion of IgG at the syncytiotrophoblast layers of the placenta. These layers represent the main location of exchange for nutrients, gases or drugs between the blood of pregnant women and of the fetus. IgG is then transported across the syncytiotrophoblast layers in coated vesicles that protect them from lysosome-mediated degradation. IgG transport from mother to neonate is mediated by the heterodimer fetal Fc receptor neonatal (FcRn) molecule, including an α-chain homologous to major histocompatibility complex class I molecules and β-2-microglobulin that both play a key role in placental IgG transport, catabolism and recycling (Figure 1). Among all the subtypes of Fcγ receptors described in human placenta, the subtype III appears to contribute mostly to IgG transfer, and its expression on the surface of the syncytiotrophoblast has been detected from 13 weeks of gestation. The subsequent active transport of biologics across the placenta starts by week 13–17 and increases gradually as the pregnancy progresses, with the highest amounts of IgG being transferred from the maternal blood stream to the fetus during the third trimester [2–4]. At 17–22 weeks of gestation, the fetal levels of IgG represented only 5–10% of those found in maternal circulation. Acceleration of the transfer of all IgG subclasses, especially IgG1, has been reported during the third trimester. Moreover, the levels of exogenously administered IgG1 therapy in umbilical cords correlate with the timing of the last dose prior to delivery [5]. Around 26 weeks of gestation, serum fetal IgG levels reached maternal concentrations and even exceeded it by threefold (sometimes higher) at term as assessed in cord blood levels in infants [4,6].

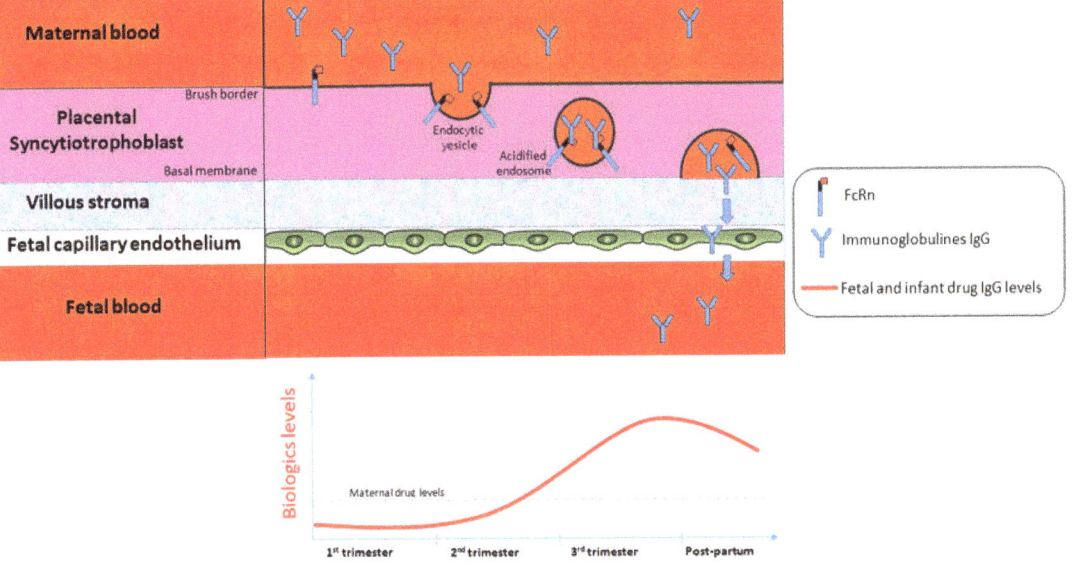

Figure 1. Placenta immunoglobulin G (IgG) transport.

Interestingly, the distribution of antibody therapies among the maternal, cord and fetal blood depends on multiple complex metabolic factors as well as on the maturation of the placenta [7]. The magnitude of maternal IgG transport depends on the isotype of IgG, and IgG1 is preferentially transported to the fetus in comparison to IgG4, IgG3 and IgG2, which is the least detected of all. For example, at 17–22 weeks of gestation, the fetal levels of IgG1 were reported to be threefold higher than those of IgG2. Moreover, cord blood drug levels vary depending on the type of anti-TNF agents, with a fetal/maternal ratio of 2.6 and 1.5, respectively, for IFX and for ADA. This active transfer of IgG during the second half of a pregnancy is clinically relevant since it results in a strong exposure of antibody therapies in fetus in utero and in early life period, which represents a critical period for development, maturation and programming of the immune system. In addition, these high drug levels in neonates during pregnancy could be, at least theoretically, associated with a higher susceptibility of infection.

1.4. Transfer of Maternal Biologics and Drugs from Breast Tissue into Breast Milk

Serum drug concentrations directly affect drug transfer from breast tissue into breast milk, and it is assumed that most drugs can be present in breast milk due to the diffusion of small chemical molecules or active transport mediated by FcRn receptors for monoclonal antibodies (a mechanism similar to the placenta). However, beyond drug levels, other factors including breast milk pH, molecule size, protein binding and breast inflammation might interfere with the transfer of drugs into breast milk. Historically, it was recommended that women receiving biologics avoid breastfeeding. However, secretory IgA represents the predominant immunoglobulin detected in breast milk, and irrespective of the biologic, drug concentrations in breast milk are very low when compared with those found in maternal serum or in the umbilical cord, and peak concentrations were seen between 24–72 h after drug administration. Although the mechanisms of intestinal absorption of immunoglobulin possibly involving FcRn remain unclear, a small fraction of ingested monoclonal antibodies by infants from breast feeding may be absorbed in the gut, as it has been well demonstrated in an infant who was not exposed to IFX during pregnancy but was exposed to the drug during breastfeeding [8]. In addition, breastfeeding while receiving biologics did not negatively interfere with the risk of infection or of fetal developmental milestones, and hence, breastfeeding in women exposed to biologics is considered to be low risk.

1.5. Pharmacokinetics of Anti-TNF Agents in IBD during Pregnancy
Study Selection

According to our study selection, 12 studies using biologics were included, nine concerning IFX, four ADA and one golimumab (GLM), and 173 participants, including 112 (70%) with Crohn's disease (CD), 46 (29%) ulcerative colitis (UC) and 2 (1%) unspecified IBD, were enrolled.

1.6. Maternal Infliximab Trough Concentrations during Pregnancy

Four studies investigated serum drug trough levels in pregnant women with IBD treated with IFX. By pooling all patients (except those in the study from Bortlik M et al. [9]), all the women had detectable serum infliximab, but infliximab was detected neither in the breast milk of nursing mothers nor in the serum of breast-fed newborns in the first study analyzing this [10]. Seow et al. [11] included prospectively twenty-five pregnant women treated with IFX or ADA maintenance therapies from the University of Calgary IBD pregnancy clinic with serum bio-banking collected each trimester. Fifteen women (8 CD, 7 UC) were treated with IFX. In this cohort, the median serum trough IFX concentrations were 8.50 µg/mL (IQR: 7.23–10.07 µg/mL) during the first trimester, 10.31 µg/mL (IQR: 7.66–15.63 µg/mL) during the second trimester and 21.02 µg/mL (IQR: 16.01–26.70 µg/mL) during the last trimester. After adjusting for various parameters involved in drug clearance (albumin, body mass index and CRP levels), serum IFX trough levels increased significantly by 4.2 µg/mL per trimester during pregnancy [12]. IFX levels were measured pre-conception, in each trimester, at delivery and postpartum in maternal serum in 23 pregnant women with IBD under IFX therapy in a prospective observational study [12]. Modelling showed an increase in IFX levels of 0.16 µg/L/week (95% CI: 0.08–0.24) ($p < 0.001$), similar to the previous findings from Seow [11]. Van Eliesen et al. [13] measured placental drug transfer and exposure to IFX and etanercept in six women with autoimmune diseases (in which two had CD). Healthy term placentas were infused with 100 µg/mL IFX (n = 4) or etanercept (n = 5) for 6 h. IFX was detectable both in the cord blood and in the placenta with a cord-to-maternal ratio and a placenta-to-maternal ratio of 1.6 ± 0.4 and 0.3 ± 0.1, respectively. From experiments using ex vivo placenta drug infusion, the magnitude of drug transfer into the placenta was not different between the drugs. Fetal drug concentrations in the blood for IFX and etanercept were 0.3 ± 0.3 µg/mL and 0.2 ± 0.2 µg/mL, respectively. However, IFX drug levels were significantly superior compared to those of etanercept (19 ± 6 µg/g versus 1 ± 3 µg/g, $p < 0.001$) in the placenta. Therefore, a higher tissue drug exposure was found with IFX than with etanercept in both in vivo and in ex vivo drug-infused placentas. In line with previous studies, a retrospective study enrolling 23 pregnant IBD patients with IFX reported that drug clearance decreased significantly during the second and the last trimester, leading to an increase in maternal IFX concentration irrespective of the drug regimen [14].

Altogether, using the TDM guidance, maternal IFX drug levels may remain constant in a de-intensified regimen, despite a de-intensified drug regimen being administered to pregnant women with IBD.

1.7. IFX and Maternal Trough Concentration before, during and after Pregnancy

Seow et al. and Flanagan et al. have showed that drug levels after delivery were higher compared to those during the pre-pregnancy period (10.17 µg/mL versus 6.9 µg/mL and 10.3 versus 7.9 µg/mL, respectively, in contrast with data from the study of Grišic et al.) (5.9 µg/mL versus 7.3 µg/mL) [11,12,14]. Overall, when comparing the IFX levels during and after pregnancy, they were all higher during pregnancy. Figure 2 reports the dynamics of drug levels before, during and after pregnancy.

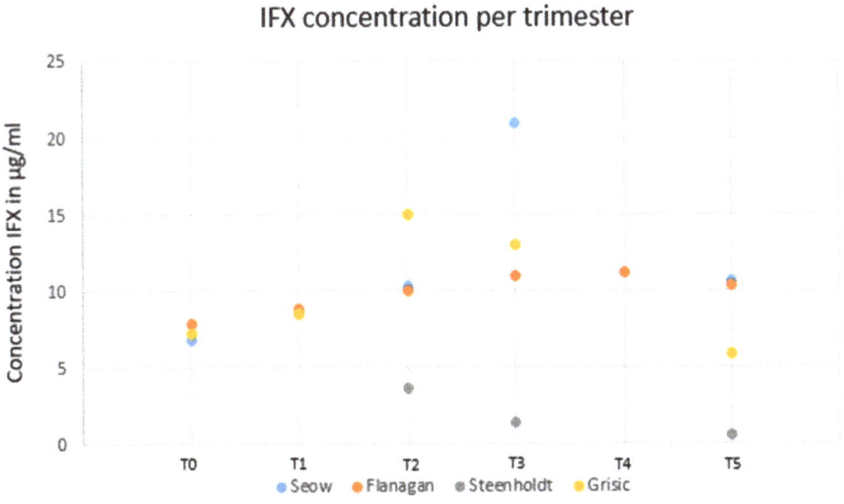

Figure 2. Infliximab concentration per trimester from all available studies.

1.8. Placenta Drug Transfer in Pregnant Women Treated with Infliximab

Two studies have reported some small case reports investigating drug levels in the blood of breast-fed infants from mothers exposed to IFX. In the first case, the breast-fed infant's serum IFX level was 39.5 microg/mL at 6 weeks after birth [15]. In this case, a last infusion of IFX (10 mg/kg) was administered to the mother two weeks before delivery. In another study, a woman with UC receiving a common dose of IFX infusions until gestation week 31 gave birth to a healthy child at gestation week 37 [16]. Relatively high maternal serum drug levels were reported during pregnancy. In addition, detectable IFX drug levels were found in the infant's blood at week 16 after birth, but not at reassessment at week 28. In 11 IBD pregnant patients treated with IFX, drug concentrations in the cord blood and in the blood of an infant at birth were compared with those of the mother [15]. Not only was IFX detectable in the blood of the infants for as long as 6 months, but also the median level of IFX in the cord was 160% higher compared with that of the mother. In a study including 32 CD pregnant patients treated with IFX, there was a relationship between IFX cord levels and the gestational week of last exposure as well as maternal serum levels [9]. In fact, anti-TNF drug levels in the cord blood at birth depend on the type of anti-TNF type. In a recent prospective single-center study, including 131 pregnancies that resulted in a live birth in women with IBD treated with IFX (n = 52) and ADA (n = 58). At birth, drug levels in the 94 cord blood samples were significantly higher for women treated with IFX than those treated with ADA. Interestingly, whereas the transport of ADA across the placenta was relatively limited and increased in a linear fashion during the third trimester, IFX transportation increased exponentially [17].

1.9. IFX Drug Levels during Breastfeeding

In a large prospective multicenter study analyzing the drug concentrations in 72 breast milk samples from patients treated with IFX therapy, drug was detected in breast milk in 19 out of 29 exposed women (with a maximum drug concentration of 0.74 µg/mL) [18].

1.10. Duration of IFX Detection in Newborns

In a prospective multicentric study involving 44 pregnant women treated with IFX, the authors investigated the drug concentrations in cord blood of newborns and drug clearance after birth, and the relationships between these factors and IFX levels in mothers at birth and the subsequent risk of infection in infants during the first year of life. The time from the last exposure to IFX during pregnancy was found inversely associated with drug levels in the umbilical cord (IFX: $r = -0.77$, $p < 0.0001$) and in the blood of women at time of birth (IFX, $r = -0.80$; $p < 0.0001$ for both). The median ratio of infant/mother drug concentration at birth was 1.97 (95% CI, 1.50–2.43). The mean drug clearance time in infants was 7.3 months (95% CI, 6.2–8) In this study, 4 (5%) and 16 (20%) infants experienced bacterial infections and non-serious viral infections, respectively. Infants whose mothers received a combination of an anti-TNF agent and thiopurine had a 2.7-fold higher risk of infection compared with those treated with an anti-TNF monotherapy (95% CI, 1.09–6.78; $p = 0.02$). Drugs were not detected in infant blood after the age of 12 months [5]. In a prospective study including 107 infants exposed to anti-TNF during pregnancy (in which 66 were under IFX), the authors proposed a pharmacokinetic model to predict time for drug clearance after birth in infants exposed during pregnancy. All infants with detectable drug levels in cord blood at birth and with at least one additional blood sample within the first year were enrolled. Drugs were detectable in the blood of 25 infants (23%) at 6 months. At 12 months, IFX was detected in three infants (4%) whereas ADA was undetectable. Using a Bayesian forecasting method based on a one-compartment PK model, the predicted drug clearing time was related with the measured observations [19]. In a recent study [20], the authors proposed a physiologically based pharmacokinetic (PBPK) model for anti-TNF therapies in adults and extrapolated the results to pregnant women, fetuses and infants with the objective to identify the best timing for the last dosing of IFX, ADA and GLM during pregnancy in IBD, and with the objective to study the recommended vaccine schedules for infants exposed to these drugs. The main results are reported in Tables 1 and 2 and are of interest for clinical practice. The timing of the last dosing of IFX and ADA was defined by the lowest limit of the therapeutic range. Optimal IFX trough concentrations were considered between 3–7 µg/mL [21]. However, IFX trough concentrations over 15 µg/mL increase the likelihood of infection [22]. For pregnant women exposed to ADA, numerous studies failed to demonstrate a link between ADA trough concentrations and the increased risks of infection. Hence, to adjust optimal drug level, taking blood samples throughout pregnancy in women with IBD is recommended, as shown by Mahadevan et al. [23].

Table 1. Recommended timing of last dosing.

Drug	Dose and Frequency	Timing of Last Dose (Weeks before Delivery)
Adalimumab	40 mg/2 W	0–2
	40 mg/W	0–3
	80 mg/2 W	0–4
Infliximab	5 mg/kg/8 W	5–11
	5 mg/kg/6 W	6–13
	7.5 mg/kg/8 W	8–13
	8 mg/kg/8 W	8–13

Table 2. Recommended timing of vaccine.

Drug	Dose and Frequency	Timing of Vaccination (Months after Delivery)
Adalimumab	40 mg/2 W	8
	40 mg/W	9
	80 mg/2 W	9
Infliximab	5 mg/kg/8 W	11
	5 mg/kg/6 W	12
	7.5 mg/kg/8 W	12
	8 mg/kg/8 W	12

1.11. TNF-α Inhibitors—ADA and Maternal Trough Concentration during Pregnancy

Two studies analyzed adalimumab serum levels during pregnancy in IBD patients. Seow et al. analyzed 11 pregnant patients with IBD treated with ADA. After adjusting for albumin, BMI and CRP, drug levels remained stable ($p > 0.05$) during pregnancy [11]. Flanagan et al. [12] included 15 IBD patients treated with IFX (n = 23) and with ADA (n = 15) and with vedolizumab (n = 12) with at least two intrapartum observations. Conversely, when compared to IFX, modelling showed no change in ADA levels. These results are reported in Figure 3.

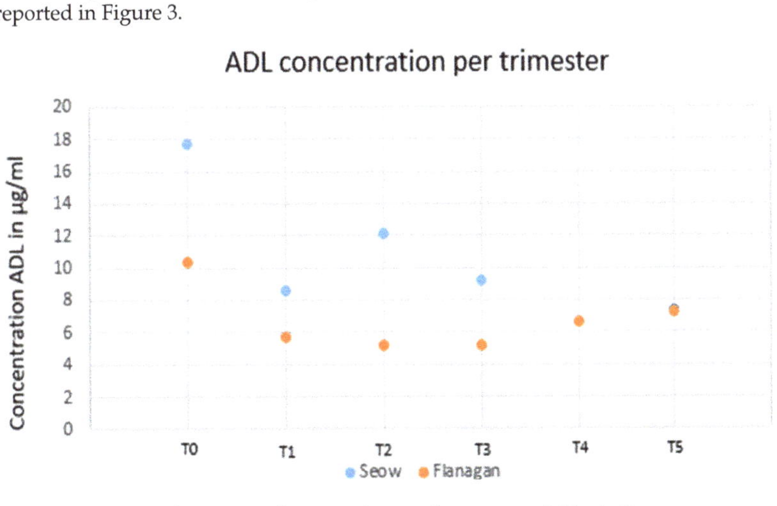

Figure 3. Adalimumab concentrations per trimester from two available studies.

1.12. Placental Transfer of ADA

Two studies analyzed placental transfer of adalimumab. Mahadevan et al. [6] investigated it in 10 pregnant women with IBD treated with ADA. Serum drug levels were compared at birth in the mother, infant and cord blood, and then monthly in the infant until the drugs were undetectable. The median level of ADA in the cord was 153% than that measured in blood of the mother. In addition, the drug remained detectable in the infants for as long as 6 months. Borthlik et al. [9] analyzed the correlation between serum anti-TNF-α concentrations in the blood of infants and mothers at delivery with gestational age at the last exposure. Conversely, when compared to IFX, no correlation was found in the case of ADA for this.

1.13. ADA and Breast Milk (Table 3)

In a large and prospective multicenter study, among the 72 breast milk samples, ADA was detected in 2 of the 21 women under treatment with a maximal drug concentration of 0.71 μg/mL [18]. As with IFX, the maternal use of ADA appears to be compatible with breastfeeding.

Table 3. Breast milk drug levels.

Drug	Total Patients	Total Patients with a Detectable Level, n (%)	Peak Time Range, h	Peak (Range), μg/mL
Adalimumab	21	2 (9.5)	12–24	0.71 (0.45–0.71)
Infliximab	29	19 (66.0)	24–48	0.74 (0.15–0.74)
Golimumab	1	0 (0)	NA	NA
Certolizumab	13	3 (23.0)	24–48	0.29 (0.27–0.29)
Ustekinumab	6	4 (66.7)	12–24	1.57 (0.72–1.57)
Natalizumab	2	1 (50.0)	24	0.46

NA—Not applicable.

1.14. Duration of ADA in Newborns

Through a large and prospective multicenter study including 44 pregnant women treated with ADA, the authors investigated the concentrations of IFX in umbilical cord blood of newborns and the rates of drug clearance after birth. They also analyzed the relationship between drug concentrations in mothers at birth and the risk of infection during the infant's first year of life [5]. There was a negative relationship between time from last exposure to ADA during pregnancy and drug concentration in the umbilical cord ($r = -0.64$, $p = 0.0003$) and in mothers at time of birth (ADA, $r = -0.80$; $p < 0.0001$). The median ratio of infant/mother drug concentration at birth was 1.21 for ADA (95% confidence interval (CI), 0.94–1.49), whereas the mean time of ADA clearance in infants was 4.0 months (95% CI, 2.9–5.0), and contrarily, IFX was cleared slower than ADA.

1.15. TNF-α Inhibitors—GLM Maternal Trough Concentration during Pregnancy, in Breast Milk and in Children

Very little data about maternal drug trough concentration are available with GLM therapy during pregnancy. Only one case study [24] covered GLM, reporting data exclusively at delivery (6.6 mcg/mL). For GLM, no advice on dosage was provided by the authors. Currently, no data are published about the evolution of serum levels of GLM during pregnancy, and thus, we do not know if the pharmacokinetics are similar to that of IFX or ADA.

Data on the use of GLM therapy during breastfeeding remain scarce (Table 3). Given the high molecular weight of GLM (around 150,000 Da), it is likely that a very low amount of drug is detected in milk samples during breastfeeding. In addition to low GLM concentration in milk, it is also likely to be partially degraded during digestion, leading to a very low drug exposure to the breastfed infant. However, we need more information on this topic, and in the meanwhile, GLM should be used with caution during breastfeeding, especially if nursing a newborn or preterm infant. Drug transfer to an infant may be minimized by waiting for at least 2 weeks postpartum. Matro et al. [18] have reported the case of one mother treated with GLM, and they failed to detect GLM in breast milk samples.

No publication is available about the exposure duration of GLM in children from mothers using GLM during pregnancy. Based on very little data reporting very low drug concentration in children post-birth, we can speculate a similar management of live vaccines in newborns as with the other anti-TNF drugs.

1.16. Outcomes of Pregnancy and Children When Using Anti-TNF during Pregnancy

In a recent meta-analysis pooling wight studies with a total of 527 pregnant women with IBD. A total of 343 were treated with IFX and 184 with ADA [25]. Compared to ADA, adverse pregnancy outcomes including congenital malformations and spontaneous abortion were not increased in case of exposure to IFX. Another meta-analysis has reported adverse pregnancy outcomes (APOs), congenital abnormalities (CAs), preterm birth (PTB) and low birth weight (LBW) to assess the risks associated with anti-TNFα therapy for pregnancy outcomes [26]. Anti-TNFα agents were not associated with an increased risk of APOs, CAs, PTB or LBW in comparison with disease-matched controls. Moreover, when comparing with the risk of CAs in the general population, there was no increased risk under anti-TNF therapy. Altogether, these data provide some reassurance for IBD patients and clinicians in terms of safety profile of anti-TNFα therapy during pregnancy. Finally, a separate recent meta-analysis [27] included 48 studies to assess the prevalence of adverse pregnancy outcomes in women with IBD exposed to biologic therapy. They failed to detect any difference in terms of adverse pregnancy outcomes amongst pregnant women with IBD exposed to biological therapy compared with that of the general population. In all studies, TDM was not analyzed to identify an association between serum drug levels and adverse events.

Moreover, some studies analyzed the impact of monoclonal antibody therapy use during pregnancy and the response to vaccination in newborns. In a large study including 179 women exposed to biologics, when measuring antibody titers after vaccination against HiB and tetanus toxin, the vaccine efficacy in their infants of at least 7 months of age did not appear to be affected by in utero drug exposure [28]. Julssgaard et al. [5] analyzed the concentrations of anti-TNFα in mothers and newborns and reported the risk of infections during the time. They reported bacterial and viral infections in 4 (5%) and 16 (20%) infants, respectively, and all were infectious events with benign courses. They estimated the relative risk for infection to 2.7 in infants whose mothers were treated with a combotherapy (anti-TNF agent and thiopurine), compared with anti-TNF monotherapy (95% CI, 1.09–6.78; $p = 0.02$). A prospective cohort study [29] including 191 children (IFX (67 [35%] of 191) and ADA (49 [26%])) investigated whether live rotavirus vaccine could be administered safely to infants exposed to biologic agents. They did not report severe adverse events after immunization except for three (2%) infants requiring medical attention. So, according to the authors, rotavirus vaccination is safe and can be proposed to infants exposed to anti-TNF agents in utero. A systematic bibliographic search was performed recently to assess the effectiveness and safety of vaccines in children exposed to biological drugs in utero and/or those whose mothers received biological agents during lactation [30]. Vaccines were considered to be effective in infants exposed to anti-TNF agents in utero. In contrast to live-attenuated vaccines which should be avoided while drug levels are detectable in the infants, inactivated vaccines are likely safe. All vaccines (including live-attenuated and inactivated) are possibly safe in children breastfed by mothers treated with anti-TNF therapy. However, drug levels during pregnancy or in cord blood were not concomitantly measured in this study in order to look for an association with the very low drug concentrations found in breast milk.

When can we resume IFX and ADA during pregnancy?

Firstly, studies have reported the increased levels of IFX concentrations during the third trimester of pregnancy, contrary to ADA. So, using TDM, we can speculate the possibility of decreasing the dose of IFX during this time to obtain therapeutic concentrations. The IFX concentrations in Figure 2 report discrepancies at T5 for two studies [10,15]. These discordances at T5 may possibly be explained by various time-points of drug measurement after delivery. Kane et al. and Vasilauskas et al. provided drug measurements at 14 weeks, whereas Seow et al. [11] and Flanagan et al. [12] considered post-pregnancy measurements up to 6 months [14,15]. Grisic et al. [14] reported drug assessments up to 250 weeks after conception, and Steenholdt et al. [16] proposed their last measurement at 28 weeks after delivery. However, we think that it would be interesting to measure TDM of IFX and ADA after delivery, using a proactive strategy.

For breast milk, anti-TNF concentrations are very low, and breast feeding during IFX or ADA administration is recommended to be safe. The more important point is about serum levels in newborns. Mahadevan et al. suggested performing biologic therapy for weeks before delivery. Indeed, no effects in pregnant women and newborns were reported in all studies, except for serum anti-TNF concentrations in newborns. Finally, the important question is to identify the best timing for the last dosage of IFX, ADA and GLM in pregnant women with IBD, as well as to propose the recommended vaccine schedules for infants exposed to these drugs. A PK model to predict time-to-clearance in infants exposed to anti-TNF agents during pregnancy has been developed by Liu et al. [19]. According to their online results, they can predict the duration of anti-TNF in the child and can adapt the date of live vaccination [31]. Chen et al. [20] recommend more stringent points for timing the last dose and vaccine according to the regimen used for pregnant women. However, for practitioners not using TDM, it would be easier to time live vaccines at an age of one year for the child or to discuss vaccination before the completion of one year in case no drug is detected in blood.

1.17. Serum Ustekinumab Levels during Pregnancy and Breastfeeding (Figure 4)

Ustekinumab is an entirely humanized IgG1 monoclonal antibody blocking the p40 subunit of interleukin (IL) IL-12 and IL-23 and is currently approved for the treatment of CD and UC. Interleukin-12 targeted by ustekinumab contributes to uterine physiology (uterine angiogenesis), the regulation of trophoblast invasion and local vascular remodeling during implantation of an embryo [32]. Notably, both high and low levels of IL-12 in pregnancy have been associated with early spontaneous abortions. In addition, IL-23 regulates the critical functions of human decidual immune cells, which play a key role in the tolerance of genetically different (allogenic) cells while aiding the mother's immune function in early pregnancy [33]. These findings raise the concern of the potential interference of ustekinumab exposure on pregnancy. However, clinical results from a large registry comparing the pregnancy events occurring in IBD patients exposed and not exposed to ustekinumab are reassuring and did not show any unexpected adverse outcomes on pregnancy and child growth. Data in the literature on ustekinumab PK during pregnancy remain unclear, limited to small case series, and concern exclusively drug measurement in maternal, cord and infant blood and not drug concentrations in intestinal tissues. Sako M et al. investigated drug concentrations at delivery in maternal peripheral and cord blood from a patient with CD treated with ustekinumab and in infants' blood at six months [34]. Similar to anti-TNF agents, the level of ustekinumab in cord blood was 2.8-fold higher compared with that measured in maternal serum, but drug concentration was undetectable in the baby's bloodstream after six months [34–36]. Similar findings were reported in three other case reports, one in a pregnant women with CD treated until 33 weeks of gestation with the dose interval of ustekinumab shortened to every 4 weeks, another in a woman with refractory CD treated with ustekinumab until week 30 of pregnancy [35], and finally, in a patient with UC under usual maintenance therapy with a 2–2.5 times higher drug concentration in cord blood than in contemporaneous maternal serum. In the last case, the drug was still detectable in infant serum more than 2 months after the last maternal dose [37]. Interestingly, maternal drug serum trough levels which were monitored at induction therapy and throughout pregnancy were found to be stable [38].

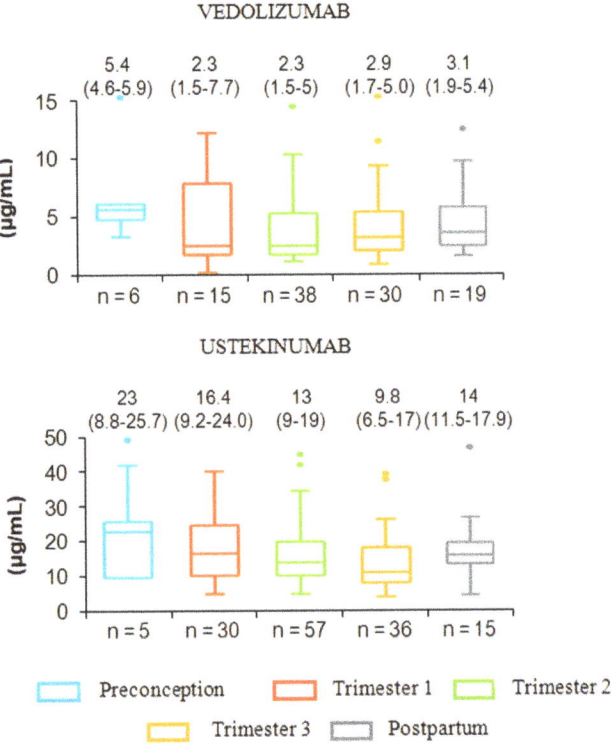

Figure 4. Pharmacokinetics of pregnant women with IBD.

Recently, several larger prospective observational cohort studies investigated the pharmacokinetics of ustekinumab during pregnancy. The first one from Mitrova K et al. reported drug levels in 15 infant–mother pairs during pregnancy in IBD patients [39]. At the time of delivery, drug levels in the cord and in the maternal blood were strongly correlated with a median infant-to-maternal ratio of 1.7, concordant with those previously observed in the precedent small case series. The second study presented during the last ECCO Congress which is not yet published reported the Australian experience of PK of ustekinumab and vedolizumab in pregnant women with IBD. This multicenter prospective cohort study included 35 pregnant patients treated with the maintenance dose of ustekinumab. They investigated both infant and maternal drug levels at delivery, as well as drug concentrations in infants at various time-points until drug clearance. They reported a strong positive correlation between drug levels in maternal and infant sera at time of delivery, and the infant/maternal drug level ratio was 1.74 (IQR 1.24–3.5) in accordance with that previously reported in the previous case series [40]. Time to drug clearance in infants was 13 weeks (IQR 9–22), and serum ustekinumab was not detected 15 weeks after delivery in two-third of infants. Interestingly, in this cohort, time to clearance in infants did not differ between women who received the last dose of ustekinumab during the second and those that received it during the third trimester of pregnancy. The third prospective study included 15 women with CD under ustekinumab treatment and confirmed previous data with infant drug levels at delivery that were 1.79 (IQR 1.26–3.1) fold higher than maternal levels with a median clearance time of 9 weeks (range 6–19) in nine infants in whom drugs levels were measured over time [36]. In the Pregnancy in Inflammatory Bowel Disease and Neonatal

Outcomes, PIANO registry, a prospective observational study that included pregnant women with IBD in 30 US centers, similar pharmacokinetics findings of ustekinumab during pregnancy were observed in a small subgroup of patients [6].

Altogether, few studies determined ustekinumab PK during pregnancy; however, their results are in line with the overall stable concentrations of maternal serum drug levels throughout pregnancy and in infants. A lack of correlation was seen between ustekinumab concentrations in the umbilical cord blood with the gestational week during which the drug was administered. In addition, drug clearance time was not different regardless of the time of the last ustekinumab injection during the second half of pregnancy.

1.18. Ustekinumab Levels during Breastfeeding (Table 3)

Limited data on breast milk transfer of ustekinumab from women to their infants are available. Drug exposure of infants to ustekinumab during breastfeeding and whether drug exposure in infants has an impact on the risk of infection and developmental milestones remains unclear and controversial. A recent case report of a 36-year-old female with UC treated with a maintenance regimen of ustekinumab (90 mg/8 weeks) has provided information on drug concentrations in breast milk which were substantially lower compared with those found in cord blood (ratio 1 to 100) or in maternal serum (ration 1 to 20) and decreased gradually thereafter. When comparing serum maternal ustekinumab levels with those in breast milk, the ratio of area under the time–concentration curves of the drug was very low (0.0008) [37]. Ustekinumab was also detected in low concentration in breast milk from a small case report including three nursing mothers with CD exposed to treatment (90 mg/8 weeks for two of them and intensified dose of 90 mg/4 weeks for the latter) [41].

Notably, the low drug concentrations measured in breast milk samples collected one hour after the completion of drug administration were two-fold lower compared with pre-dose serum levels. A multicenter prospective observational study investigated breast milk samples from six women with IBD treated with ustekinumab. The low levels of ustekinumab in breast milk were detected in four out of six patients with a peak concentration of 1.57 µg/mL (ranging from 0.72–1.57). This was seen 12–72 h post-injection and was followed by a gradual decrease thereafter. In addition, infection rates and developmental delay at 12 months did not differ between drug-exposed and non-exposed breastfed infants [18].

Altogether, our knowledge on the usefulness of monitoring serum ustekinumab or vedolizumab maternal levels during pregnancy remains unclear and is currently not recommended in patients with IBD. TDM during pregnancy and proactive dose adjustment are not necessary since their impact on making clinical decisions has not been demonstrated in routine clinical practice. Overall, drug concentrations at birth in blood infant cord and in serum after birth, due to placental drug transfer, may have a greater impact on the risk of infection and development outcomes than drug transfer during lactation.

1.19. Serum Vedolizumab Trough Levels during Pregnancy (Figure 4)

Vedolizumab (a humanized monoclonal antibody antagonizing $\alpha 4\beta 7$ integrin receptors) was approved for the treatment of IBD patients. The receptor targeted by vedolizumab inhibits leukocyte trafficking into the gut and subsequently reduces the recruitment of immune and inflammatory cells. It is also involved in placental development which has caused apprehension about its use in pregnant women. Data about the potential impact of vedolizumab exposure during pregnancy are limited and are mainly results from the European retrospective multicenter case–control observational CONCEIVE study. The study reports pregnancy and child developmental outcomes in 73 women with IBD exposed to vedolizumab. Additionally, a retrospective cohort study from the GETAID including 44 drug-exposed women with IBD during pregnancy and a few cases from the PIANO registry also contribute to the available data [42,43]. There was no clear evidence of a negative safety signal although further larger, prospective and dedicated studies are required to confirm these reassuring findings.

At the time of delivery, vedolizumab was detectable in the serum of infants. Although the mechanisms of transfer of vedolizumab across the placenta to the fetal blood stream are similar to the IgG antibodies, placental pharmacokinetic studies have reported substantial differences between vedolizumab and other biologics including anti-TNF agents and ustekinumab. A comparative study investigating the placental pharmacokinetics of vedolizumab and ustekinumab in women with IBD (15 exposed to ustekinumab and 16 to vedolizumab) found lower drug concentrations of vedolizumab in the cord blood than in the maternal blood. This is in contrast with concentrations measured in mothers exposed to ustekinumab during pregnancy. In this cohort, the median vedolizumab concentrations in maternal and in cord blood samples from mothers with IBD was 7.3 mg/L and 4.5 mg/L with a median infant-to-maternal ratio of 0.66 (compared with 1.7 in the cohort of pregnant mothers exposed to ustekinumab) [39]. Moreover, there was a positive relationship between drug levels in the cord blood and the gestational week of the last vedolizumab infusion.

1.20. Serum Vedolizumab Trough Levels during Breastfeeding (Table 3)

There are limited data regarding the impact of vedolizumab exposure in women with IBD during breastfeeding on infant outcomes. All data available during pregnancy and breastfeeding concern intravenous vedolizumab administration, and no data are available with the recently approved subcutaneous injection of vedolizumab.

Vedolizumab is detected in breast milk at low concentrations. Drug levels in breast milk from five vedolizumab-treated lactating women with IBD were investigated in a short report. Breast milk samples were collected prior to infusion, 30 min post-infusion and then twice daily for up to 14 days. Vedolizumab was detected in all breast milk samples with varying concentrations which were very low based on the corresponding serum concentration (less than 1%). The peak drug concentration was 0.318 µg/mL in this cohort and was raised from 3–7 days after infusion. Taking into account the maximal vedolizumab concentrations in milk samples and the overall amount of milk ingested by the infants (around 150 mL per kilogram of body weight), it is estimated that the infants could receive 0.048 mg per kilogram body weight per day [5].

Altogether, we should keep in mind that vedolizumab is detected in maternal and cord blood, and drug concentrations in the cord blood are lower than in maternal blood in the majority of cases, in contrast to those measured for ustekinumab. Safety data on the use of vedolizumab during pregnancy and breastfeeding do not indicate any negative effects. Ustekinumab and vedolizumab exposure during pregnancy and lactation are both considered low risk by the recent ECCO guidelines despite the limited available data [44]. However, we require more prospective, real-life and larger dedicated studies to confirm these reassuring findings.

2. Conclusions

It is actually well established among clinicians to resume the treatment of pregnant women with IBD. The benefit/risk ratio of the drug is evaluated, taking into account both the mother and the fetus. It is of great interest to maintain IBD control in remission and to minimize the subsequent risks on pregnancy outcomes, such as miscarriages and pre-term birth. Recent guidelines of the European Crohn's and Colitis Organization (ECCO) as well as recommendations from the American Gastroenterological Association (AGA) are available and both state that maintaining IBD in remission is central to reduce adverse outcomes. Both consider biologic therapy to be safe when used for maintenance regimen during pregnancy. However, there is no clear recommendation on the use of TDM during pregnancy or in the management of newborns from mothers exposed to biologics during pregnancy. However, in contrast to other biologics, given the reduced IFX clearance during pregnancy, the use of TDM in pregnant mothers treated with IFX might help clinicians to adjust the therapeutic dose of IFX during this period. During lactation, low drug concentrations are detected in breast milk, and subsequently, breast feeding can be considered safe with the administration of anti-TNF agents. Limited data on breast milk transfer of ustekinumab, vedolizumab and golimumab from women to their infants are available. However, preliminary results are safe with very low levels of the drug. So, for anti-TNF drugs, breast feeding can be considered safe with the administration of these biologics. The essential question is to determine the best timing for the last dosing of all anti-TNF agents available for pregnant women with IBD, as well as to assess the recommended vaccine schedules for infants exposed to these drugs. Using models, the duration of anti-TNF drug persistence in a child post-birth can be predicted, allowing the identification of the optimal date to inject life vaccines in infants in a personalized manner. However, for physicians not using TDM in a daily practice, it should be easier to time live vaccines at an age of one year for the child or to discuss vaccination before the completion of one year in the absence of drug detection in the blood.

Author Contributions: X.R., S.P., M.B., L.A., A.R., M.F. and S.N., performed the research; X.R., S.P., S.N. and M.B., study concept and design. S.P., X.R., S.N. and M.B., data analysis and interpretation. S.N., X.R., S.P. and M.B., manuscript writing. All authors have read and agreed to the published version of the manuscript.

Funding: This research received no external funding.

Institutional Review Board Statement: Not applicable.

Informed Consent Statement: Not applicable.

Data Availability Statement: Data in this review of articles are contained within the article.

Conflicts of Interest: X.R.: abbvie, Pfizer, Celltrion, Janssen, Takeda, Theradiag. S.N.: Abbvie, Amgen, Celltrion, Janssen, Takeda. S.P.: Abbvie, Takeda, Jansen, Theradiag. The other authors declare no conflict of interest.

References

1. Kane, S.V.; Acquah, L.A. Placental transport of immunoglobulins: A clinical review for gastroenterologists who prescribe therapeutic monoclonal antibodies to women during conception and pregnancy. *Am. J. Gastroenterol.* **2009**, *104*, 228–233. [CrossRef]
2. Gusdon, J.P. Fetal and maternal immunoglobulin levels during pregnancy. *Am. J. Obstet. Gynecol.* **1969**, *103*, 895–900. [CrossRef] [PubMed]
3. Garty, B.Z.; Ludomirsky, A.; Danon, Y.L.; Peter, J.B.; Douglas, S.D. Placental transfer of immunoglobulin G subclasses. *Clin. Diagn. Lab. Immunol.* **1994**, *1*, 667–669. [CrossRef] [PubMed]
4. Malek, A.; Sager, R.; Kuhn, P.; Nicolaides, K.H.; Schneider, H. Evolution of Maternofetal Transport of Immunoglobulins During Human Pregnancy. *Am. J. Reprod. Immunol.* **1996**, *36*, 248–255. [CrossRef]
5. Julsgaard, M.; Christensen, L.A.; Gibson, P.R.; Gearry, R.B.; Fallingborg, J.; Hvas, C.L.; Bibby, B.M.; Uldbjerg, N.; Connell, W.R.; Rosella, O.; et al. Concentrations of Adalimumab and Infliximab in Mothers and Newborns, and Effects on Infection. *Gastroenterology* **2016**, *151*, 110–119. [CrossRef] [PubMed]
6. Mahadevan, U.; Long, M.D.; Kane, S.V.; Roy, A.; Dubinsky, M.C.; Sands, B.E.; Cohen, R.D.; Chambers, C.D.; Sandborn, W.J.; Crohn's Colitis Foundation Clinical Research Alliance. Pregnancy and Neonatal Outcomes after Fetal Exposure to Biologics and Thiopurines among Women with Inflammatory Bowel Disease. *Gastroenterology* **2021**, *160*, 1131–1139. [CrossRef] [PubMed]
7. Palmeira, P.; Quinello, C.; Silveira-Lessa, A.L.; Zago, C.A.; Carneiro-Sampaio, M. IgG placental transfer in healthy and pathological pregnancies. *Clin. Dev. Immunol.* **2012**, *2012*, 985646. [CrossRef]
8. Fritzsche, J.; Pilch, A.B.; Mury, D.; Schaefer, C.; Weber-Schoendorfer, C. Infliximab and Adalimumab Use During Breastfeeding. *J. Clin. Gastroenterol.* **2012**, *46*, 718–719. [CrossRef]
9. Bortlik, M.; Machkova, N.; Duricova, D.; Malickova, K.; Hrdlicka, L.; Lukas, M.; Kohout, P.; Shonova, O.; Lukas, M. Pregnancy and newborn outcome of mothers with inflammatory bowel diseases exposed to anti-TNF-α therapy during pregnancy: Three-center study. *Scand. J. Gastroenterol.* **2013**, *48*, 951–958. [CrossRef]
10. Kane, S.; Ford, J.; Cohen, R.; Wagner, C. Absence of infliximab in infants and breast milk from nursing mothers receiving therapy for crohn's disease before and after delivery. *J. Clin. Gastroenterol.* **2009**, *43*, 613–616. [CrossRef]
11. Seow, C.H.; Leung, Y.; Casteele, N.V.; Afshar, E.E.; Tanyingoh, D.; Bindra, G.; Stewart, M.J.; Beck, P.L.; Kaplan, G.G.; Ghosh, S.; et al. The effects of pregnancy on the pharmacokinetics of infliximab and adalimumab in inflammatory bowel disease. *Aliment. Pharmacol. Ther.* **2017**, *45*, 1329–1338. [CrossRef]
12. Flanagan, E.; Gibson, P.R.; Wright, E.K.; Moore, G.T.; Sparrow, M.P.; Connell, W.; Kamm, M.A.; Begun, J.; Christensen, B.; De Cruz, P.; et al. Infliximab, adalimumab and vedolizumab concentrations across pregnancy and vedolizumab concentrations in infants following intrauterine exposure. *Aliment. Pharmacol. Ther.* **2020**, *52*, 1551–1562. [CrossRef] [PubMed]

13. Eliesen, G.A.M.; van Drongelen, J.; van Hove, H.; Kooijman, N.I.; van den Broek, P.; de Vries, A.; Roeleveld, N.; Russel, F.G.M.; Greupink, R. Assessment of Placental Disposition of Infliximab and Etanercept in Women with Autoimmune Diseases and in the Ex Vivo Perfused Placenta. *Clin. Pharmacol. Ther.* **2020**, *108*, 99–106. [CrossRef] [PubMed]
14. Grišić, A.M.; Dorn-Rasmussen, M.; Ungar, B.; Brynskov, J.; Ilvemark, J.F.K.F.; Bolstad, N.; Warren, D.J.; Ainsworth, M.A.; Huisinga, W.; Ben-Horin, S.; et al. Infliximab clearance decreases in the second and third trimesters of pregnancy in inflammatory bowel disease. *United Eur. Gastroenterol. J.* **2021**, *9*, 91–101. [CrossRef] [PubMed]
15. Vasiliauskas, E.A.; Church, J.A.; Silverman, N.; Barry, M.; Targan, S.R.; Dubinsky, M.C. Case Report: Evidence for Transplacental Transfer of Maternally Administered Infliximab to the Newborn. *Clin. Gastroenterol. Hepatol.* **2006**, *4*, 1255–1258. [CrossRef]
16. Steenholdt, C.; Al-Khalaf, M.; Ainsworth, M.A.; Brynskov, J. Therapeutic infliximab drug level in a child born to a woman with ulcerative colitis treated until gestation week 31. *J. Crohn's Colitis* **2012**, *6*, 358–361. [CrossRef] [PubMed]
17. Kanis, S.L.; de Lima-Karagiannis, A.; van der Ent, C.; Rizopoulos, D.; van der Woude, C.J. Anti-TNF Levels in Cord Blood at Birth are Associated with Anti-TNF Type. *J. Crohn's Colitis* **2018**, *12*, 939–947. [CrossRef]
18. Matro, R.; Martin, C.F.; Wolf, D.; Shah, S.A.; Mahadevan, U. Exposure Concentrations of Infants Breastfed by Women Receiving Biologic Therapies for Inflammatory Bowel Diseases and Effects of Breastfeeding on Infections and Development. *Gastroenterology* **2018**, *155*, 696–704. [CrossRef] [PubMed]
19. Liu, Z.; Julsgaard, M.; Zhu, X.; Martin, J.; Barclay, M.L.; Cranswick, N.; Gibson, P.R.; Gearry, R.B.; van der Giessen, J.; Connor, S.J.; et al. Timing of Live Attenuated Vaccination in Infants Exposed to Infliximab or Adalimumab in Utero: A Prospective Cohort Study in 107 Children. *J. Crohns. Colitis* **2022**, *16*, 1835–1844. [CrossRef]
20. Chen, J.; Lin, R.; Guo, G.; Wu, W.; Ke, M.; Ke, C.; Huang, P.; Lin, C. Physiologically-Based Pharmacokinetic Modeling of Anti-Tumor Necrosis Factor Agents for Inflammatory Bowel Disease Patients to Predict the Withdrawal Time in Pregnancy and Vaccine Time in Infants. *Clin. Pharmacol. Ther.* **2023**, *114*, 1254–1263. [CrossRef]
21. Papamichael, K.; Vogelzang, E.H.; Lambert, J.; Wolbink, G.; Cheifetz, A.S. Therapeutic drug monitoring with biologic agents in immune mediated inflammatory diseases. *Expert Rev. Clin. Immunol.* **2019**, *15*, 837–848. [CrossRef] [PubMed]
22. Bejan-Angoulvant, T.; Ternant, D.; Daoued, F.; Medina, F.; Bernard, L.; Mammou, S.; Paintaud, G.; Mulleman, D. Relationship Between Serum Infliximab Concentrations and Risk of Infections in Patients Treated for Spondyloarthritis. *Arthritis Rheumatol.* **2017**, *69*, 108–113. [CrossRef]
23. Mahadevan, U.; Robinson, C.; Bernasko, N.; Boland, B.; Chambers, C.; Dubinsky, M.; Friedman, S.; Kane, S.; Manthey, J.; Sauberan, J.; et al. Inflammatory Bowel Disease in Pregnancy Clinical Care Pathway: A Report from the American Gastroenterological Association IBD Parenthood Project Working Group. *Gastroenterology* **2019**, *156*, 1508–1524. [CrossRef] [PubMed]
24. Benoit, L.; Mir, O.; Berveiller, P. Treating Ulcerative Colitis During Pregnancy: Evidence of Materno–Fetal Transfer of Golimumab. *J. Crohn's Colitis* **2019**, *13*, 669–670. [CrossRef] [PubMed]
25. Wang, H.; Hu, Y.; Chen, F.; Shen, M. Comparative safety of infliximab and adalimumab on pregnancy outcomes of women with inflammatory bowel diseases: A systematic review & meta-analysis. *BMC Pregnancy Childbirth* **2022**, *22*, 854.
26. Shihab, Z.; Yeomans, N.D.; De Cruz, P. Anti-Tumour Necrosis Factor α Therapies and Inflammatory Bowel Disease Pregnancy Outcomes: A Meta-analysis. *J. Crohn's Colitis* **2016**, *10*, 979–988. [CrossRef]
27. Nielsen, O.H.; Gubatan, J.M.; Juhl, C.B.; Streett, S.E.; Maxwell, C. Biologics for Inflammatory Bowel Disease and Their Safety in Pregnancy: A Systematic Review and Meta-analysis. *Clin. Gastroenterol. Hepatol.* **2022**, *20*, 74–87. [CrossRef]
28. Beaulieu, D.B.; Ananthakrishnan, A.N.; Martin, C.; Cohen, R.D.; Kane, S.V.; Mahadevan, U. Use of Biologic Therapy by Pregnant Women with Inflammatory Bowel Disease Does Not Affect Infant Response to Vaccines. *Clin. Gastroenterol. Hepatol.* **2017**, *16*, 99–105. [CrossRef]
29. Fitzpatrick, T.; Alsager, K.; Sadarangani, M.; Pham-Huy, A.; Murguía-Favela, L.; Morris, S.K.; Seow, C.H.; Piché-Renaud, P.-P.; Jadavji, T.; Vanderkooi, O.G.; et al. Immunological effects and safety of live rotavirus vaccination after antenatal exposure to immunomodulatory biologic agents: A prospective cohort study from the Canadian Immunization Research Network. *Lancet Child Adolesc. Health* **2023**, *7*, 648–656. [CrossRef]
30. Gisbert, J.P.; Chaparro, M. Vaccines in Children Exposed to Biological Agents In Utero and/or During Breastfeeding: Are They Effective and Safe? *J. Crohn's Colitis* **2023**, *17*, 995–1009. [CrossRef]
31. Selinger, C.P.; Nelson-Piercy, C.; Fraser, A.; Hall, V.; Limdi, J.; Smith, L.; Smith, M.; Nasur, R.; Gunn, M.; King, A.; et al. IBD in pregnancy: Recent advances, practical management. *Frontline Gastroenterol.* **2020**, *12*, 214–224. [CrossRef]
32. Lédée-Bataille, N.; Dubanchet, S.; Coulomb-L'Hermine, A.; Durand-Gasselin, I.; Frydman, R.; Chaouat, G. A new role for natural killer cells, interleukin (IL)-12, and IL-18 in repeated implantation failure after in vitro fertilization. *Fertil. Steril.* **2004**, *81*, 59–65. [CrossRef] [PubMed]
33. Cai, J.-Y.; Li, M.-J. Interleukin 23 regulates the functions of human decidual immune cells during early pregnancy. *Biochem. Biophys. Res. Commun.* **2016**, *469*, 340–344. [CrossRef] [PubMed]
34. Sako, M.; Yoshimura, N.; Sonoda, A.; Okano, S.; Ueda, M.; Tezuka, M.; Mine, M.; Yamanishi, S.; Hashimoto, K.; Kobayashi, K.; et al. Safety Prediction of Infants Born to Mothers with Crohn's Disease Treated with Biological Agents in the Late Gestation Period. *J. Anus Rectum Colon* **2021**, *5*, 426–432. [CrossRef] [PubMed]
35. Klenske, E.; Osaba, L.; Nagore, D.; Rath, T.; Neurath, M.F.; Atreya, R. Drug Levels in the Maternal Serum, Cord Blood and Breast Milk of a Ustekinumab-Treated Patient with Crohn's Disease. *J. Crohns. Colitis* **2019**, *13*, 267–269. [CrossRef]

36. Flanagan, E.; Prentice, R.; Wright, E.K.; Gibson, P.R.; Ross, A.L.; Begun, J.; Sparrow, M.P.; Goldberg, R.; Rosella, O.; Burns, M.; et al. Ustekinumab levels in pregnant women with inflammatory bowel disease and infants exposed in utero. *Aliment. Pharmacol. Ther.* **2022**, *55*, 700–704. [CrossRef] [PubMed]
37. Saito, J.; Kaneko, K.; Kawasaki, H.; Hayakawa, T.; Yakuwa, N.; Suzuki, T.; Sago, H.; Yamatani, A.; Murashima, A. Ustekinumab during pregnancy and lactation: Drug levels in maternal serum, cord blood, breast milk, and infant serum. *J. Pharm. Health Care Sci.* **2022**, *8*, 18. [CrossRef]
38. Rowan, C.R.; Cullen, G.; Mulcahy, H.E.; Keegan, D.; Byrne, K.; Murphy, D.J.; Sheridan, J.; Doherty, G.A. Ustekinumab Drug Levels in Maternal and Cord Blood in a Woman with Crohn's Disease Treated Until 33 Weeks of Gestation. *J. Crohn's Colitis* **2017**, *12*, 376–378. [CrossRef]
39. Mitrova, K.; Pipek, B.; Bortlik, M.; Bouchner, L.; Brezina, J.; Douda, T.; Drasar, T.; Drastich, P.; Falt, P.; Klvana, P.; et al. Differences in the placental pharmacokinetics of vedolizumab and ustekinumab during pregnancy in women with inflammatory bowel disease: A prospective multicentre study. *Therap. Adv. Gastroenterol.* **2021**, *14*, 17562848211032790. [CrossRef]
40. Prentice, R.; Flanagan, E.; Wright, E.K.; Gibson, P.R.; Rosella, S.; Godberg, R.; Prideaux, L.; Kiburg, K.; Ross, A.L.; Burns, M.; et al. Pharmacokinetics of vedolizumab and ustekinumab in pregnant womeen with inflammatory bowel disease and their infants exposed in utero. *J. Crohn's Colitis* **2023**, *17* (Suppl. S1), 508–510. [CrossRef]
41. Avni-Biron, I.; Mishael, T.; Zittan, E.; Livne-Margolin, M.; Zinger, A.; Tzadok, R.; Goldenberg, R.; Kopylov, U.; Ron, Y.; Hadar, E.; et al. Ustekinumab during pregnancy in patients with inflammatory bowel disease: A prospective multicentre cohort study. *Aliment. Pharmacol. Ther.* **2022**, *56*, 1361–1369. [CrossRef] [PubMed]
42. Wils, P.; Seksik, P.; Stefanescu, C.; Nancey, S.; Allez, M.; de Chambrun, G.P.; Altwegg, R.; Gilletta, C.; Vuitton, L.; Viennot, S.; et al. Safety of ustekinumab or vedolizumab in pregnant inflammatory bowel disease patients: A multicentre cohort study. *Aliment. Pharmacol. Ther.* **2020**, *53*, 460–470. [CrossRef] [PubMed]
43. Moens, A.; van der Woude, C.J.; Julsgaard, M.; Humblet, E.; Sheridan, J.; Baumgart, D.C.; Gilletta De Saint-Joseph, C.; Nancey, S.; Rahier, J.F.; Bossuyt, P.; et al. Pregnancy outcomes in inflammatory bowel disease patients treated with vedolizumab, anti-TNF or conventional therapy: Results of the European CONCEIVE study. *Aliment. Pharmacol. Ther.* **2020**, *51*, 129–138. [CrossRef] [PubMed]
44. Torres, J.; Chaparro, M.; Julsgaard, M.; Katsanos, K.; Zelinkova, Z.; Agrawal, M.; Ardizzone, S.; Campmans-Kuijpers, M.; Dragoni, G.; Ferrante, M.; et al. European Crohn's and Colitis Guidelines on Sexuality, Fertility, Pregnancy, and Lactation. *J. Crohn's Colitis* **2023**, *17*, 1–27. [CrossRef]

Disclaimer/Publisher's Note: The statements, opinions and data contained in all publications are solely those of the individual author(s) and contributor(s) and not of MDPI and/or the editor(s). MDPI and/or the editor(s) disclaim responsibility for any injury to people or property resulting from any ideas, methods, instructions or products referred to in the content.

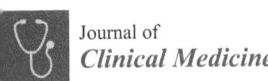

Review

A Review of Therapeutic Drug Monitoring in Patients with Inflammatory Bowel Disease Receiving Combination Therapy

Sanket Patel [1] and Andres J. Yarur [2,*]

1 Virtua Health, Voorhees, NJ 08043, USA; spatel11@virtua.org
2 Cedars-Sinai Medical Center, 8730 Alden Dr., Los Angeles, CA 90048, USA
* Correspondence: andres.yarur@cshs.org

Abstract: Background: Inflammatory Bowel Disease (IBD) impacts millions worldwide, presenting a major challenge to healthcare providers and patients. The advent of biologic therapies has enhanced the prognosis, but many patients exhibit primary or secondary non-response, underscoring the need for rigorous monitoring and therapy optimization to improve outcomes. **Objective**: This narrative review seeks to understand the role of therapeutic drug monitoring (TDM) in optimizing treatment for IBD patients, especially for those on combination therapies of biologics and immunomodulators. **Methods**: A comprehensive synthesis of the current literature was undertaken, focusing on the application, benefits, limitations, and future directions of TDM in patients receiving a combination of biologic therapies and immunomodulators. **Results**: While biological therapies have improved outcomes, rigorous monitoring and therapy optimization are needed. TDM has emerged as a pivotal strategy, enhancing outcomes cost-effectively while reducing adverse events. While most data pertain to monotherapies, TDM's applicability also extends to combination therapy. **Conclusion**: TDM plays a crucial role in the treatment optimization of IBD patients on combination therapies. Further research is needed to fully understand its potential and limitations in the broader context of IBD management.

Keywords: inflammatory bowel disease; ulcerative colitis; Crohn's disease; therapeutic drug monitoring; combination therapy; biologics; immunomodulators

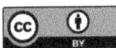

1. Introduction

Inflammatory Bowel Disease (IBD) is a chronic condition of the gastrointestinal tract, classically differentiated into Crohn's disease (CD) or ulcerative colitis (UC) based on the location, behavior, and histopathologic characteristics. The disease can manifest in periods of flare-ups and remission, potentially leading to severe complications, diminished quality of life, and increased mortality if not adequately managed. Optimal management strategies are essential to alleviate symptoms, prevent complications, and enhance long-term prognosis, ultimately aiming to improve patients' quality of life.

A growing number of options are available in the therapeutic armamentarium of IBD, with the first biologic being approved more than twenty years ago [1]. While infliximab was the first anti-tumor necrosis factor (TNF) agent approved, several other anti-TNF therapies have since become available for use in IBD, such as adalimumab, certolizumab, and golimumab. Vedolizumab, ustekinumab, and risankizumab are newer biologics with an alternative mechanism of action that have been shown to be effective and have been approved for Crohn's disease (CD) and/or ulcerative colitis (UC). Even though these are effective drugs at inducing and maintaining remission in IBD, a high number of patients do not respond or develop a loss of response over time [1–11].

Given the need for effective strategies in this complex therapeutic landscape, combination therapy with biologics and immunomodulators is commonly employed. Within this context, therapeutic drug monitoring (TDM) has emerged as a valuable tool to optimize treatment, and while its use in combination therapy can be beneficial, there are nuances and limitations that warrant a closer look. In general, TDM aims to recapture the response to biologic therapy or prevent the loss of response. It involves measuring drug concentrations and anti-drug antibodies (ADAs) in specific clinical settings. In patients with a partial or loss of response to anti-TNF therapy, it allows for the identification of those who may benefit from dose adjustment as opposed to those who are likely to benefit from a switch to another agent with either the same or an alternative mechanism of action. Importantly, TDM can effectively guide the use and optimization of combination therapies with immunomodulators like thiopurines and methotrexate [12]. Patients needing combination therapy usually have a higher disease burden and more aggressive phenotype; hence, the optimization of treatment regimens in this population becomes even more important. In addition to the association between improved clinical outcomes and higher drug concentrations, cost-effectiveness has been demonstrated through this approach [13,14].

Overall, TDM has gained traction as a potential tool to tailor treatment regimens, minimize adverse effects, and cost-effectively improve drug efficacy. This review aims to provide an overview of TDM's role in patients with IBD receiving combination therapy, highlighting available evidence and discussing practical aspects, benefits, limitations, and future directions.

2. Methodology

Our search strategy involved identifying relevant studies on TDM in IBD patients treated with combination therapy. Electronic databases, including PubMed, MEDLINE, and EMBASE, were queried for the appropriate studies published up to 2023. Keywords such as "ulcerative colitis", "Crohn's disease", "inflammatory bowel disease", "therapeutic drug monitoring", "combination therapy", "biologics", and "immunomodulators" were applied to identify relevant studies. We included studies discussing TDM in the context of IBD treatment with combination therapy, studies examining the impact of TDM on clinical outcomes, studies presenting data on drug levels of biologics concerning treatment outcomes, and studies available in the English language (Figure 1). Studies without direct relevance to the topic were excluded. To ensure the integrity of our review and minimize bias, two independent reviewers screened titles and abstracts. The full-text articles were reviewed based on inclusion criteria to identify the appropriate studies; any disagreements were resolved through discussion, and no automation tools were employed during the screening and inclusion process. Our review considered various factors, including participants' characteristics; study design; TDM methodologies; clinical outcomes; key findings; and intervention details, such as the type of therapy, dosage, durations, levels, and specific combinations. Our findings are presented in a narrative synthesis, highlighting the variations and trends observed in the literature regarding TDM in IBD combination therapy.

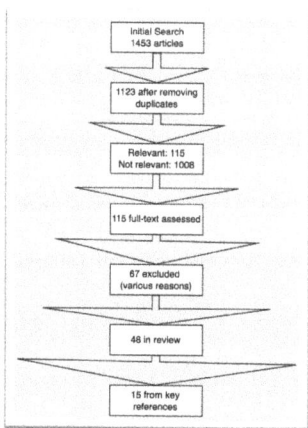

Figure 1. Flowchart of selection of review articles.

3. Therapeutic Drug Monitoring Strategies in Inflammatory Bowel Disease

The observations that led to TDM in IBD as a strategy were paved by an era of monotherapy thiopurine use as the capabilities to measure its sub-metabolites in red blood cells emerged [15]. Thiopurines are available as pro-drugs that undergo a series of enzymatic pathways leading to the production of several sub-metabolites. Among those, two have been found to have clinical relevance and are used to monitor and optimize the clinical care of patients receiving thiopurines. Of the two, higher 6-thioguanine nucleotide (6-TGN) concentrations have been associated with higher rates of efficacy but also a higher risk of myelotoxicity, while higher 6-methylmercaptopurine nucleotide (6-MMP) concentrations are linked with an increased risk of developing hepatotoxicity [16,17]. Due to its low cost, thiopurine monotherapy can still play an important role in the treatment of IBD, even though it is currently mainly used in the setting of combination therapy with biologics [16,18–20].

The use of TDM In IBD really surged with the wide use of anti-TNF and the relatively high rates of primary and secondary non-response seen with these drugs. Observational studies have found a clear association between higher serum concentrations of anti-TNFs and better outcomes, such as clinical remission, biochemical response, and endoscopic improvement [21–23]. Higher anti-TNF concentrations are also associated with histologic remission [24]. Despite this dose–response relationship, increasing exposure to the drug (e.g., increasing the dose) does not always translate into a better response, highlighting the complex pharmacokinetic and pharmacodynamic mechanisms of these agents and IBD [25,26]. Conversely, the development of ADAs is associated with a higher drug clearance, a loss of response, and the development of adverse events.

Several interconnected factors potentially influence the pharmacokinetics of anti-TNF. Inflammatory burden, obesity, genetics, immunogenicity, and the concomitant use of immunomodulators are all associated with anti-TNF pharmacokinetics (Figure 2).

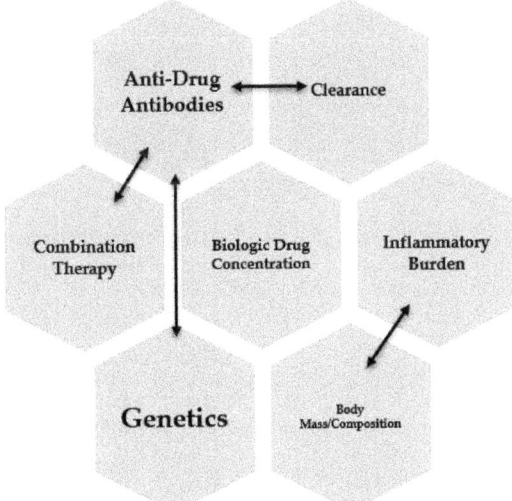

Figure 2. Interconnected factors influencing biologic drug levels.

Two strategies for applying TDM in IBD patients receiving anti-TNFs are currently well recognized. Reactive TDM involves measuring drug levels and ADAs in those experiencing non-response to therapy. Patients with low drug levels and no significant immunogenicity are more likely to benefit from dose escalation, while those with either high drug levels or the presence of high ADA titers are more likely to profit from a change in therapy.

Proactive TDM involves monitoring drug levels irrespective of the response to therapy while optimizing the dosage to maintain an "optimal" drug level. The main goal of proactive TDM is to maintain optimal exposure to the drug, avoiding under-exposure and the development of immunogenicity, ultimately preventing the loss of response [21,22,24,27]. Even though this strategy should theoretically offer significant advantages, the evidence is conflicting. Table 1 shows select studies comparing proactive and reactive monitoring.

Table 1. Select studies comparing proactive vs. reactive TDM.

Study Name/Reference	Study Design	Population	Intervention	Key Findings
TAXIT [28]	Randomized trial	IBD patients on infliximab	Proactive TDM vs. as-needed dose adjustment	Proactive TDM was not superior
TAILORIX [29,30]	Randomized trial	IBD patients on infliximab	Proactive TDM	Results similar to TAXIT
PAILOT [31]	Non-blinded RCT	Pediatric CD patients on adalimumab	Proactive dose adjustment	More efficacious than reactive approach
NOR-DRUM A and B [32,33]	Randomized study	IBD patients on various treatments	Proactive TDM	No benefit during induction but beneficial during maintenance

Both the TAXIT (Trough Concentration Adapted Infliximab Treatment) and TAILORIX (Tailored Treatment With Infliximab for Active Crohn's Disease) randomized trials looked into the effectiveness of proactive TDM in patients receiving infliximab for IBD [28–30]. Even though the overall conclusion of these studies was that proactive TDM is not better than as-needed dose adjustment, multiple factors need to be considered when interpreting the results of these studies and applying them to clinical practice. For example, there is significant heterogenicity in phenotypes (acute severe UC or perianal CD, for example), drug clearance, and other important variables among patients. Considering these differences, target infliximab levels are likely heterogeneous among patients. Factors such as body composition (particularly with higher visceral adipose tissue) and an elevated inflammatory burden may influence these goal concentrations [12,34–36]. Proactive TDM has also been studied in patients receiving adalimumab. PAILOT (Pediatric Crohn's Disease Adalimumab Level-based Optimization Treatment) was a non-blinded randomized controlled trial of pediatric patients with CD on adalimumab, and it demonstrated that proactive dose adjustment was more efficacious than a reactive approach when looking into sustained corticosteroid-free clinical remission [31]. While a large Norwegian study (NOR-DRUM A and B) showed no benefit during the induction phase, it did demonstrate the advantage of proactive TDM during the maintenance phase across IBD and other immune-mediated diseases, suggesting that the timing of proactive TDM application may be important [32,33].

TDM is a more cost-effective approach than empiric treatment adjustments. Velayos and colleagues compared the monitoring strategy and empiric drug escalation and found that TDM was more effective [37]. A randomized control trial in Denmark found that TDM-based treatment was more economical without a difference in clinical efficacy [38]. Proactive TDM is also slightly more cost-effective than the reactive approach, while TDM for thiopurines is significantly cost-effective [39,40].

Another strategy that could also promise a potential benefit is precision dosing, offering a more personalized approach to management. A Scandinavian study randomized a group of CD and UC patients in remission on infliximab to continue the drug with a dose based on a pharmacokinetic-modeled dashboard system to target trough levels ≥ 3 μg/mL or to continue standard dosing. After a year of follow-up, patients dosed based on the dashboard had higher rates of sustained clinical remission than those who continued standard therapy [41]. Even though the current evidence is conflicting, proactive TDM could potentially evolve into a personalized approach that considers individual patient factors, such as disease severity, comorbidities, pharmacokinetic variability, and phenotypic and genetic characteristics, to tailor treatment regimens to each patient. Overall, while the evidence is still equivocal, proactive TDM can be recommended, especially for patients receiving monotherapy or those with a high drug clearance, such as acute severe UC. Proactive TDM can also predict the development of immunogenicity and non-response when re-initiating infliximab after a drug holiday [42,43].

The role of TDM in biologics other than infliximab and adalimumab is less established. Most observational studies have shown a relationship between exposure and response [44–49]. Despite this, there is a lack of clinical evidence showing that dose escalation improves outcomes. The ENTERPRET study was an open-label, randomized trial that included patients with UC starting vedolizumab, who had drug clearance and non-response at week six. Patients were randomized to either continue the standard maintenance treatment (300 mg every 8 weeks) or receive a higher dose regimen (600 mg followed by 300 mg or 600 mg every 4 weeks (based on drug clearance)). After 30 weeks, there were no differences in clinical or endoscopic outcomes between the patients who were randomized to receive higher doses and those who continued standard treatment [50]. The POWER study was a double-blind, randomized, controlled trial that assessed CD patients with secondary non-response to ustekinumab who underwent dose intensification with IV re-induction or placebo followed by subcutaneous ustekinumab maintenance therapy. While inflammatory biomarkers and endoscopic outcomes did improve, the primary endpoint of clinical response at week 16 was not achieved [51]. Another important variable that distinguishes the use of TDM in anti-TNF and vedolizumab or ustekinumab is the very low rate of immunogenicity seen with these newer biologics [9–11,52].

As opposed to ustekinumab and vedolizumab, immunogenicity is commonly seen with most anti-TNF agents. ADAs can lead to low drug levels, adverse reactions, and worse outcomes [12,53]. Immunogenicity occurs in up to 65% of infliximab-treated patients, 38% of adalimumab-treated patients, 25% of certolizumab-treated patients, and 3% of golimumab-treated patients, according to a large meta-analysis [54]. Studies suggest that the risk of immunogenicity can be reduced and potentially be reversible by using anti-TNF in combination with methotrexate or thiopurines, effectively decreasing antibody formation and increasing the effective drug concentration [12,13,55–60].

4. Evidence for TDM in Combination Therapy

Combination therapy can offer improved clinical and endoscopic outcomes while maintaining an acceptable safety profile and is commonly utilized by physicians to treat refractory or severe disease [12,60,61].

Table 2 provides a summary of the key studies that have investigated the role of combination therapy in IBD patients with study design, population, and intervention, along with key findings.

Table 2. Pertinent studies on combination therapy in IBD.

Study Name/Reference	Study Design	Population	Intervention	Key Findings
SONIC [19]	Randomized trial	CD patients on infliximab and azathioprine	Monotherapy vs. combination	Lower immunogenicity, and combination therapy superior
UC-SUCCESS [57]	Randomized trial	UC patients on infliximab and azathioprine	Monotherapy vs. combination	Results similar to SONIC
COMMIT [58]	Randomized trial	CD patients on infliximab and methotrexate	Monotherapy vs. combination	Lower immunogenicity but no significant difference in clinical outcomes

The SONIC trial explored the efficacy of infliximab and azathioprine monotherapies compared to the combination of both drugs; it showed that patients receiving combination therapy achieved significantly higher rates of corticosteroid-free clinical remission and lower rates of immunogenicity [19]. UC-SUCCESS showed similar superiority of the combination of infliximab and azathioprine in patients with UC [57]. A subsequent post hoc analysis of SONIC also showed that, despite the fact that patients on combination therapy achieved higher infliximab concentrations, the higher rates of efficacy seen were driven by higher drug levels and not by the use of combination therapy [13]. The COMMIT trial studied the efficacy of combining infliximab and parenteral methotrexate. Even though it did show that patients receiving the combination of infliximab and methotrexate had achieved higher infliximab levels and lower rates of ADA than those receiving monotherapy, no benefit was found when comparing clinical outcomes [58].

Combination therapy plays an important role in patients who have a higher risk of achieving sub-therapeutic anti-TNF levels and in those with a higher risk of developing immunogenicity. Patients who develop anti-drug antibodies to one anti-TNF are much more likely to develop antibodies to subsequent anti-TNF use [59], and, in this scenario, TDM with combo-therapy can be helpful to prevent immunogenicity to a second anti-TNF. Roblin et al. randomized IBD patients who had a loss of response to the first anti-TNF given as monotherapy and were starting a second anti-TNF to either receive monotherapy or combination therapy. Those who received the combination had a significantly lower risk of developing clinical non-response and developing antibodies to the second agent [62].

An important novel approach when using TDM in the combination therapy of anti-TNF and a thiopurine is to optimize therapy not only by measuring the drug levels of the biologic but also by measuring 6-TGN and optimizing the thiopurine to maximize the pharmacokinetic augmentations of the biologic. This is particularly important, as optimizing thiopurines (via dose adjustment or pharmacologic manipulation) may be significantly more cost-effective than increasing the dose of the biologic. The COMBO-IBD study investigated how the use of thiopurine or methotrexate, and 6-TGN levels were correlated with the achieved infliximab concentrations. Patients with 6-TGN levels ≥ 146 pmol per 8×10^8 RBC or those receiving oral methotrexate had achieved higher drug concentrations than the patients on infliximab monotherapy or those receiving concomitant thiopurine that had 6-TGN levels < 146 pmol per 8×10^8 RBC [63]. Even though the study could only demonstrate an association, it reasonably suggested optimizing thiopurine in patients receiving combination treatment and that those achieving low infliximab concentrations are at a high risk of developing immunogenicity. Interestingly, the same study also showed that this phenomenon is not seen in patients on vedolizumab or ustekinumab, and the use of combination therapy, independent of the agent or 6-TGN concentration, was not associated with higher drug levels of these two biologics [63].

As previously mentioned, it is still unclear whether the better outcomes seen with combination therapy are mainly driven by a pharmacokinetic augmentation or whether there is a synergistic mechanism when combining both drugs [18–20,57]. While more studies are warranted, if the positive outcomes are really due to the better pharmacokinetics, it would be interesting to see whether a comparable efficacy can be achieved by using infliximab monotherapy and proactively adjusting dosing without the need for combo-therapy.

5. Role of TDM When Restarting Anti-TNFs after a Drug Holiday

Circumstances arise where patients may discontinue anti-TNF and are subsequently restarted after a drug holiday. TDM can be useful in identifying patients who are more likely to develop infusion reactions and non-responses. A practical approach is to perform proactive TDM one to two weeks following re-exposure to anti-TNF therapy; the presence of ADAs suggests a higher likelihood of an infusion reaction occurring with continued dosing and warrants a treatment change [64–66]. The use of combination therapy can decrease the risk of developing ADAs in these patients, and while checking thiopurine metabolites soon after restarting therapy may be too early, optimizing the thiopurine after induction aiming to achieve adequate 6-TGN levels is reasonable [64–66]. In situations where an adequate level is present without ADAs after anti-TNF re-exposure, proactive TDM may also help to avoid combo-therapy.

Genetics, specifically the HLA-DQA1*05 variant, has been associated with a higher risk of immunogenicity [67]. However, its role in clinical practice is still unclear. In a post hoc analysis of the precision infliximab trial, HLA-DQA1*05 carriage was not associated with ADA formation or higher drug durability [68]. Another single-center retrospective cohort suggests that carriers of this genotypic variant under a proactive TDM strategy are not associated with a higher risk of treatment cessation or worse clinical outcomes [69]. Proactive TDM may be a better predictor of immunogenicity, but larger prospective studies are needed to confirm this.

TDM and De-Escalation of Combination Therapy

De-escalating treatment in patients receiving combination therapy is another strategy used in select patients, mainly aiming to decrease the risk of potential adverse events. A randomized controlled trial comparing azathioprine/6-mercaptopurine or methotrexate discontinuation vs. continuation in patients receiving a standard dose of infliximab showed that, after 6 months of combination therapy, continuing the immunosuppressant did not offer a clinical benefit. However, the patients who continued the combination therapy had higher infliximab drug levels [70,71]. A study by Sokol et al., however, did find that immunomodulator discontinuation on combo-therapy infliximab led to disease exacerbation, the development of complications, and the need to switch therapies [72]. Overall, it is reasonable to use TDM when considering de-escalation [42]. Roblin et al. demonstrated in an open-label, prospective, randomized trial that a reduction in the dose of thiopurine after 6 months of stable remission (>1 year of treatment) on combo-therapy with infliximab was as effective as full-dose azathioprine, but discontinuation led to a significant drop in the infliximab trough level, even though no major impact on clinical outcomes was observed [73]. In the patients who underwent the thiopurine dose reduction, 6-TGN < 146 pmol per 8×10^8 RBC was associated with worsening infliximab pharmacokinetics. In this setting, it is reasonable to use TDM not only when completely discontinuing the immunosuppressant but also when reducing the azathioprine dose and using 6-TGN levels to determine an optimal threshold level, ultimately aiming to concomitantly increase efficacy and safety.

From a biological standpoint, it would also be sensible to check the drug level before and after de-escalation (or dose reduction). The risk of requiring infliximab dose escalation, drug discontinuation, and IBD surgery is much lower when patients maintain a higher infliximab trough when the immunomodulator is stopped [71].

TDM data specific to golimumab use in UC and certolizumab in CD in the setting of combination therapy are lacking. A subgroup analysis of observational data suggests that a lower number of patients develop immunogenicity with these drugs than with infliximab and adalimumab. More data are needed to draw meaningful conclusions regarding TDM, immunogenicity risk, and combo-therapy de-escalation [74,75].

6. Discussion

While the combination therapy of anti-TNF and immunomodulators can offer higher effectiveness, a relatively high number of patients still do not respond to treatment or lose response. A large and evolving body of evidence has shown that the use of TDM in patients receiving monotherapy and combination therapy of anti-TNF can be tremendously useful. Since reactive and proactive TDM strategies are also cost-effective, their increased utilization can help treat IBD patients in a more cost-effective way. Another benefit of using a monitored approach includes the avoidance of potential adverse effects seen with combo-therapy.

While the findings in this review have significant implications for clinical practice, unfortunately, the widespread adoption of TDM remains an important barrier. For example, most centers rely on external laboratories, and there might be a significant lag time from sampling and laboratory processing until the clinician receives an actionable result. Furthermore, there is a lack of consensus on optimal target concentrations, which likely vary based on the type of assay used, phenotype of the disease, inflammatory burden, and timing through the dose cycle [76]. The implementation of commercially available point-of-care testing could reduce the lag time, while the standardization of assays to enhance reliability and quality control could help to minimize some of these issues [77,78]. Nevertheless, factors like cost, accessibility, and external validation need careful consideration before recognizing the impact of real-time value on clinical decision making.

As more data become available, personalized TDM strategies and their use in combination with treat-to-target strategies are becoming a standard in IBD management. We might see elements of pharmacogenetics and pharmacokinetic-modeled dashboards aided by artificial intelligence where dosing and monitoring are tailored to each patient [79]. Future studies looking into precision medicine considering multiple patient-centered variables are needed. Furthermore, studies looking into the optimization of newer biologics and small molecules used in the treatment of IBD are also warranted.

7. Conclusions

The TDM of anti-TNFs in patients with IBD has been proven to be a useful tool. In patients receiving combination therapy, it can also provide an opportunity to further optimize therapies, especially in patients with non-response to drugs and those not achieving the desired pharmacokinetic effect despite concomitant thiopurine use, and to help guide treatment de-escalation or re-initiation. Conversely, the use of combination therapy and the use of TDM in patients receiving vedolizumab or ustekinumab do not seem to offer a clear benefit.

Limitations

It is important to acknowledge the limitations inherent in the available literature, as the quality and consistency of reporting across the included studies may vary, potentially affecting the generalizability of the findings. First, overall, there is a limited amount of evidence regarding the use of TDM in combination therapy. Also, our review included articles published in English, which may have omitted relevant studies published in other languages. Second, the heterogeneity of the included studies, in terms of study design, population, and intervention, might have influenced the overall conclusions. The review process may also have inherent biases, such as a potential selection bias in the studies included.

Author Contributions: Writing—original draft preparation, S.P.; writing—review and editing, S.P. and A.J.Y.; supervision, A.J.Y. All authors have read and agreed to the published version of the manuscript.

Funding: This research received no external funding.

Institutional Review Board Statement: Not applicable.

Informed Consent Statement: Not applicable.

Conflicts of Interest: AJY is a consultant for Bristol Myers Squibb, Arena, Pfizer, and Celltrion.

References

1. Targan, S.R.; Hanauer, S.B.; van Deventer, S.J.H.; Mayer, L.; Present, D.H.; Braakman, T.; DeWoody, K.L.; Schaible, T.F.; Rutgeerts, P.J. A Short-Term Study of Chimeric Monoclonal Antibody CA2 to Tumor Necrosis Factor α for Crohn's Disease. *N. Engl. J. Med.* **1997**, *337*, 1029–1036. [CrossRef]
2. Sandborn, W.J.; Rutgeerts, P.; Enns, R.; Hanauer, S.B.; Colombel, J.-F.; Panaccione, R.; D'Haens, G.; Li, J.; Rosenfeld, M.R.; Kent, J.D.; et al. Adalimumab Induction Therapy for Crohn Disease Previously Treated with Infliximab. *Ann. Intern. Med.* **2007**, *146*, 829. [CrossRef]
3. Hanauer, S.B.; Sandborn, W.J.; Rutgeerts, P.; Fedorak, R.N.; Lukas, M.; MacIntosh, D.; Panaccione, R.; Wolf, D.; Pollack, P. Human Anti–Tumor Necrosis Factor Monoclonal Antibody (Adalimumab) in Crohn's Disease: The CLASSIC-I Trial. *Gastroenterology* **2006**, *130*, 323–333. [CrossRef]

4. Hanauer, S.B.; Feagan, B.G.; Lichtenstein, G.R.; Mayer, L.F.; Schreiber, S.; Colombel, J.F.; Rachmilewitz, D.; Wolf, D.C.; Olson, A.; Bao, W.; et al. Maintenance Infliximab for Crohn's Disease: The ACCENT I Randomised Trial. *Lancet* 2002, *359*, 1541–1549. [CrossRef]
5. Colombel, J.; Sandborn, W.J.; Rutgeerts, P.; Enns, R.; Hanauer, S.B.; Panaccione, R.; Schreiber, S.; Byczkowski, D.; Li, J.; Kent, J.D.; et al. Adalimumab for Maintenance of Clinical Response and Remission in Patients with Crohn's Disease: The CHARM Trial. *Gastroenterology* 2007, *132*, 52–65. [CrossRef]
6. Sandborn, W.J.; Feagan, B.G.; Stoinov, S.; Honiball, P.J.; Rutgeerts, P.; Mason, D.; Bloomfield, R.; Schreiber, S. Certolizumab Pegol for the Treatment of Crohn's Disease. *N. Engl. J. Med.* 2007, *357*, 228–238. [CrossRef] [PubMed]
7. Schreiber, S.; Khaliq-Kareemi, M.; Lawrance, I.C.; Thomsen, O.Ø.; Hanauer, S.B.; McColm, J.; Bloomfield, R.; Sandborn, W.J. Maintenance Therapy with Certolizumab Pegol for Crohn's Disease. *N. Engl. J. Med.* 2007, *357*, 239–250. [CrossRef]
8. Feagan, B.G.; Rutgeerts, P.; Sands, B.E.; Hanauer, S.; Colombel, J.-F.; Sandborn, W.J.; Van Assche, G.; Axler, J.; Kim, H.-J.; Danese, S.; et al. Vedolizumab as Induction and Maintenance Therapy for Ulcerative Colitis. *N. Engl. J. Med.* 2013, *369*, 699–710. [CrossRef]
9. Sandborn, W.J.; Feagan, B.G.; Rutgeerts, P.; Hanauer, S.; Colombel, J.-F.; Sands, B.E.; Lukas, M.; Fedorak, R.N.; Lee, S.; Bressler, B.; et al. Vedolizumab as Induction and Maintenance Therapy for Crohn's Disease. *N. Engl. J. Med.* 2013, *369*, 711–721. [CrossRef]
10. Sands, B.E.; Sandborn, W.J.; Panaccione, R.; O'Brien, C.D.; Zhang, H.; Johanns, J.; Adedokun, O.J.; Li, K.; Peyrin-Biroulet, L.; Van Assche, G.; et al. Ustekinumab as Induction and Maintenance Therapy for Ulcerative Colitis. *N. Engl. J. Med.* 2019, *381*, 1201–1214. [CrossRef]
11. Feagan, B.G.; Sandborn, W.J.; Gasink, C.; Jacobstein, D.; Lang, Y.; Friedman, J.R.; Blank, M.A.; Johanns, J.; Gao, L.-L.; Miao, Y.; et al. Ustekinumab as Induction and Maintenance Therapy for Crohn's Disease. *N. Engl. J. Med.* 2016, *375*, 1946–1960. [CrossRef] [PubMed]
12. Kennedy, N.A.; Heap, G.A.; Green, H.D.; Hamilton, B.; Bewshea, C.; Walker, G.J.; Thomas, A.; Nice, R.; Perry, M.H.; Bouri, S.; et al. Predictors of Anti-TNF Treatment Failure in Anti-TNF-Naive Patients with Active Luminal Crohn's Disease: A Prospective, Multicentre, Cohort Study. *Lancet Gastroenterol. Hepatol.* 2019, *4*, 341–353. [CrossRef] [PubMed]
13. Colombel, J.-F.; Adedokun, O.J.; Gasink, C.; Gao, L.-L.; Cornillie, F.J.; D'Haens, G.R.; Rutgeerts, P.J.; Reinisch, W.; Sandborn, W.J.; Hanauer, S.B. Combination Therapy with Infliximab and Azathioprine Improves Infliximab Pharmacokinetic Features and Efficacy: A Post Hoc Analysis. *Clin. Gastroenterol. Hepatol.* 2019, *17*, 1525–1532.e1. [CrossRef]
14. Marquez-Megias, S.; Nalda-Molina, R.; Sanz-Valero, J.; Más-Serrano, P.; Diaz-Gonzalez, M.; Candela-Boix, M.R.; Ramon-Lopez, A. Cost-Effectiveness of Therapeutic Drug Monitoring of Anti-TNF Therapy in Inflammatory Bowel Disease: A Systematic Review. *Pharmaceutics* 2022, *14*, 1009. [CrossRef]
15. Dubinsky, M.C.; Lamothe, S.; Yang, H.Y.; Targan, S.R.; Sinnett, D.; Théorêt, Y.; Seidman, E.G. Pharmacogenomics and Metabolite Measurement for 6-Mercaptopurine Therapy in Inflammatory Bowel Disease. *Gastroenterology* 2000, *118*, 705–713. [CrossRef]
16. Dart, R.J.; Irving, P.M. Optimising Use of Thiopurines in Inflammatory Bowel Disease. *Expert Rev. Clin. Immunol.* 2017, *13*, 877–888. [CrossRef] [PubMed]
17. Lim, S.Z.; Chua, E.W. Revisiting the Role of Thiopurines in Inflammatory Bowel Disease Through Pharmacogenomics and Use of Novel Methods for Therapeutic Drug Monitoring. *Front. Pharmacol.* 2018, *9*, 1107. [CrossRef]
18. Mao, R.; Guo, J.; Luber, R.; Chen, B.-L.; He, Y.; Zeng, Z.-R.; Ben-Horin, S.; Sparrow, M.P.; Roblin, X.; Chen, M.-H. 6-Thioguanine Nucleotide Levels Are Associated with Mucosal Healing in Patients with Crohn's Disease. *Inflamm. Bowel Dis.* 2018, *24*, 2621–2627. [CrossRef]
19. Colombel, J.F.; Sandborn, W.J.; Reinisch, W.; Mantzaris, G.J.; Kornbluth, A.; Rachmilewitz, D.; Lichtiger, S.; d'Haens, G.; Diamond, R.H.; Broussard, D.L.; et al. Infliximab, Azathioprine, or Combination Therapy for Crohn's Disease. *N. Engl. J. Med.* 2010, *362*, 1383–1395. [CrossRef] [PubMed]
20. Yarur, A.J.; Kubiliun, M.J.; Czul, F.; Sussman, D.A.; Quintero, M.A.; Jain, A.; Drake, K.A.; Hauenstein, S.I.; Lockton, S.; Deshpande, A.R.; et al. Concentrations of 6-Thioguanine Nucleotide Correlate with Trough Levels of Infliximab in Patients with Inflammatory Bowel Disease on Combination Therapy. *Clin. Gastroenterol. Hepatol.* 2015, *13*, 1118–1124.e3. [CrossRef] [PubMed]
21. Maser, E.A.; Villela, R.; Silverberg, M.S.; Greenberg, G.R. Association of Trough Serum Infliximab to Clinical Outcome After Scheduled Maintenance Treatment for Crohn's Disease. *Clin. Gastroenterol. Hepatol.* 2006, *4*, 1248–1254. [CrossRef] [PubMed]
22. Yarur, A.J.; Jain, A.; Hauenstein, S.I.; Quintero, M.A.; Barkin, J.S.; Deshpande, A.R.; Sussman, D.A.; Singh, S.; Abreu, M.T. Higher Adalimumab Levels Are Associated with Histologic and Endoscopic Remission in Patients with Crohns Disease and Ulcerative Colitis. *Inflamm. Bowel Dis.* 2016, *22*, 409–415. [CrossRef]
23. Vande Casteele, N.; Feagan, B.G.; Vermeire, S.; Yassine, M.; Coarse, J.; Kosutic, G.; Sandborn, W.J. Exposure-Response Relationship of Certolizumab Pegol Induction and Maintenance Therapy in Patients with Crohn's Disease. *Aliment. Pharmacol. Ther.* 2017, *47*, 229–237. [CrossRef]
24. Papamichael, K.; Cheifetz, A.S.; Melmed, G.Y.; Irving, P.M.; Vande Casteele, N.; Kozuch, P.L.; Raffals, L.E.; Baidoo, L.; Bressler, B.; Devlin, S.M.; et al. Appropriate Therapeutic Drug Monitoring of Biologic Agents for Patients with Inflammatory Bowel Diseases. *Clin. Gastroenterol. Hepatol.* 2019, *17*, 1655–1668.e3. [CrossRef] [PubMed]

25. Battat, R.; Lukin, D.; Scherl, E.J.; Pola, S.; Kumar, A.; Okada, L.; Yang, L.; Jain, A.; Siegel, C.A. Immunogenicity of Tumor Necrosis Factor Antagonists and Effect of Dose Escalation on Anti-Drug Antibodies and Serum Drug Concentrations in Inflammatory Bowel Disease. *Inflamm. Bowel Dis.* **2020**, *27*, 1443–1451. [CrossRef]
26. Afif, W.; Loftus, E.V.; Faubion, W.A.; Kane, S.V.; Bruining, D.H.; Hanson, K.A.; Sandborn, W.J. Clinical Utility of Measuring Infliximab and Human Anti-Chimeric Antibody Concentrations in Patients with Inflammatory Bowel Disease. *Am. J. Gastroenterol.* **2010**, *105*, 1133–1139. [CrossRef]
27. Vermeire, S.; Dreesen, E.; Papamichael, K.; Dubinsky, M.C. How, When, and for Whom Should We Perform Therapeutic Drug Monitoring? *Clin. Gastroenterol. Hepatol.* **2020**, *18*, 1291–1299. [CrossRef]
28. Vande Casteele, N.; Ferrante, M.; Van Assche, G.; Ballet, V.; Compernolle, G.; Van Steen, K.; Simoens, S.; Rutgeerts, P.; Gils, A.; Vermeire, S. everine Trough Concentrations of Infliximab Guide Dosing for Patients with Inflammatory Bowel Disease. *Gastroenterology* **2015**, *148*, 1320–1329.e3. [CrossRef] [PubMed]
29. D'Haens, G.; Vermeire, S.; Lambrecht, G.; Baert, F.; Bossuyt, P.; Pariente, B.; Buisson, A.; Bouhnik, Y.; Filippi, J.; vander Woude, J.; et al. Increasing Infliximab Dose Based on Symptoms, Biomarkers, and Serum Drug Concentrations Does Not Increase Clinical, Endoscopic, and Corticosteroid-Free Remission in Patients with Active Luminal Crohn's Disease. *Gastroenterology* **2018**, *154*, 1343–1351.e1. [CrossRef]
30. Laharie, D.; D'Haens, G.; Nachury, M.; Lambrecht, G.; Bossuyt, P.; Bouhnik, Y.; Louis, E.; Janneke van der Woude, C.; Buisson, A.; Van Hootegem, P.; et al. Steroid-Free Deep Remission at One Year Does Not Prevent Crohn's Disease Progression: Long-Term Data From the TAILORIX Trial. *Clin. Gastroenterol. Hepatol.* **2022**, *20*, 2074–2082. [CrossRef] [PubMed]
31. Assa, A.; Matar, M.; Turner, D.; Broide, E.; Weiss, B.; Ledder, O.; Guz-Mark, A.; Rinawi, F.; Cohen, S.; Topf-Olivestone, C.; et al. Proactive Monitoring of Adalimumab Trough Concentration Associated with Increased Clinical Remission in Children with Crohn's Disease Compared with Reactive Monitoring. *Gastroenterology* **2019**, *157*, 985–996.e2. [CrossRef]
32. Syversen, S.W. Effect of Therapeutic Drug Monitoring vs Standard Therapy During Infliximab Induction on Disease Remission In. *JAMA* **2021**, *325*, 1744–1754. [CrossRef] [PubMed]
33. Syversen, S.W. Effect of Therapeutic Drug Monitoring vs Standard Therapy During Maintenance Infliximab Therapy on Disease. *JAMA* **2021**, *326*, 2375–2384. [CrossRef] [PubMed]
34. Yarur, A.J.; Abreu, M.T.; Deepak, P.; Beniwal-Patel, P.; Papamichail, K.; Vaughn, B.; Bruss, A.; Sekhri, S.; Moosreiner, A.; Gu, P.; et al. Patients with Inflammatory Bowel Diseases and Higher Visceral Adipose Tissue Burden May Benefit from Higher Infliximab Concentrations to Achieve Remission. *Am. J. Gastroenterol.* **2023**, 10-14309, in press. [CrossRef]
35. Magro, F.; Rodrigues-Pinto, E.; Santos-Antunes, J.; Vilas-Boas, F.; Lopes, S.; Nunes, A.; Camila-Dias, C.; Macedo, G. High C-Reactive Protein in Crohn's Disease Patients Predicts Nonresponse to Infliximab Treatment. *J. Crohn's Colitis* **2014**, *8*, 129–136. [CrossRef]
36. Hibi, T.; Sakuraba, A.; Watanabe, M.; Motoya, S.; Ito, H.; Sato, N.; Yoshinari, T.; Motegi, K.; Kinouchi, Y.; Takazoe, M.; et al. C-Reactive Protein Is an Indicator of Serum Infliximab Level in Predicting Loss of Response in Patients with Crohn's Disease. *J. Gastroenterol.* **2013**, *49*, 254–262. [CrossRef]
37. Velayos, F.S.; Kahn, J.G.; Sandborn, W.J.; Feagan, B.G. A Test-Based Strategy Is More Cost Effective Than Empiric Dose Escalation for Patients with Crohn's Disease Who Lose Responsiveness to Infliximab. *Clin. Gastroenterol. Hepatol.* **2013**, *11*, 654–666. [CrossRef] [PubMed]
38. Steenholdt, C.; Brynskov, J.; Thomsen, O.Ø.; Munck, L.K.; Fallingborg, J.; Christensen, L.A.; Pedersen, G.; Kjeldsen, J.; Jacobsen, B.A.; Oxholm, A.S.; et al. Individualised Therapy Is More Cost-Effective than Dose Intensification in Patients with Crohn's Disease Who Lose Response to Anti-TNF Treatment: A Randomised, Controlled Trial. *Gut* **2014**, *63*, 919–927. [CrossRef]
39. Negoescu, D.M.; Enns, E.A.; Swanhorst, B.; Baumgartner, B.; Campbell, J.P.; Osterman, M.T.; Papamichael, K.; Cheifetz, A.S.; Vaughn, B.P. Proactive Vs Reactive Therapeutic Drug Monitoring of Infliximab in Crohn's Disease: A Cost-Effectiveness Analysis in a Simulated Cohort. *Inflamm. Bowel Dis.* **2020**, *26*, 103–111. [CrossRef]
40. McNeill, R.P.; Barclay, M.L. Cost-Effectiveness of Therapeutic Drug Monitoring in Inflammatory Bowel Disease. *Curr. Opin. Pharmacol.* **2020**, *55*, 41–46. [CrossRef]
41. Strik, A.S.; Löwenberg, M.; Mould, D.R.; Berends, S.E.; Ponsioen, C.I.; van den Brande, J.M.H.; Jansen, J.M.; Hoekman, D.R.; Brandse, J.F.; Duijvestein, M.; et al. Efficacy of Dashboard Driven Dosing of Infliximab in Inflammatory Bowel Disease Patients; a Randomized Controlled Trial. *Scand. J. Gastroenterol.* **2020**, *56*, 145–154. [CrossRef]
42. Cheifetz, A.S.; Abreu, M.T.; Afif, W.; Cross, R.K.; Dubinsky, M.C.; Loftus, E.V.; Osterman, M.T.; Saroufim, A.; Siegel, C.A.; Yarur, A.J.; et al. A Comprehensive Literature Review and Expert Consensus Statement on Therapeutic Drug Monitoring of Biologics in Inflammatory Bowel Disease. *Am. J. Gastroenterol.* **2021**, *116*, 2014–2025. [CrossRef]
43. Sethi, S.; Dias, S.; Kumar, A.; Blackwell, J.; Brookes, M.J.; Segal, J.P. Metaanalysis: The Efficacy of Therapeutic Drug Monitoring of Anti TNF Therapy in Inflammatory Bowel Disease. *Aliment. Pharmacol. Ther.* **2022**, *57*, 1362–1374. [CrossRef] [PubMed]
44. Singh, S.; Dulai, P.S.; Vande Casteele, N.; Battat, R.; Fumery, M.; Boland, B.S.; Sandborn, W.J. Systematic Review with Meta-Analysis: Association between Vedolizumab Trough Concentration and Clinical Outcomes in Patients with Inflammatory Bowel Diseases. *Aliment. Pharmacol. Ther.* **2019**, *50*, 848–857. [CrossRef] [PubMed]
45. Dreesen, E.; Verstockt, B.; Bian, S.; de Bruyn, M.; Compernolle, G.; Tops, S.; Noman, M.; Van Assche, G.; Ferrante, M.; Gils, A.; et al. Evidence to Support Monitoring of Vedolizumab Trough Concentrations in Patients with Inflammatory Bowel Diseases. *Clin. Gastroenterol. Hepatol.* **2018**, *16*, 1937–1946.e8. [CrossRef] [PubMed]

46. Adedokun, O.J.; Xu, Z.; Gasink, C.; Jacobstein, D.; Szapary, P.; Johanns, J.; Gao, L.-L.; Davis, H.M.; Hanauer, S.B.; Feagan, B.G.; et al. Pharmacokinetics and Exposure Response Relationships of Ustekinumab in Patients with Crohn's Disease. *Gastroenterology* **2018**, *154*, 1660–1671. [CrossRef] [PubMed]
47. Battat, R.; Kopylov, U.; Bessissow, T.; Bitton, A.; Cohen, A.; Jain, A.; Martel, M.; Seidman, E.; Afif, W. Association Between Ustekinumab Trough Concentrations and Clinical, Biomarker, and Endoscopic Outcomes in Patients with Crohn's Disease. *Clin. Gastroenterol. Hepatol. Off. Clin. Pract. J. Am. Gastroenterol. Assoc.* **2017**, *15*, 1427–1434. [CrossRef] [PubMed]
48. Yarur, A.J.; Bruss, A.; Naik, S.; Beniwal-Patel, P.; Fox, C.; Jain, A.; Berens, B.; Patel, A.; Ungaro, R.; Bahur, B.; et al. Vedolizumab Concentrations Are Associated with Long-Term Endoscopic Remission in Patients with Inflammatory Bowel Diseases. *Dig. Dis. Sci.* **2019**, *64*, 1651–1659. [CrossRef]
49. Yarur, A.J.; Digestive Disease Week ePoster Library 2022. Higher Serum Ustekinumab Levels Correlate with Higher Rates of Steroid-Free Deep Remission and Endoscopic Healing in Patients with IBD. Available online: https://eposters.ddw.org/ddw/2022/ddw-2022/353592/ (accessed on 29 April 2023).
50. Osterman, M.T.; Jairath, V.; Rana-Khan, Q.; James, A.; Balma, D.; Mehrotra, S.; Yang, L.; Lasch, K.; Yarur, A.J. 791: A randomized trial of vedolizumab dose optimization in patients with moderate to severe ulcerative colitis who have early nonresponse and high drug clearance: The enterpret trial. *Gastroenterology* **2022**, *162*, S-190–S-191. [CrossRef]
51. Admin, S. European Crohn's and Colitis Organisation-ECCO-P436 Efficacy and Safety of Intravenous Ustekinumab Re-Induction Therapy in Crohn's Disease Patients with Secondary Loss of Response to Ustekinumab Maintenance Therapy: Week 16 Results from the POWER Trial. Available online: https://www.ecco-ibd.eu/publications/congress-abstracts/item/p436-efficacy-and-safety-of-intravenous-ustekinumab-re-induction-therapy-in-crohn-s-disease-patients-with-secondary-loss-of-response-to-ustekinumab-maintenance-therapy-week-16-results-from-the-power-trial.html (accessed on 21 May 2023).
52. Yarur, A.J.; Deepak, P.; Vande Casteele, N.; Battat, R.; Jain, A.; Okada, L.; Osterman, M.; Regueiro, M. Between Vedolizumab Levels, Anti-Vedolizumab Antibodies, and Endoscopic Healing Index in a Large Population of Patients with Inflammatory Bowel Diseases. *Dig. Dis. Sci.* **2020**, *66*, 3563–3569. [CrossRef]
53. Vande Casteele, N.; Khanna, R.; Levesque, B.G.; Stitt, L.; Zou, G.Y.; Singh, S.; Lockton, S.; Hauenstein, S.; Ohrmund, L.; Greenberg, G.R.; et al. The Relationship between Infliximab Concentrations, Antibodies to Infliximab and Disease Activity in Crohn's Disease. *Gut* **2014**, *64*, 1539–1545. [CrossRef] [PubMed]
54. Vermeire, S.; Gils, A.; Accossato, P.; Lula, S.; Marren, A. Immunogenicity of Biologics in Inflammatory Bowel Disease. *Ther. Adv. Gastroenterol.* **2018**, *11*, 1756283X1775035. [CrossRef]
55. Stallhofer, J.; Guse, J.; Kesselmeier, M.; Grunert, P.C.; Lange, K.; Stalmann, R.; Eckardt, V.; Stallmach, A. Immunomodulator Comedication Promotes the Reversal of Anti-Drug Antibody-Mediated Loss of Response to Anti-TNF Therapy in Inflammatory Bowel Disease. *Int. J. Color. Dis.* **2023**, *38*, 54. [CrossRef] [PubMed]
56. Ungar, B.; Kopylov, U.; Engel, T.; Yavzori, M.; Fudim, E.; Picard, O.; Lang, A.; Williet, N.; Paul, S.; Chowers, Y.; et al. Addition of an Immunomodulator Can Reverse Antibody Formation and Loss of Response in Patients Treated with Adalimumab. *Aliment. Pharmacol. Ther.* **2017**, *45*, 276–282. [CrossRef] [PubMed]
57. Panaccione, R.; Ghosh, S.; Middleton, S.; Márquez, J.R.; Scott, B.B.; Flint, L.; van Hoogstraten, H.J.F.; Chen, A.C.; Zheng, H.; Danese, S.; et al. Combination Therapy with Infliximab and Azathioprine Is Superior to Monotherapy with Either Agent in Ulcerative Colitis. *Gastroenterology* **2014**, *146*, 392–400.e3. [CrossRef]
58. Feagan, B.G.; McDonald, J.W.D.; Panaccione, R.; Enns, R.A.; Bernstein, C.N.; Ponich, T.P.; Bourdages, R.; MacIntosh, D.G.; Dallaire, C.; Cohen, A.; et al. Methotrexate in Combination with Infliximab Is No More Effective Than Infliximab Alone in Patients with Crohn's Disease. *Gastroenterology* **2014**, *146*, 681–688.e1. [CrossRef] [PubMed]
59. Vande Casteele, N.; Abreu, M.T.; Flier, S.; Papamichael, K.; Rieder, F.; Silverberg, M.S.; Khanna, R.; Okada, L.; Yang, L.; Jain, A.; et al. Patients with Low Drug Levels or Antibodies to a Prior Anti-Tumor Necrosis Factor Are More Likely to Develop Antibodies to a Subsequent Anti-Tumor Necrosis Factor. *Clin. Gastroenterol. Hepatol.* **2022**, *20*, 465–467.e2. [CrossRef]
60. Vermeire, S.; Noman, M.; Assche, G.V.; Baert, F.; D'Haens, G.; Rutgeerts, P. Effectiveness of Concomitant Immunosuppressive Therapy in Suppressing the Formation of Antibodies to Infliximab in Crohn's Disease. *Gut* **2007**, *56*, 1226–1231. [CrossRef]
61. Privitera, G.; Pugliese, D.; Onali, S.; Petito, V.; Scaldaferri, F.; Gasbarrini, A.; Danese, S.; Armuzzi, A. Combination Therapy in Inflammatory Bowel Disease–from Traditional Immunosuppressors towards the New Paradigm of Dual Targeted Therapy. *Autoimmun. Rev.* **2021**, *20*, 102832. [CrossRef] [PubMed]
62. Roblin, X.; Williet, N.; Boschetti, G.; Phelip, J.-M.; Del Tedesco, E.; Berger, A.-E.; Vedrines, P.; Duru, G.; Peyrin-Biroulet, L.; Nancey, S.; et al. Addition of Azathioprine to the Switch of Anti-TNF in Patients with IBD in Clinical Relapse with Undetectable Anti-TNF Trough Levels and Antidrug Antibodies: A Prospective Randomised Trial. *Gut* **2020**, *69*, 1206–1212. [CrossRef]
63. Yarur, A.J.; McGovern, D.; Abreu, M.T.; Cheifetz, A.; Papamichail, K.; Deepak, P.; Bruss, A.; Beniwal-Patel, P.; Dubinsky, M.; Targan, S.R.; et al. Combination Therapy with Immunomodulators Improves the Pharmacokinetics of Infliximab But Not Vedolizumab or Ustekinumab. *Clin. Gastroenterol. Hepatol.* **2022**, *21*, 2908–2917. [CrossRef] [PubMed]
64. Baert, F.; Drobne, D.; Gils, A.; Vande Casteele, N.; Hauenstein, S.; Singh, S.; Lockton, S.; Rutgeerts, P.; Vermeire, S. Early Trough Levels and Antibodies to Infliximab Predict Safety and Success of Reinitiation of Infliximab Therapy. *Clin. Gastroenterol. Hepatol.* **2014**, *12*, 1474–1481.e2. [CrossRef] [PubMed]
65. Normatov, I. Mo1890–Using Therapeutic Drug Monitoring to Predict Success of Restarting Infliximab Therapy After a Drug Holiday in Inflammatory Bowel Disease. *Gastroenterology* **2019**, *156*, S-876. [CrossRef]

66. Louis, E.; Mary, J.-Y.; Vernier-Massouille, G.; Grimaud, J.-C.; Bouhnik, Y.; Laharie, D.; Dupas, J.-L.; Pillant, H.; Picon, L.; Veyrac, M.; et al. Maintenance of Remission among Patients with Crohn's Disease on Antimetabolite Therapy after Infliximab Therapy Is Stopped. *Gastroenterology* **2012**, *142*, 63–70.e5, quiz e31. [CrossRef]
67. Sazonovs, A.; Kennedy, N.A.; Moutsianas, L.; Heap, G.A.; Rice, D.L.; Reppell, M.; Bewshea, C.M.; Chanchlani, N.; Walker, G.J.; Perry, M.H.; et al. HLA-DQA1*05 Carriage Associated with Development of Anti-Drug Antibodies to Infliximab and Adalimumab in Patients with Crohn's Disease. *Gastroenterology* **2020**, *158*, 189–199. [CrossRef]
68. Spencer, E.A.; Stachelski, J.; Dervieux, T.; Dubinsky, M.C. Failure to Achieve Target Drug Concentrations During Induction and Not HLA-DQA1∗05 Carriage Is Associated with Antidrug Antibody Formation in Patients with Inflammatory Bowel Disease. *Gastroenterology* **2022**, *162*, 1746–1748.e3. [CrossRef]
69. Fuentes-Valenzuela, E.; García-Alonso, F.J.; Maroto-Martín, C.; Juan Casamayor, L.; Garrote, J.A.; Almendros Muñoz, R.; De Prado, Á.; Vara Castrodeza, A.; Marinero, M.Á.; Calleja Carbajosa, R.; et al. Influence of *HLADQA1*05* Genotype in Adults with Inflammatory Bowel Disease and Anti-TNF Treatment with Proactive Therapeutic Drug Monitoring: A Retrospective Cohort Study. *Inflamm. Bowel Dis.* **2023**, *29*, 1586–1593. [CrossRef] [PubMed]
70. Van Assche, G.; Magdelaine–Beuzelin, C.; D'Haens, G.; Baert, F.; Noman, M.; Vermeire, S.; Ternant, D.; Watier, H.; Paintaud, G.; Rutgeerts, P. Withdrawal of Immunosuppression in Crohn's Disease Treated with Scheduled Infliximab Maintenance: A Randomized Trial. *Gastroenterology* **2008**, *134*, 1861–1868. [CrossRef]
71. Drobne, D.; Bossuyt, P.; Breynaert, C.; Cattaert, T.; Vande Casteele, N.; Compernolle, G.; Jürgens, M.; Ferrante, M.; Ballet, V.; Wollants, W.-J.; et al. Withdrawal of Immunomodulators After Co-Treatment Does Not Reduce Trough Level of Infliximab in Patients with Crohn's Disease. *Clin. Gastroenterol. Hepatol.* **2015**, *13*, 514–521.e4. [CrossRef]
72. Sokol, H.; Seksik, P.; Carrat, F.; Nion-Larmurier, I.; Vienne, A.; Beaugerie, L.; Cosnes, J. Usefulness of Co-Treatment with Immunomodulators in Patients with Inflammatory Bowel Disease Treated with Scheduled Infliximab Maintenance Therapy. *Gut* **2010**, *59*, 1363–1368. [CrossRef]
73. Roblin, X.; Boschetti, G.; Williet, N.; Nancey, S.; Marotte, H.; Berger, A.; Phelip, J.M.; Peyrin-Biroulet, L.; Colombel, J.F.; Del Tedesco, E.; et al. Azathioprine Dose Reduction in Inflammatory Bowel Disease Patients on Combination Therapy: An Open-Label, Prospective and Randomised Clinical Trial. *Aliment. Pharmacol. Ther.* **2017**, *46*, 142–149. [CrossRef] [PubMed]
74. Dulai, P.S.; Siegel, C.A.; Colombel, J.-F.; Sandborn, W.J.; Peyrin-Biroulet, L. Systematic Review: Monotherapy with Antitumour Necrosis Factor α Agents versus Combination Therapy with an Immunosuppressive for IBD. *Gut* **2014**, *63*, 1843–1853. [CrossRef] [PubMed]
75. Dai, C.; Huang, Y.-H.; Jiang, M. Combination Therapy in Inflammatory Bowel Disease: Current Evidence and Perspectives. *Int. Immunopharmacol.* **2023**, *114*, 109545. [CrossRef] [PubMed]
76. Papamichael, K.; Afif, W.; Drobne, D.; Dubinsky, M.C.; Ferrante, M.; Irving, P.M.; Kamperidis, N.; Kobayashi, T.; Kotze, P.G.; Lambert, J.; et al. Therapeutic Drug Monitoring of Biologics in Inflammatory Bowel Disease: Unmet Needs and Future Perspectives. *Lancet Gastroenterol. Hepatol.* **2022**, *7*, 171–185. [CrossRef] [PubMed]
77. Laserna-Mendieta, E.J.; Salvador-Martín, S.; Arias-González, L.; Ruiz-Ponce, M.; Menchén, L.A.; Sánchez, C.; López-Fernández, L.A.; Lucendo, A.J. Comparison of a New Rapid Method for the Determination of Adalimumab Serum Levels with Two Established ELISA Kits. *Clin. Chem. Lab. Med.* **2019**, *57*, 1906–1914. [CrossRef]
78. Nasser, Y.; Labetoulle, R.; Harzallah, I.; Berger, A.-E.; Roblin, X.; Paul, S. Comparison of Point-of-Care and Classical Immunoassays for the Monitoring Infliximab and Antibodies Against Infliximab in IBD. *Dig. Dis. Sci.* **2018**, *63*, 2714–2721. [CrossRef]
79. Irving, P.M.; Gecse, K.B. Optimizing Therapies Using Therapeutic Drug Monitoring: Current Strategies and Future Perspectives. *Gastroenterology* **2022**, *162*, 1512–1524. [CrossRef]

Disclaimer/Publisher's Note: The statements, opinions and data contained in all publications are solely those of the individual author(s) and contributor(s) and not of MDPI and/or the editor(s). MDPI and/or the editor(s) disclaim responsibility for any injury to people or property resulting from any ideas, methods, instructions or products referred to in the content.

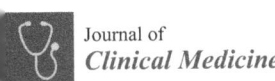

Review

Therapeutic Drug Monitoring of Subcutaneous Infliximab in Inflammatory Bowel Disease—Understanding Pharmacokinetics and Exposure Response Relationships in a New Era of Subcutaneous Biologics

Robert D. Little [1], Mark G. Ward [1], Emily Wright [2], Asha J. Jois [3], Alex Boussioutas [1], Georgina L. Hold [4], Peter R. Gibson [1] and Miles P. Sparrow [1,*]

1. Department of Gastroenterology, Alfred Health and Monash University, Melbourne 3004, Australia
2. Department of Gastroenterology, St. Vincent's Hospital, Melbourne University, Melbourne 3004, Australia
3. Department of Gastroenterology & Clinical Nutrition, Royal Children's Hospital, Melbourne 3052, Australia
4. Microbiome Research Centre, St. George Hospital, University of New South Wales, Sydney 2217, Australia
* Correspondence: m.sparrow@alfred.org.au; Tel.: +61-3-9076-2223

Abstract: CT-P13 is the first subcutaneous infliximab molecule approved for the management of inflammatory bowel disease (IBD). Compared to intravenous therapy, SC infliximab offers a range of practical, micro- and macroeconomic advantages. Data from the rheumatological literature suggest that subcutaneous CT-P13 may lead to superior disease outcomes in comparison to intravenous infliximab. Existing studies in IBD have focussed on pharmacokinetic comparisons and are inadequately powered to evaluate efficacy and safety differences between the two modes of administration. However, emerging clinical trial and real-world data support comparable clinical, biochemical, endoscopic and safety outcomes between subcutaneous and intravenous infliximab in both luminal Crohn's disease and ulcerative colitis. Across the available data, subcutaneous CT-P13 provides relative pharmacokinetic stability and higher trough drug levels when compared to intravenous administration. The clinical impact of this observation on immunogenicity and treatment persistence is yet to be determined. Trough levels between the two methods of administration should not be compared in isolation as any subcutaneous advantage must be considered in the context of comparable total drug exposure and the theoretical disadvantage of lower peak concentrations compared to intravenous therapy. Furthermore, target drug levels for subcutaneous CT-P13 associated with remission are not known. In this review, we present the available literature surrounding the pharmacokinetics of subcutaneous CT-P13 in the context of therapeutic drug monitoring and highlight the potential significance of these observations on the clinical management of patients with IBD.

Keywords: infliximab; CT-P13; subcutaneous; therapeutic drug monitoring

1. Introduction

Inflammatory bowel disease (IBD) comprises a group of chronic, immune-mediated disorders including both ulcerative colitis (UC) and Crohn's disease (CD) [1,2]. Anti-tumour necrosis factor (anti-TNF) biologics such as infliximab and adalimumab are effective in the induction and maintenance of remission in IBD, with primary response rates of 40–70% [3–8]. Infliximab, a chimeric IgG1 monoclonal antibody, has over 25 years of post-marketing efficacy and safety data in IBD [9]. After expiry of the patent for originator infliximab, a number of biosimilars have been developed, allowing market competition and consequent cost savings [10,11]. CT-P13 was the first infliximab biosimilar to be approved for UC and CD in Europe and the USA [12]. Intravenous CT-P13 has demonstrated non-inferior pharmacokinetics, efficacy and safety outcomes in both rheumatological conditions [13,14] and IBD [15–21]. Adherence to intravenous administration is measurable and

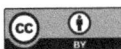

may be superior to that of self-administered biologic or oral therapy [22–24]. Furthermore, drug storage conditions are likely to be more regulated within hospital pharmacy departments in contrast to the variability and inadequacy reported with home-based biologic storage [22,23,25,26]. However, subcutaneous rather than intravenous biologic therapy is preferable to many patients and clinicians [27–30]. In comparison to intravenous therapy, de-centralising care provision may allow greater patient flexibility, convenience and a range of individual and macroeconomic healthcare benefits [31–35]. The COVID-19 pandemic highlighted the advantages of transitioning care away from the hospital setting [36]. In this context, a number of guidelines have suggested considering the prioritisation of subcutaneous biologics in IBD management [37,38].

The subcutaneous formulation of CT-P13 attained European Medicines Agency (EMA) approval for IBD in 2020 on the basis of two small randomised controlled trials (RCTs) reporting comparable pharmacokinetics, efficacy and safety of subcutaneous CT-P13 as compared to intravenous CT-P13 in both rheumatoid arthritis and active CD [39,40]. A subsequent meta-analysis comparing subcutaneous CT-P13 with historical intravenous infliximab outcomes in patients with moderate-severe rheumatoid arthritis suggests a potential efficacy benefit with subcutaneous therapy [41]. Similarly, a network meta-regression pooling individual patient data from two RCTs comparing subcutaneous and intravenous CT-P13 in rheumatoid arthritis patients supports subcutaneous CT-P13 providing superior clinical response and improvements in functional disability [42]. The available interventional controlled studies of subcutaneous CT-P13 in IBD to date are inadequately powered to assess efficacy and safety differences between the two methods of administration and are limited to outpatient moderate-severe UC and luminal CD. The pivotal RCT evaluating subcutaneous CT-P13 in IBD was conducted in two parts. Part 1, published in abstract form only, was a phase I, open-label dose-finding RCT in 44 patients with active CD. Following intravenous infliximab induction at week 0 and week 2, patients were randomised to receive either standard maintenance intravenous infliximab 5 mg/kg 8-weekly or 120 mg, 180 mg or 240 mg of subcutaneous CT-P13 2-weekly [40]. Part 2 was an open-label, non-inferiority trial involving 131 anti-TNF naïve patients with active CD or UC across 50 centres. Following intravenous induction, patients were randomised to receive maintenance intravenous infliximab 5 mg/kg 8-weekly or subcutaneous CT-P13 at a dose of 120 mg (if <80 kg) or 240 mg ($\geq$80 kg) 2-weekly [43]. The primary outcomes were pharmacokinetic and will be discussed in detail. Consistent with emerging real-world data, there were comparable clinical, biochemical, endoscopic and safety outcomes between subcutaneous and intravenous infliximab formulations [40,43]. Across all indications, trough drug levels are consistently higher in patients receiving subcutaneous CT-P13 than those treated with intravenous infliximab.

However, comparing drug levels at these time points does not adequately reflect total drug exposure between the two formulations. The significance of this observation on pharmacokinetics, disease activity, immunogenicity and treatment persistence in IBD is yet to be determined and requires further studies incorporating therapeutic drug monitoring (TDM). TDM of intravenous infliximab has been shown to be cost-effective and to improve clinical and objective outcomes in IBD [44,45]. There is a well-established exposure-response relationship for intravenous infliximab, with multiple studies having demonstrated that higher trough drug levels are associated with improved patient outcomes [44–47]. Evidence supporting TDM of other biologics is less robust, particularly for adalimumab, ustekinumab and vedolizumab [46,48].

There is an unmet need to confirm the value of TDM of subcutaneous infliximab, interpret the significance of elevated trough drug levels and determine concentration thresholds associated with remission. Furthermore, the potential disadvantages of lower peak concentrations with subcutaneous therapy requires evaluation. This review aims to appraise the literature surrounding subcutaneous CT-P13 TDM, highlight the current knowledge gaps, and provide guidance for clinical practice.

2. Search Strategy

A literature search was conducted using PubMed Online and the Cochrane Library databases. The search was performed using the following linked search terms: 'CT-P13 OR infliximab;' AND 'subcutaneous;' AND 'Crohn's disease (CD) OR ulcerative colitis (UC) OR inflammatory bowel disease (IBD).' The search was restricted to English language original research including both full-text and abstract publications presenting TDM data from 1 January 2010 to 22 August 2022. After exclusion of duplicates, 146 articles were identified and imported into a systematic review platform (www.rayan.ai, accessed on 22 August 2022). Titles and abstracts were screened and approved independently by two reviewers (RDL and AJJ) to ensure relevance and availability of drug level data. Reference lists of selected articles were reviewed with additional publications selected as appropriate. Seven original publications were chosen for discussion (Figure 1), with a further three post hoc analyses included.

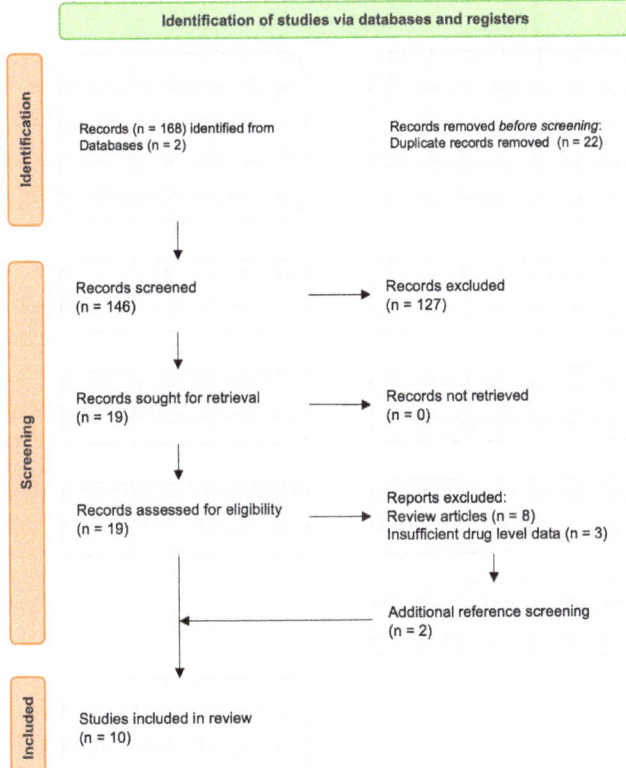

Figure 1. Search strategy outlining screening and eligibility assessment.

3. Pharmacokinetics of Subcutaneous CT-P13

The pharmacokinetics of intravenous infliximab are well described [49–52]. In short, administration via the intravenous route leads to early and rapid peak concentration followed by a steady decline to trough. Subcutaneously administered biologics have slower absorption, lower bioavailability, lower peak concentration and smaller differences between peak and trough concentrations. To date, there has only been one original, peer-reviewed published article defining the pharmacokinetics of subcutaneous CT-P13. Using patient data including a total of 2772 infliximab drug levels from the pivotal IBD CT-P13 Part 1 [40] and Part 2 [43] studies, Hanzel et al. constructed a population pharmacokinetic model incorporating the effect of body weight, anti-drug antibodies and serum albumin, given their known influence on clearance of intravenous infliximab [53]. The bioavailability of subcutaneous CT-P13 was reported as 79%, half-life 10.8 days and drug clearance estimated at 0.355 L/d in a typical patient weighing 70 kg, with a serum albumin of 44 g/L and no anti-drug antibodies. A prior subcutaneous CT-P13 Assessment Report by the EMA describing three separate population pharmacokinetic models based on clinical trials across healthy volunteers, rheumatological and gastroenterological indications calculated a bioavailability of between 58% and 72% [54]. It is important to note that many of these data are published in abstract form only or included in non-peer reviewed product reports. The estimated half-life and clearance of subcutaneous CT-P13 is comparable to findings from previous studies of intravenous infliximab in IBD, albeit with non-matched disease activity, weight, albumin and immunomodulator use between the models [49,50]. The calculated bioavailability of subcutaneous CT-P13 is comparable to that of adalimumab (64%) [55] and golimumab (52%) [56].

4. Impact of Dosing on Exposure-Response Relationship

Data from Part 1 of the pivotal subcutaneous CT-P13 RCT in patients with CD investigated the exposure-response relationship of 120 mg, 180 mg and 240 mg fortnightly subcutaneous CT-P13 doses in comparison to maintenance 5 mg/kg 8-weekly intravenous infliximab. At week 22–30, median subcutaneous infliximab drug levels incremented proportionally according to increasing subcutaneous dosing regimens (120 mg 2-weekly 13.3 µg/mL; 180 mg 2-weekly 19.9 µg/mL; 240 mg subcutaneous 2-weekly 26.5 µg/mL) and were significantly higher than those observed with intravenous infliximab (5 mg/kg 8-weekly 2.3 µg/mL) [40]. Similarly, in the Supplementary Materials of Part 2 of the pivotal RCT, mean trough levels at week 22 were higher in the 15 patients receiving 240 mg subcutaneous CT-P13 compared with 44 patients receiving 120 mg subcutaneous CT-P13 (mean [standard deviation; SD] 26.2 µg/mL [13.65] vs. 19.8 µg/mL [7.75], respectively) despite belonging to a higher weight category (80–115 kg vs. <80 kg, respectively) [43]. Despite allowing escalation to 240 mg 2-weekly from week 30 in patients with loss of response, data on the frequency of this event and subsequent changes in drug level are not presented. In contrast, escalating to a dose of 240 mg 2-weekly was strikingly effective in recapturing response in REMSWITCH, an observational, post-switch cohort of 133 patients [57]. Of the 22 patients who relapsed during the 6-month study period, 15 were escalated to 240 mg 2-weekly infliximab with recapture of clinical and combined clinical and biochemical remission in 93% and 80%, respectively. TDM data for this group of patients were not shown either at the time of relapse or following dose-intensification, as previously discussed [58].

In contrast, shortening the dose interval to weekly 120 mg subcutaneous CT-P13 may have less impact on drug levels. In a subgroup of 50 patients on prior dose-intensified intravenous infliximab from uncontrolled, real-world data by Smith et al., patients who switched to subcutaneous CT-P13 with a shortened dosing interval of 120 mg weekly had equivalent serum drug levels as patients switched to 120 mg 2-weekly at 3, 6 and 12 months despite not having worse baseline C-reactive protein (CRP) or faecal calprotectin (FCP) activity (median 16 vs. 16 µg/mL, $p > 0.05$ at all time points) [59]. Furthermore, receiving weekly vs. fortnightly dosing was not associated with trough infliximab drug levels on a linear regression analysis when controlled for multiple independent variables including disease activity, concomitant immunomodulator, anti-drug antibodies and body mass index (BMI) [59]. In summary, amongst patients requiring dose-intensified subcutaneous CT-P13, higher doses given fortnightly may achieve greater drug level increments than shortening the interval using standard 120 mg dosing, although more data are needed. The mechanism for this preliminary observation is unclear and not consistent with TDM data in adalimumab showing no difference in trough drug level between patients receiving 40 mg weekly and 80 mg fortnightly doses [60].

5. Comparing Drug Levels between Intravenous and Subcutaneous Infliximab

There are subcutaneous infliximab TDM data from a total of 465 individual patients across four published full-text articles [43,57,59,61] with additional data provided by 75 patients published in abstract or letter form [40,62,63] (Table 1). The majority of these studies compare drug levels between the two formulations taken at trough. However, trough drug levels between the two modes of administration are not directly comparable and do not reflect total drug exposure over a matched treatment period. This section will first outline available through TDM data, then contextualise these observations by discussing differing peak concentrations, relative drug level stability and comparable total drug exposure. Lastly, preliminary evidence supporting an exposure-response relationship will be presented.

Following intravenous induction at week 0 and week 2, receiving subcutaneous CT-P13 is associated with higher trough drug levels compared to continuing intravenous infliximab across the two available RCTs [40,43]. Data from Part 2 of the pivotal CT-P13 study in 131 patients show mean (SD) week 22 trough drug levels of 21.5 (9.9) µg/mL compared with 2.9 (2.6) µg/mL in the intravenous arm. When comparing geometric least squares mean (LSM), a more accurate estimate of true population mean, and adjusting for immunomodulator use, disease type, response status at week 6, and weight class, patients receiving subcutaneous CT-P13 had a trough drug level of 21.0 µg/mL compared to 1.8 µg/mL in the intravenous arm. As the lower bound of the 90% confidence interval for ratio of the geometric LSMs exceeded 80%, the primary outcome of pharmacokinetic non-inferiority of subcutaneous compared with intravenous CT-P13 was met. In addition, following switch to subcutaneous administration at week 30 in the original intravenous arm, the trough drug concentrations increased to comparable levels to those in the original subcutaneous arm. Similarly, when compared with pre-switch intravenous trough levels, both prospective and retrospective observational data confirm higher median trough drug levels following subcutaneous CT-P13 across time points ranging from 4 weeks to 6 months, except in patients requiring 10 mg/kg 4 weekly intravenous infliximab at the time of switching (Table 1).

Pharmacokinetic parameters that best predict optimal efficacy for infliximab are uncertain. As presented in Figure 2, possible predictors might be total drug exposure, maintenance of drug level stability, peak concentrations and trough concentrations, all of which differ between the two modes of administration. For intravenous infliximab therapy, TDM is performed at trough with a number of established concentration thresholds associated with varying depths of remission [46,47]. However, TDM performed earlier in the treatment cycle has also shown promising predictive potential, and the magnitude of these earlier drug levels may be important for severely active IBD [64,65]. Comparing only trough drug levels between subcutaneous and intravenous formulations does not accurately reflect differing peak concentrations. The most informative data regarding complementary pharmacokinetic parameters arise from Supplementary Materials of Part 2 of the pivotal RCT [43]. During the 8-week intensive TDM at steady state, the mean concentrations of subcutaneous CT-P13 are relatively stable when compared to the immediate peak and predictable decline of intravenous administration (Figure 3). Data generated by population pharmacokinetic modelling provide further detail. Whilst higher trough drug levels with subcutaneous infliximab are observed, the maximum peak drug level with subcutaneous infliximab is lower than with intravenous administration (mean 29.8 µg/mL vs. 105.6 µg/mL, respectively).

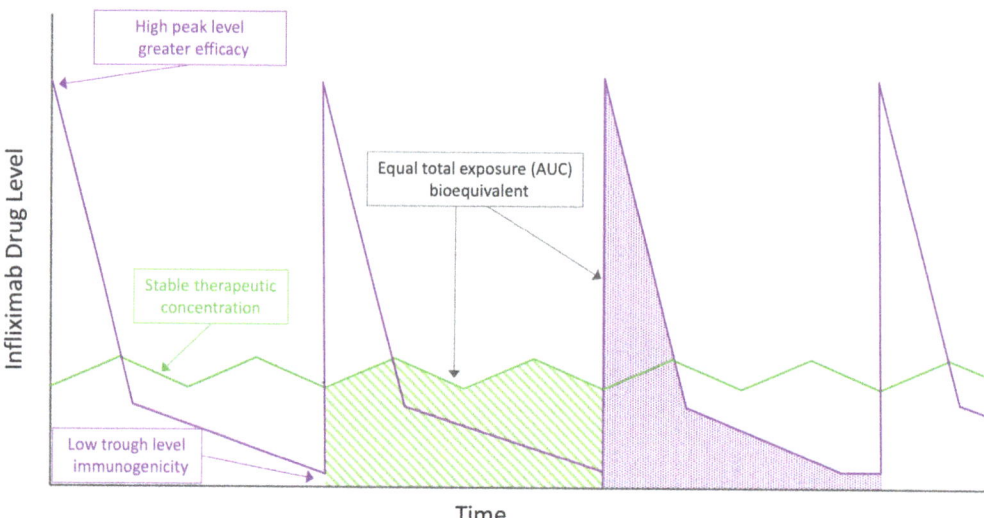

Figure 2. Visual representation of proposed theoretical pharmacokinetic advantages and disadvantages between intravenous (purple) and subcutaneous (green) infliximab. AUC = area under the curve.

Comparable total drug exposure between subcutaneous and intravenous infliximab using the area under the curve (AUC) over an 8-week treatment period reflects the trade-off between trough and peak drug levels in the two formulations—graphically depicted in Figure 2. Using the same non-linear mixed-effect model, the mean AUC was slightly higher in the subcutaneous as compared with intravenous CT-P13 arms (35,467 µg·h/mL versus 28,284 µg·h/mL). Prospective, uncontrolled TDM data from 20 CD patients and a total of 120 drug levels taken across two fortnightly treatment cycles supports subcutaneous drug level stability both within and across cycles [61]. Similar to prior adalimumab data [66, 67], a more stable steady state concentration-time profile offered by subcutaneous CT-P13 may allow greater flexibility with timing of TDM across the 14-day treatment cycle. However, more intensive pharmacokinetic analysis of adalimumab has demonstrated marked interpatient variability in subcutaneous absorption [68]. More data, ideally arising from a population pharmacokinetic analysis incorporating variables known to affect drug levels are required to translate these observations into clinical practice for subcutaneous CT-P13 [69]. Until these data emerge, we advise continuing to perform TDM of subcutaneous infliximab at trough where practicable.

Table 1. Summary of original research reporting drug levels and disease outcomes in patients with inflammatory bowel disease (IBD) receiving subcutaneous infliximab (IFX; CT-P13) including full text and published abstracts.

Study	Design	Objectives	n	Characteristics	Drug Levels (μg/mL) and Anti-Drug Antibodies (μg/mL)		Disease Outcomes
					Intravenous (IV)	Subcutaneous (SC)	
Schreiber (2021) [43]	Multicentre (n = 50) randomised, open-label, non-inferiority trial.	Primary: to compare week 22 trough drug levels in patients exposed to IV or SC infliximab following IV induction. Secondary: to compare clinical outcomes between IV and SC infliximab.	131	41% CD, 60% UC 0% in remission Anti-TNF naïve Immunomodulator use: 44%	*Drug levels*: Mean (SD) W22 level: 2.9 (2.6) Adjusted geometric LSM W22 level: 1.8 *Anti-drug antibodies*: W22 ADA: 32 (49%) W22 nADA: 12 (19%)	*Drug levels*: Mean (SD) W22 level: 21.5 (9.9) Adjusted geometric LSM W22 level: 21 *Anti-drug antibodies*: W22 ADA: 21 (32%) W22 nADA: 4 (6%) *Laboratory assays*: Infliximab: ECLIA ADA: Drug-tolerant ECLIA with ACE	Comparable W30 and W54 clinical, biochemical, endoscopic response rates between IV and SC arms.
Smith (2022) [59]	Retrospective, multicentre (n = 3) cohort study.	Primary: to evaluate treatment persistence post-switch from IV to SC infliximab. Secondary: to compare clinical outcomes and drug levels between IV and SC infliximab.	181	64% CD, 33% UC, 3% IBD-U 87% in remission Prior IV infliximab: −131 5 mg/kg q8W −50 5 mg/kg q4 or q6W Immunomodulator use: 59%	*Drug levels*: Median (range) level: 8.9 (0.4–16)	*Drug levels*: Median level: 16 at 3, 6 and 12 months *Anti-drug antibodies*: Throughout study: 14 (8%) *Laboratory assays*: Drug-tolerant ELISA for infliximab levels plus free and bound ADA OR Drug-sensitive in-house ELISA for infliximab levels and ADA, dependent on centre.	Treatment persistence 92% No significant difference in clinical or biochemical activity between baseline and at 3, 6, or 12 months post-switch to SC infliximab.

Table 1. Cont.

Study	Design	Objectives	n	Characteristics	Drug Levels (µg/mL) and Anti-Drug Antibodies (µg/mL)		Disease Outcomes
					Intravenous (IV)	Subcutaneous (SC)	
Buisson (2022) [57]	Prospective, multicentre (n = 3) cohort study.	Primary: to assess clinical and pharmacological outcomes post-switch from IV to SC infliximab in IBD patients according to different IV infliximab regimens.	133	72% CD, 28% UC Perianal lesions (42%) 100% in remission Prior IV infliximab: – 44% 5 mg/kg q8W – 31% 10 mg/kg q8W – 14% 10 mg/kg q6W – 11% 10 mg/kg q4W Immunomodulator use: 26%	Drug levels: Median (IQR) baseline level: – 5 mg/kg q8W 4.7 (2.4–6.8) – 10 mg/kg q8W 7.2 (4.4–11.9) – 10 mg/kg q6W 8.1 (6.2–15.1) – 10 mg/kg q4W 18.5 (11.9–20) Anti-drug antibodies: 2 (2%) positive ADAs	Drug levels: Median (IQR) level at W16–24: – Prior 5 mg/kg q8W 15.1 (11.2–18.2) – Prior 10 mg/kg q8W 18.7 (8–20) – Prior 10 mg/kg q6W 14.3 (11.9–17.6) – Prior 10 mg/kg q4W 20 (17.7–20) Anti-drug antibodies: No positive ADAs Laboratory assays: Infliximab: ELISA ADA: drug-sensitive ELISA	By W16–24 a clinical or faecal calprotectin recurrence occurred in: – 10.2% 5 mg/kg q8W – 7.3% 10mg/kg q8W – 16.7% 10mg/kg q6W – 66.7% 10mg/kg q4W Intensification to 240 mg q2W, recaptured clinical remission in 93% (14/15).
Roblin (2022) [61]	Prospective, single centre cohort study.	Primary: to investigate the intra-individual variations of infliximab drug levels across and between 2 cycles of SC infliximab.	20	100% CD 100% in remission Immunomodulator use: 40%	Drug levels: Median (IQR) level: 3.9 (1.2–7.9) Anti-drug antibodies: No ADAs	Drug levels: Median (IQR) W8 level 11 (7.5–15.1) Similar level independent of sampling period (day 3–6, day 7–9, day 14). Anti-drug antibodies: No ADAs. Laboratory assays: Infliximab: ELISA ADA: drug-sensitive ELISA	No clinical relapse.

Table 1. *Cont.*

Study	Design	Objectives	n	Characteristics	Drug Levels (μg/mL) and Anti-Drug Antibodies (μg/mL) Intravenous (IV)	Drug Levels (μg/mL) and Anti-Drug Antibodies (μg/mL) Subcutaneous (SC)	Disease Outcomes
Abstracts and Letters:							
Schreiber (2018) [40]	Randomised, open-label controlled trial	Primary: find the optimal dose of SC infliximab in patients with active CD following IV induction at W0, W2 and randomisation 1:1:1:1 to: - IV 5 mg/kg q8W - 120 mg SC q2W - 180 mg SC q2W - 240 mg SC q2W Secondary: evaluate clinical outcomes and pharmacokinetics.	44	100% CD 0% in remission Immunomodulator use: not reported	*Drug levels:* Median W30 level (predicted interval 5th–95th percentile): 2.3 (0.1–8.6) *Anti-drug antibodies:* 7 (58%) positive ADAs	*Drug levels:* Median W30 TL (predicted interval 5th-95th percentile): - 120 mg SC: 13.3 (5.6–26.8) - 180 mg SC: 19.9 (8.4–40) - 240 mg SC: 26.5 (11.2–53.2) *Anti-drug antibodies:* 3 (10%) positive ADAs *Laboratory assays:* Not specified	Similar rates of clinical remission and response between SC and IV infliximab arms.
Chivato Martin-Falquina (2022) [62]	Retrospective, single-centre cohort study.	Primary: to report rates of remission and treatment persistence in IBD patients post-switch from IV to SC infliximab.	14	29% CD, 71% UC 100% in remission 79% prior intensified IV infliximab. Doses not specified Immunomodulator use: 64%	*Drug levels:* Median (IQR) level: 7 (2.4–10.5) *Anti-drug antibodies:* Not reported	*Drug levels:* W8 (IQR) level: 14.1 (IQR 12.2–22.7) *Anti-drug antibodies:* Not reported *Laboratory assays:* Not specified	Treatment persistence 93% 93% remained in clinical remission at 8 weeks.
Argüelles-Arias (2022) [63]	Retrospective, single centre, cohort study.	To assess efficacy and safety post-switch from IV to SC infliximab.	17	71% CD, 29% UC 100% in remission Immunomodulator use: 53%	*Drug levels:* Median (IQR) level: 6.1 (3.5–8.9) *Anti-drug antibodies:* Not reported	*Drug levels:* Median (IQR) W24 level: 19.9 (12.3–21.6) *Anti-drug antibodies:* Not reported *Laboratory assays:* Not specified	No clinical relapse but a reduced faecal calprotectin at W24 following switch to SC infliximab.

Abbreviations: UC (ulcerative colitis), CD (Crohn's disease), IFX or CT-P13 (infliximab), SC (subcutaneous), IV (intravenous), ADA (antidrug antibody), nADA (neutralising ADA), SD (standard deviation), IQR (interquartile range), ELISA (enzyme-linked immunosorbent assay), ECLIA (electrochemiluminescence), ACE (affinity capture elution), W (week), q_W (_-weekly dosing).

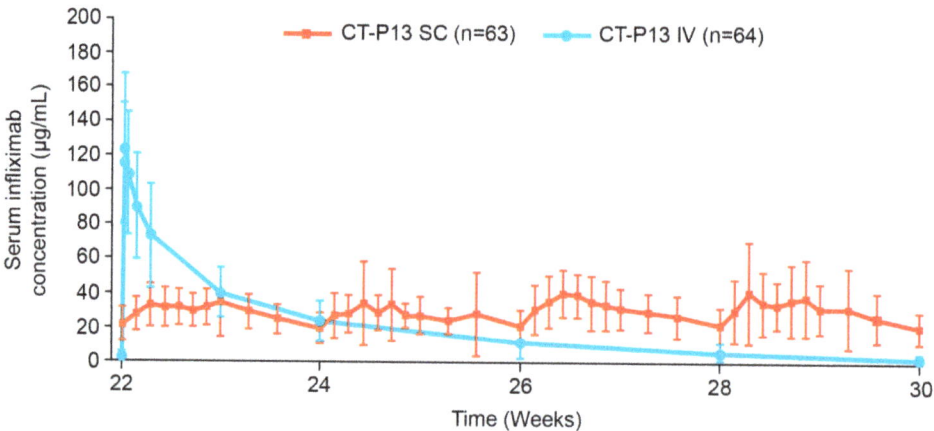

IV, intravenous; PK, pharmacokinetic; SC, subcutaneous; SD, standard deviation.

Note: Concentrations below the lower limit of quantification were set to the lower limit of quantification.

Figure 3. Mean (±SD) serum infliximab concentration for CT-P13 subcutaneous and CT-P13 intravenous arms during the more intensive 8-week sampling interval at steady state (PK monitoring period; PK population). Reprinted from: Gastroenterology, 2021; Schreiber S. et al. Randomized Controlled Trial: Subcutaneous vs. Intravenous Infliximab CT-P13 Maintenance in Inflammatory Bowel Disease (online Supplementary Materials, Figure S7, p. 31), Copyright (2021), with permission from Elsevier.

Further studies are also required to determine target concentration thresholds for subcutaneous infliximab. In a post hoc analysis of 55 patients receiving subcutaneous CT-P13 in the Part 2 RCT, Ye et al. report preliminary data supporting an exposure-response relationship [70]. In this analysis, a higher proportion of patients with drug levels in the 4th quartile (≥26.7 µg/mL) achieved clinical remission and a faecal calprotectin ≤250 µg/g at week 54, as compared to patients with drug levels in the 1st quartile (<16.4 µg/mL) (79% vs. 46% and 91% vs. 62%, respectively). More data are needed to determine optimal drug level targets associated with depth of remission across a broader range of IBD phenotypes.

6. Predictors of Infliximab Drug Levels

Increasing body weight, presence of anti-drug antibodies, hypoalbuminaemia, absence of concomitant immunomodulation and increased disease activity are covariates that are associated with increase clearance of intravenous IFX, adalimumab and golimumab [49–52,56,68]. Similar data are accruing for subcutaneous CT-P13.

6.1. Body Weight

Evaluation of the effect of body weight on drug levels in the pivotal part 2 trial is limited by both exclusion of patients with obesity and the weight-based dosing regimen [43]. However, in their population pharmacokinetic model, Hanzel et al. reported body weight as a covariate affecting drug clearance by up to 43% between weights of 70 to 120 kg. In contrast, bioavailability of subcutaneous infliximab did not appear to be affected by body weight. Using Monte Carlo weight-based exposure simulations, receiving subcutaneous CT-P13 led to higher drug exposure in patients weighing 50 kg, comparable exposure in patients weighing 70 kg and lower exposure in patients weighing 120 kg in comparison to intravenous administration [53]. However, in the largest published real-world cohort of 181 patients post-switch from intravenous to subcutaneous IFX, trough drug levels were not affected by BMI, despite utilising non-weight-based dosing of subcutaneous CT-P13. Similarly, in a prospective drug sampling study evaluating TDM stability across the 14-day treatment cycle, Roblin et al. demonstrated that BMI had no association with low subcutaneous IFX drug levels (HR 0.83 95% CI 0.46–4.21; $p = 0.69$), although the number of patients who were overweight was small. Buisson et al. found that neither body weight nor BMI were associated with disease relapse amongst real-world switch data in 133 patients [57]. These findings may again be limited by low median BMI in the cohort. Clarification of the effect of body weight and body composition on pharmacokinetics and clinical outcomes is paramount given that obesity may modestly increase the odds of non-response to both fixed-dose and weight-based anti-TNF therapy [71], however, results are conflicting [72–74].

6.2. Serum Albumin

Hanzel et al. found that subcutaneous CT-P13 clearance was 30% greater when the serum albumin concentration was 32 g/L compared with that at 44 g/L [53]. Despite the limited pharmacokinetic understanding, hypoalbuminaemia is associated with lower intravenous infliximab drug levels [51]. Commonly proposed hypotheses include a correlation with increased inflammatory disease activity, protein catabolism and increased mucosal losses [75]. In healthy states, individuals with low albumin have lower neonatal Fc receptor (FcRn) activity and therefore accelerated clearance of IgG, including monoclonal antibodies [76,77]. How this relationship is altered in active IBD and the subsequent effect on monoclonal antibody clearance is unclear. In their comprehensive modelling study, Hanzel et al. found that no other biochemical parameters of disease activity (CRP, faecal calprotectin, platelet count) had a clinically relevant effect on drug clearance beyond the effect of hypoalbuminaemia [53]. In contrast, uncontrolled data from Roblin et al. showed no association between albumin and subcutaneous CT-P13 drug levels. However, numbers were small and all patients were in clinical and biochemical remission with a consequent homogenous and normal mean (SD) albumin of 39.6 (2.5) g/L at recruitment [61].

6.3. Immunomodulator Use

In IBD patients receiving intravenous infliximab, combination therapy with immunomodulators is associated with higher drug levels, less immunogenicity and subsequent greater disease control compared with those treated with anti-TNF monotherapy [66,78–82]. The benefit of concomitant immunomodulator use in patients receiving subcutaneous CT-P13 is less clear. In a post hoc analysis of 66 patients in the subcutaneous arm of the pivotal Part 2 CT-P13 trial, D'Haens et al. found comparable median (IQR) trough week 54 drug levels between those who received combination therapy with immunomodulators and those that received infliximab monotherapy (21.7 [19–25.3] vs. 20.8 [16.1–29.1] µg/mL, respectively) [83]. Similarly, there were no differences in clinical response rates (85% in combination therapy vs. 74% monotherapy; $p = 0.3582$) or development of neutralising anti-drug antibodies between the two groups (16% combination therapy vs. 7% monotherapy; $p = 0.40$) [83]. On a multivariate model evaluating a cohort of 181 patients switched to subcutaneous CT-P13 (58% on combination therapy), immunomodulator use was not associated with higher infliximab trough levels [59]. There was also no association between risk of disease relapse and immunomodulator use from the REMSWITCH cohort of 133 patients, of which 57% were receiving dose-intensified intravenous infliximab and 26% were on combination therapy at baseline. Further data, over a longer period of follow up are required to clarify the role of immunomodulators in subcutaneous CT-P13 therapy.

6.4. Immunogenicity

Immunogenicity to anti-TNFs is common, particularly in the first 12 months of therapy [66,80,81,84,85]. Detection of anti-drug antibodies is dependent on the type of laboratory assay, the dilution accuracy and the positivity thresholds. Drug-sensitive ELISA, electrochemiluminescence immunoassay (ECLIA) or radioimmunoassays can detect anti-drug antibodies only in the absence of drug, whereas drug-tolerant assays, such as homogenous mobility-shift assays (HMSAs) and newer ELISAs, can detect anti-drug antibodies in the presence of detectable drug [86–88]. Unsurprisingly, lowering the anti-drug antibody-positivity threshold increases the rate of detection of both transient anti-drug antibody and low-titre persistent, non-neutralising anti-drug antibodies [89]. The natural history and clinical relevance of these phenomena in comparison to the pharmacodynamic inactivation induced by neutralising anti-drug antibodies remain unclear [84,86,89,90]. Attention to laboratory methods must be made when interpreting immunogenicity data in IBD. In Part 2 of the pivotal subcutaneous CT-P13 RCT, total anti-drug antibodies and neutralising anti-drug antibodies were analysed using a drug-tolerant ECLIA platform with an affinity capture elution able to detect titres ≥ 25 and ≥ 1000 ng/mL, respectively. As Part 1 was only published in abstract form, there are no details on the assay used. In this study, 7/12 (58%) CD patients in the intravenous arm compared to just 3/30 (10%) in the subcutaneous arms developed anti-drug antibodies by week 30 [40]. In contrast, in the much larger Part 2 study, a similar proportion of patients in each arm converted to anti-drug antibody positive status over the 54 weeks (70% in subcutaneous vs. 64% in intravenous) but a smaller proportion of patients in the subcutaneous arm had positive neutralising anti-drug antibodies compared to the intravenous arm (18% vs. 37%, respectively; $p = 0.019$) [43]. No anti-drug antibody titres were presented in either study and there was no apparent impact of differing binary neutralising anti-drug antibody positivity rates on disease control and drug levels between the two groups. In four pharmacokinetic models examining intravenous infliximab in IBD patients, anti-drug antibodies have been observed to affect drug clearance by between 29% and 72% [49,50,52,91]. In their evaluation of drug levels from the pivotal Part 1 and Part 2 subcutaneous CT-P13 trials, Hanzel et al. estimated a congruent increase in clearance of 39% in patients with anti-drug antibodies. In the largest published real-world post-switch cohort of 181 patients, only 14 patients (8%) developed anti-drug antibodies [59]. Consistent with the prior modelling, anti-drug antibodies in these patients were strongly inversely associated with subcutaneous infliximab levels on multivariate analysis (OR -13.34, 95% CI $-15.41\text{x}-11.33$; $p < 0.001$) [59]. Interpretation of immunogenicity data from the available uncontrolled cohorts is limited by varying assay use (including across centres within the same study [59]) and the lack of comparator groups (Table 1).

Whilst the above results are preliminary, the potential for lower rates of immunogenicity reflects a promising theoretical advantage of subcutaneous infliximab. Traditionally, subcutaneously administered biologics were considered to be more immunogenic than intravenous therapy due to theoretical exposure to antigen-presenting cells within the epidermis and dermis [92], although objective evidence supporting higher antibody formation are conflicting [93–95]. There are several unproven hypotheses for subcutaneous infliximab being less immunogenic than intravenous administration. Low drug levels seen at the more pronounced concentration troughs with both maintenance [80,86] and episodic [96,97] intravenous therapy are associated with antibody formation. Comparing representative concentration-time curves, the drug level stability of subcutaneous dosing may avoid exposure to the more immunogenic concentration thresholds of intravenous therapy as depicted graphically in Figure 2. In addition, it has been suggested [43,59,98] that the higher circulating drug levels seen with subcutaneous CT-P13 may both reduce formation of immunogenic drug-antigen immune complexes and induce 'high-zone tolerance'. Whilst infliximab-TNF complexes have been demonstrated to drive anti-drug antibody formation [99], how this relates to the varying drug level exposure pattern of subcutaneous relative to intravenous infliximab is not clear. In 'high-zone tolerance,' exposure to high concentrations of an antigen may induce tolerance via blunting of the immune response [93,100–102]. Once again, it is not clear why this mechanism would be preferentially activated by the stable moderate drug levels of subcutaneous therapy and not the high peak concentrations of intravenous infliximab therapy. Further prospective, controlled trials with a longer duration of follow up are required to confirm a difference in anti-drug antibody formation, the antibody subtype and whether there are meaningful clinical consequences.

7. Conclusions and Future Directions

The available evidence suggests comparable efficacy and safety of subcutaneous infliximab for adult patients with UC or luminal CD, despite differences in pharmacokinetics such as bioavailability and the concentration-time profile. The economic advantages of biosimilar molecules are complemented by practical benefits such as patient convenience, reduced risk of in-hospital exposure to nosocomial infection, and alleviation of hospital resources and staffing pressures. However, potential disadvantages regarding adherence or inadequacy of drug storage require consideration. The most promising biological advantage of subcutaneous infliximab may be the stability of drug levels, as compared with the marked differences between peak and trough concentrations with intravenous therapy. Maintaining drug level stability may avoid the prolonged low trough levels associated with intravenous infliximab with a subsequent reduction in immunogenicity and a greater treatment persistence. On the other hand, the immediacy and magnitude of peak concentrations after intravenous infliximab may be the most relevant pharmacokinetic parameters to induce remission in highly active disease such as acute severe UC or severe, complex CD including perianal CD. Two ongoing large superiority RCTs in moderate-severe CD and moderate-severe UC have been powered to compare disease and safety outcomes (ClinicalTrials.gov Identifiers: NCT04205643 and NCT03945019, respectively) and may reveal the clinical significance of these differing pharmacokinetic profiles. Of importance, trough drug levels between the two modes of administration are not directly comparable and should not be considered in isolation. Future work should aim to clarify whether TDM has a role with subcutaneously administered infliximab and, if so, to define therapeutic concentration targets. Additional future directions include clarifying the role of immunomodulators, establishment of efficacy in paediatric IBD, examining adequacy of drug exposure for acute severe colitis and perianal disease and the optimal dosing regimen in patients previously requiring dose-intensified intravenous infliximab. More complete post-marketing data and real-world experience across the range of IBD phenotypes, distributions and severities will allow more precise positioning and optimisation of subcutaneous infliximab in the management of IBD.

Author Contributions: All authors have made substantive contributions to the manuscript and have approved the submitted version. Specific author contributions include: conceptualisation, R.D.L., M.G.W., A.B. and M.P.S.; methodology, R.D.L., M.G.W., E.W., G.L.H., A.J.J. and M.P.S.; literature search and screening, R.D.L. and A.J.J.; data interpretation, R.D.L., M.G.W., E.W., G.L.H., A.J.J., P.R.G. and M.P.S.; original draft preparation, R.D.L. and A.J.J.; review and editing, R.D.L., M.G.W., E.W., G.L.H., A.J.J., A.B., P.R.G. and M.P.S.; supervision, M.G.W., E.W., G.L.H., A.B., P.R.G. and M.P.S. All authors have read and agreed to the published version of the manuscript.

Funding: This research received no external funding.

Conflicts of Interest: R.D.L. has received educational support from Celltrion Healthcare and Janssen. M.G.W. has received educational grants or research support from Ferring, GESA and Abbvie, speaker fees from Janssen, Abbvie, Ferring, Takeda, Pfizer and MSD and served on advisory boards for Janssen and Abbvie. EW has received speaker fees from Celltrion Healthcare. A.J.J., G.L.H. and A.B. have no relevant conflicts of interest to declare. P.R.G. has served as a consultant or advisory board member for Anatara, Atmo Biosciences, Immunic Therapeutics, Novozymes, Novoviah, Intrinsic Medicine and Comvita. He has received research grants for investigator-driven studies from Atmo Biosciences. He is a shareholder with Atmo Biosciences. MPS has received educational grants or research support from Ferring, Orphan and Gilead, speaker fees from Janssen, Abbvie, Ferring, Takeda, Pfizer and Shire, and has served on advisory boards for Janssen, Takeda, Pfizer, Celgene, Abbvie, MSD, Emerge Health, Gilead and BMS.

References

1. Ungaro, R.; Mehandru, S.; Allen, P.B.; Peyrin-Biroulet, L.; Colombel, J.F. Ulcerative colitis. *Lancet* **2017**, *389*, 1756–1770. [CrossRef]
2. Torres, J.; Mehandru, S.; Colombel, J.F.; Peyrin-Biroulet, L. Crohn's disease. *Lancet* **2017**, *389*, 1741–1755. [CrossRef]
3. Hanauer, S.B.; Sandborn, W.J.; Rutgeerts, P.; Fedorak, R.N.; Lukas, M.; MacIntosh, D.; Panaccione, R.; Wolf, D.; Pollack, P. Human anti-tumor necrosis factor monoclonal antibody (adalimumab) in Crohn's disease: The CLASSIC-I trial. *Gastroenterology* **2006**, *130*, 323–333. [CrossRef] [PubMed]
4. Sandborn, W.J.; Hanauer, S.B.; Rutgeerts, P.; Fedorak, R.N.; Lukas, M.; MacIntosh, D.G.; Panaccione, R.; Wolf, D.; Kent, J.D.; Bittle, B.; et al. Adalimumab for maintenance treatment of Crohn's disease: Results of the CLASSIC II trial. *Gut* **2007**, *56*, 1232–1239. [CrossRef] [PubMed]
5. Hanauer, S.B.; Feagan, B.G.; Lichtenstein, G.R.; Mayer, L.F.; Schreiber, S.; Colombel, J.F.; Rachmilewitz, D.; Wolf, D.C.; Olson, A.; Bao, W.; et al. Maintenance infliximab for Crohn's disease: The ACCENT I randomised trial. *Lancet* **2002**, *359*, 1541–1549. [CrossRef]
6. Colombel, J.F.; Sandborn, W.J.; Rutgeerts, P.; Enns, R.; Hanauer, S.B.; Panaccione, R.; Schreiber, S.; Byczkowski, D.; Li, J.; Kent, J.D.; et al. Adalimumab for maintenance of clinical response and remission in patients with Crohn's disease: The CHARM trial. *Gastroenterology* **2007**, *132*, 52–65. [CrossRef]
7. Rutgeerts, P.; Sandborn, W.J.; Feagan, B.G.; Reinisch, W.; Olson, A.; Johanns, J.; Travers, S.; Rachmilewitz, D.; Hanauer, S.B.; Lichtenstein, G.R.; et al. Infliximab for induction and maintenance therapy for ulcerative colitis. *N. Engl. J. Med.* **2005**, *353*, 2462–2476. [CrossRef]
8. Sands, B.E.; Anderson, F.H.; Bernstein, C.N.; Chey, W.Y.; Feagan, B.G.; Fedorak, R.N.; Kamm, M.A.; Korzenik, J.R.; Lashner, B.A.; Onken, J.E.; et al. Infliximab maintenance therapy for fistulizing Crohn's disease. *N. Engl. J. Med.* **2004**, *350*, 876–885. [CrossRef]
9. D'Haens, G.R.; van Deventer, S. 25 years of anti-TNF treatment for inflammatory bowel disease: Lessons from the past and a look to the future. *Gut* **2021**, *70*, 1396–1405. [CrossRef]
10. Ben-Horin, S.; Vande Casteele, N.; Schreiber, S.; Lakatos, P.L. Biosimilars in Inflammatory Bowel Disease: Facts and Fears of Extrapolation. *Clin. Gastroenterol. Hepatol.* **2016**, *14*, 1685–1696. [CrossRef]
11. Jha, A.; Upton, A.; Dunlop, W.C.; Akehurst, R. The Budget Impact of Biosimilar Infliximab (Remsima(R)) for the Treatment of Autoimmune Diseases in Five European Countries. *Adv. Ther.* **2015**, *32*, 742–756. [CrossRef] [PubMed]
12. Parigi, T.L.; D'Amico, F.; Peyrin-Biroulet, L.; Danese, S. Evolution of infliximab biosimilar in inflammatory bowel disease: From intravenous to subcutaneous CT-P13. *Expert Opin. Biol. Ther.* **2021**, *21*, 37–46. [CrossRef] [PubMed]
13. Park, W.; Hrycaj, P.; Jeka, S.; Kovalenko, V.; Lysenko, G.; Miranda, P.; Mikazane, H.; Gutierrez-Urena, S.; Lim, M.; Lee, Y.A.; et al. A randomised, double-blind, multicentre, parallel-group, prospective study comparing the pharmacokinetics, safety, and efficacy of CT-P13 and innovator infliximab in patients with ankylosing spondylitis: The PLANETAS study. *Ann. Rheum. Dis.* **2013**, *72*, 1605–1612. [CrossRef] [PubMed]
14. Yoo, D.H.; Hrycaj, P.; Miranda, P.; Ramiterre, E.; Piotrowski, M.; Shevchuk, S.; Kovalenko, V.; Prodanovic, N.; Abello-Banfi, M.; Gutierrez-Urena, S.; et al. A randomised, double-blind, parallel-group study to demonstrate equivalence in efficacy and safety of CT-P13 compared with innovator infliximab when coadministered with methotrexate in patients with active rheumatoid arthritis: The PLANETRA study. *Ann. Rheum. Dis.* **2013**, *72*, 1613–1620. [CrossRef]
15. Goll, G.L.; Jorgensen, K.K.; Sexton, J.; Olsen, I.C.; Bolstad, N.; Haavardsholm, E.A.; Lundin, K.E.A.; Tveit, K.S.; Lorentzen, M.; Berset, I.P.; et al. Long-term efficacy and safety of biosimilar infliximab (CT-P13) after switching from originator infliximab: Open-label extension of the NOR-SWITCH trial. *J. Intern. Med.* **2019**, *285*, 653–669. [CrossRef]
16. Jorgensen, K.K.; Olsen, I.C.; Goll, G.L.; Lorentzen, M.; Bolstad, N.; Haavardsholm, E.A.; Lundin, K.E.A.; Mork, C.; Jahnsen, J.; Kvien, T.K.; et al. Switching from originator infliximab to biosimilar CT-P13 compared with maintained treatment with originator infliximab (NOR-SWITCH): A 52-week, randomised, double-blind, non-inferiority trial. *Lancet* **2017**, *389*, 2304–2316. [CrossRef]
17. Komaki, Y.; Yamada, A.; Komaki, F.; Micic, D.; Ido, A.; Sakuraba, A. Systematic review with meta-analysis: The efficacy and safety of CT-P13, a biosimilar of anti-tumour necrosis factor-alpha agent (infliximab), in inflammatory bowel diseases. *Aliment. Pharmacol. Ther.* **2017**, *45*, 1043–1057. [CrossRef]
18. Ebada, M.A.; Elmatboly, A.M.; Ali, A.S.; Ibrahim, A.M.; Fayed, N.; Faisal, A.F.; Alkanj, S. An updated systematic review and meta-analysis about the safety and efficacy of infliximab biosimilar, CT-P13, for patients with inflammatory bowel disease. *Int. J. Colorectal Dis.* **2019**, *34*, 1633–1652. [CrossRef]
19. Smits, L.J.T.; van Esch, A.A.J.; Derikx, L.; Boshuizen, R.; de Jong, D.J.; Drenth, J.P.H.; Hoentjen, F. Drug Survival and Immunogenicity after Switching from Remicade to Biosimilar CT-P13 in Inflammatory Bowel Disease Patients: Two-year Follow-up of a Prospective Observational Cohort Study. *Inflamm. Bowel Dis.* **2019**, *25*, 172–179. [CrossRef]
20. Ye, B.D.; Pesegova, M.; Alexeeva, O.; Osipenko, M.; Lahat, A.; Dorofeyev, A.; Fishman, S.; Levchenko, O.; Cheon, J.H.; Scribano, M.L.; et al. Efficacy and safety of biosimilar CT-P13 compared with originator infliximab in patients with active Crohn's disease: An international, randomised, double-blind, phase 3 non-inferiority study. *Lancet* **2019**, *393*, 1699–1707. [CrossRef]
21. Strik, A.S.; van de Vrie, W.; Bloemsaat-Minekus, J.P.J.; Nurmohamed, M.; Bossuyt, P.J.J.; Bodelier, A.; Rispens, T.; van Megen, Y.J.B.; D'Haens, G.R.; SECURE study group. Serum concentrations after switching from originator infliximab to the biosimilar CT-P13 in patients with quiescent inflammatory bowel disease (SECURE): An open-label, multicentre, phase 4 non-inferiority trial. *Lancet Gastroenterol. Hepatol.* **2018**, *3*, 404–412. [CrossRef]

22. Wentworth, B.J.; Buerlein, R.C.D.; Tuskey, A.G.; Overby, M.A.; Smolkin, M.E.; Behm, B.W. Nonadherence to Biologic Therapies in Inflammatory Bowel Disease. *Inflamm. Bowel Dis.* **2018**, *24*, 2053–2061. [CrossRef] [PubMed]
23. van der Have, M.; Oldenburg, B.; Kaptein, A.A.; Jansen, J.M.; Scheffer, R.C.; van Tuyl, B.A.; van der Meulen-de Jong, A.E.; Pierik, M.; Siersema, P.D.; van Oijen, M.G.; et al. Non-adherence to Anti-TNF Therapy is Associated with Illness Perceptions and Clinical Outcomes in Outpatients with Inflammatory Bowel Disease: Results from a Prospective Multicentre Study. *J. Crohn's Colitis* **2016**, *10*, 549–555. [CrossRef] [PubMed]
24. Degli Esposti, L.; Sangiorgi, D.; Perrone, V.; Radice, S.; Clementi, E.; Perone, F.; Buda, S. Adherence and resource use among patients treated with biologic drugs: Findings from BEETLE study. *Clin. Outcomes Res.* **2014**, *6*, 401–407. [CrossRef]
25. De Jong, M.J.; Pierik, M.J.; Peters, A.; Roemers, M.; Hilhorst, V.; van Tubergen, A. Exploring conditions for redistribution of anti-tumor necrosis factors to reduce spillage: A study on the quality of anti-tumor necrosis factor home storage. *J. Gastroenterol. Hepatol.* **2018**, *33*, 426–430. [CrossRef]
26. Rentsch, C.; Headon, B.; Ward, M.G.; Gibson, P.R. Inadequate storage of subcutaneous biological agents by patients with inflammatory bowel disease: Another factor driving loss of response? *J. Gastroenterol. Hepatol.* **2018**, *33*, 10–11. [CrossRef]
27. Huynh, T.K.; Ostergaard, A.; Egsmose, C.; Madsen, O.R. Preferences of patients and health professionals for route and frequency of administration of biologic agents in the treatment of rheumatoid arthritis. *Patient Prefer. Adherence* **2014**, *8*, 93–99. [CrossRef]
28. Asnong, K.; Hoefkens, E.; Lembrechts, N.; Van de Schoot, I.; Pouillon, L.; Bossuyt, P. N02 PREVIEW study: Factors associated with willingness to switch from intravenous to subcutaneous formulations of CT-P13 and vedolizumab in patients with Inflammatory Bowel Disease. *J. Crohn's Colitis* **2021**, *15*, S608–S609. [CrossRef]
29. Stoner, K.L.; Harder, H.; Fallowfield, L.J.; Jenkins, V.A. Intravenous versus Subcutaneous Drug Administration. Which Do Patients Prefer? A Systematic Review. *Patient Patient-Cent. Outcomes Res.* **2015**, *8*, 145–153. [CrossRef]
30. Vavricka, S.R.; Bentele, N.; Scharl, M.; Rogler, G.; Zeitz, J.; Frei, P.; Straumann, A.; Binek, J.; Schoepfer, A.M.; Fried, M.; et al. Systematic assessment of factors influencing preferences of Crohn's disease patients in selecting an anti-tumor necrosis factor agent (CHOOSE TNF TRIAL). *Inflamm. Bowel Dis.* **2012**, *18*, 1523–1530. [CrossRef]
31. Tetteh, E.K.; Morris, S. Evaluating the administration costs of biologic drugs: Development of a cost algorithm. *Health Econ. Rev.* **2014**, *4*, 26. [CrossRef] [PubMed]
32. Buisson, A.; Seigne, A.L.; D'huart, M.C.; Bigard, M.A.; Peyrin-Biroulet, L. The extra burden of infliximab infusions in inflammatory bowel disease. *Inflamm. Bowel Dis.* **2013**, *19*, 2464–2467. [CrossRef]
33. Heald, A.; Bramham-Jones, S.; Davies, M. Comparing cost of intravenous infusion and subcutaneous biologics in COVID-19 pandemic care pathways for rheumatoid arthritis and inflammatory bowel disease: A brief UK stakeholder survey. *Int. J. Clin. Pr.* **2021**, *75*, e14341. [CrossRef]
34. Cronin, J.; Moore, S.; Lenihan, N.; O'Shea, M.; Woods, N. The non-drug costs associated with the administration of an intravenous biologic treatment in the hospital setting. *Ir. J. Med. Sci.* **2019**, *188*, 821–834. [CrossRef] [PubMed]
35. Byun, H.G.; Jang, M.; Yoo, H.K.; Potter, J.; Kwon, T.S. Budget Impact Analysis of the Introduction of Subcutaneous Infliximab (CT-P13 SC) for the Treatment of Rheumatoid Arthritis in the United Kingdom. *Appl. Health Econ. Health Policy* **2021**, *19*, 735–745. [CrossRef] [PubMed]
36. Clough, J.N.; Hill, K.L.; Duff, A.; Sharma, E.; Ray, S.; Mawdsley, J.E.; Anderson, S.; Irving, P.M.; Samaan, M.A. Managing an IBD Infusion Unit During the COVID-19 Pandemic: Service Modifications and the Patient Perspective. *Inflamm. Bowel Dis.* **2020**, *26*, e125–e126. [CrossRef] [PubMed]
37. Kennedy, N.A.; Jones, G.R.; Lamb, C.A.; Appleby, R.; Arnott, I.; Beattie, R.M.; Bloom, S.; Brooks, A.J.; Cooney, R.; Dart, R.J.; et al. British Society of Gastroenterology guidance for management of inflammatory bowel disease during the COVID-19 pandemic. *Gut* **2020**, *69*, 984–990. [CrossRef] [PubMed]
38. Magro, F.; Rahier, J.F.; Abreu, C.; MacMahon, E.; Hart, A.; van der Woude, C.J.; Gordon, H.; Adamina, M.; Viget, N.; Vavricka, S.; et al. Inflammatory Bowel Disease Management During the COVID-19 Outbreak: The Ten Do's and Don'ts from the ECCO-COVID Taskforce. *J. Crohn's Colitis* **2020**, *14*, S798–S806. [CrossRef]
39. Westhovens, R.; Yoo, D.H.; Jaworski, J.; Matyska-Piekarska, E.; Smiyan, S.; Ivanova, D.; Zielinska, A.; Raussi, E.-K.; Batalov, A.; Lee, S.J.; et al. THU0191 Novel formulation of ct-p13 for subcutaneous administration in patients with rheumatoid arthritis: Initial results from a phase i/iii randomised controlled trial. *Ann. Rheum. Dis.* **2018**, *77*, 315. [CrossRef]
40. Schreiber, S.; Jang, B.I.; Borzan, V.; Lahat, A.; Pukitis, A.; Osipenko, M.; Mostovoy, Y.; Ben-Horin, S.; Ye, B.D.; Lee, S.J.; et al. Tu2018—Novel Formulation of CT-P13 (Infliximab Biosimilar) for Subcutaneous Administration: Initial Results from a Phase I Open-Label Randomized Controlled Trial in Patients with Active Crohn's Disease. *Gastroenterology* **2018**, *154*, 1371. [CrossRef]
41. Caporali, R.; Allanore, Y.; Alten, R.; Combe, B.; Durez, P.; Iannone, F.; Nurmohamed, M.T.; Lee, S.J.; Kwon, T.S.; Choi, J.S.; et al. Efficacy and safety of subcutaneous infliximab versus adalimumab, etanercept and intravenous infliximab in patients with rheumatoid arthritis: A systematic literature review and meta-analysis. *Expert Rev. Clin. Immunol.* **2021**, *17*, 85–99. [CrossRef] [PubMed]
42. Combe, B.; Allanore, Y.; Alten, R.; Caporali, R.; Durez, P.; Iannone, F.; Nurmohamed, M.T.; Toumi, M.; Lee, S.J.; Kwon, T.S.; et al. Comparative efficacy of subcutaneous (CT-P13) and intravenous infliximab in adult patients with rheumatoid arthritis: A network meta-regression of individual patient data from two randomised trials. *Arthritis Res. Ther.* **2021**, *23*, 119. [CrossRef] [PubMed]

43. Schreiber, S.; Ben-Horin, S.; Leszczyszyn, J.; Dudkowiak, R.; Lahat, A.; Gawdis-Wojnarska, B.; Pukitis, A.; Horynski, M.; Farkas, K.; Kierkus, J.; et al. Randomized Controlled Trial: Subcutaneous vs Intravenous Infliximab CT-P13 Maintenance in Inflammatory Bowel Disease. *Gastroenterology* **2021**, *160*, 2340–2353. [CrossRef] [PubMed]
44. Adedokun, O.J.; Sandborn, W.J.; Feagan, B.G.; Rutgeerts, P.; Xu, Z.; Marano, C.W.; Johanns, J.; Zhou, H.; Davis, H.M.; Cornillie, F.; et al. Association between serum concentration of infliximab and efficacy in adult patients with ulcerative colitis. *Gastroenterology* **2014**, *147*, 1296–1307. [CrossRef] [PubMed]
45. Steenholdt, C.; Brynskov, J.; Thomsen, O.O.; Munck, L.K.; Fallingborg, J.; Christensen, L.A.; Pedersen, G.; Kjeldsen, J.; Jacobsen, B.A.; Oxholm, A.S.; et al. Individualised therapy is more cost-effective than dose intensification in patients with Crohn's disease who lose response to anti-TNF treatment: A randomised, controlled trial. *Gut* **2014**, *63*, 919–927. [CrossRef]
46. Papamichael, K.; Cheifetz, A.S.; Melmed, G.Y.; Irving, P.M.; Vande Casteele, N.; Kozuch, P.L.; Raffals, L.E.; Baidoo, L.; Bressler, B.; Devlin, S.M.; et al. Appropriate Therapeutic Drug Monitoring of Biologic Agents for Patients with Inflammatory Bowel Diseases. *Clin. Gastroenterol. Hepatol.* **2019**, *17*, 1655–1668. [CrossRef]
47. Cheifetz, A.S.; Abreu, M.T.; Afif, W.; Cross, R.K.; Dubinsky, M.C.; Loftus, E.V., Jr.; Osterman, M.T.; Saroufim, A.; Siegel, C.A.; Yarur, A.J.; et al. A Comprehensive Literature Review and Expert Consensus Statement on Therapeutic Drug Monitoring of Biologics in Inflammatory Bowel Disease. *Am. J. Gastroenterol.* **2021**, *116*, 2014–2025. [CrossRef]
48. Gibson, D.J.; Ward, M.G.; Rentsch, C.; Friedman, A.B.; Taylor, K.M.; Sparrow, M.P.; Gibson, P.R. Review article: Determination of the therapeutic range for therapeutic drug monitoring of adalimumab and infliximab in patients with inflammatory bowel disease. *Aliment. Pharmacol. Ther.* **2020**, *51*, 612–628. [CrossRef]
49. Fasanmade, A.A.; Adedokun, O.J.; Blank, M.; Zhou, H.; Davis, H.M. Pharmacokinetic properties of infliximab in children and adults with Crohn's disease: A retrospective analysis of data from 2 phase III clinical trials. *Clin. Ther.* **2011**, *33*, 946–964. [CrossRef]
50. Fasanmade, A.A.; Adedokun, O.J.; Ford, J.; Hernandez, D.; Johanns, J.; Hu, C.; Davis, H.M.; Zhou, H. Population pharmacokinetic analysis of infliximab in patients with ulcerative colitis. *Eur. J. Clin. Pharmacol.* **2009**, *65*, 1211–1228. [CrossRef]
51. Brandse, J.F.; Mould, D.; Smeekes, O.; Ashruf, Y.; Kuin, S.; Strik, A.; van den Brink, G.R.; D'Haens, G.R. A Real-life Population Pharmacokinetic Study Reveals Factors Associated with Clearance and Immunogenicity of Infliximab in Inflammatory Bowel Disease. *Inflamm. Bowel Dis.* **2017**, *23*, 650–660. [CrossRef] [PubMed]
52. Dotan, I.; Ron, Y.; Yanai, H.; Becker, S.; Fishman, S.; Yahav, L.; Ben Yehoyada, M.; Mould, D.R. Patient Factors That Increase Infliximab Clearance and Shorten Half-life in Inflammatory Bowel Disease: A Population Pharmacokinetic Study. *Inflamm. Bowel Dis.* **2014**, *20*, 2247–2259. [CrossRef] [PubMed]
53. Hanzel, J.; Bukkems, L.H.; Gecse, K.B.; D'Haens, G.R.; Mathot, R.A.A. Population pharmacokinetics of subcutaneous infliximab CT-P13 in Crohn's disease and ulcerative colitis. *Aliment. Pharmacol. Ther.* **2021**, *54*, 1309–1319. [CrossRef] [PubMed]
54. European Medicines Agency. Remsima: Assessment Report on Extension(s) of Marketing Authorisation. Available online: https://www.ema.europa.eu/en/documents/variation-report/remsima-h-c-2576-x-0062-epar-assessment-report-variation_en.pdf (accessed on 18 August 2022).
55. European Medicines Agency. Humira (Adalimumab). Summary of Product Characteristics. Available online: https://www.ema.europa.eu/en/documents/product-information/humira-epar-product-information_en.pdf (accessed on 22 August 2022).
56. Adedokun, O.J.; Xu, Z.; Liao, S.; Strauss, R.; Reinisch, W.; Feagan, B.G.; Sandborn, W.J. Population Pharmacokinetics and Exposure-Response Modeling of Golimumab in Adults with Moderately to Severely Active Ulcerative Colitis. *Clin. Ther.* **2020**, *42*, 157–174. [CrossRef] [PubMed]
57. Buisson, A.; Nachury, M.; Reymond, M.; Yzet, C.; Wils, P.; Payen, K.; Laugie, M.; Manlay, L.; Mathieu, N.; Pereira, B.; et al. Effectiveness of Switching from Intravenous to Subcutaneous Infliximab in Patients with Inflammatory Bowel Diseases: The REMSWITCH Study. *Clin. Gastroenterol. Hepatol.* **2022**, in press. [CrossRef] [PubMed]
58. Little, R.D.; Ward, M.G.; Sparrow, M.P. Letter to the Editor: Can subcutaneous infliximab replace dose-intensified intravenous administration in inflammatory bowel disease? *Clin. Gastroenterol. Hepatol.* **2022**. Epub ahead of printing. [CrossRef]
59. Smith, P.J.; Critchley, L.; Storey, D.; Gregg, B.; Stenson, J.; Kneebone, A.; Rimmer, T.; Burke, S.; Hussain, S.; Teoh, W.Y.; et al. Efficacy and Safety of Elective Switching from Intravenous to Subcutaneous Infliximab (Ct-P13): A Multi-Centre Cohort Study. *J. Crohn's Colitis* **2022**, *16*, 1436–1446. [CrossRef]
60. Paul, S.; Williet, N.; Nancey, S.; Veyrard, P.; Boschetti, G.; Phelip, J.M.; Flourie, B.; Roblin, X. No Difference of Adalimumab Pharmacokinetics When Dosed at 40 mg Every Week or 80 mg Every Other Week in IBD Patients in Clinical Remission After Adalimumab Dose Intensification. *Dig. Dis. Sci.* **2021**, *66*, 2744–2749. [CrossRef]
61. Roblin, X.; Veyrard, P.; Bastide, L.; Berger, A.E.; Barrau, M.; Paucelle, A.S.; Waeckel, L.; Kwiatek, S.; Flourie, B.; Nancey, S.; et al. Subcutaneous injection of infliximab CT-P13 results in stable drug levels within 14-day treatment cycle in Crohn's disease. *Aliment. Pharmacol. Ther.* **2022**, *56*, 77–83. [CrossRef]
62. Falquina, I.C.M.; Chumillas, R.M.S.; Garcia, L.A.; González, B.V.; Cuesta, N.R.; Hernández, L.A.; Pascual, L.A.; Aladrén, B.S. P617 Switching from an intensified regimen of infliximab to a subcutaneous standard dose in adults with Inflammatory Bowel Disease: Our experience in a tertiary hospital. *J. Crohn's Colitis* **2022**, *16*, i544–i545. [CrossRef]
63. Arguelles-Arias, F.; Alvarez, P.F.; Laria, L.C.; Perez, B.M.; Jimenez, M.B.; Merino-Bohorquez, V.; Alvarez, A.C.; Hernandez, M.A.C. Switch to subcutaneous infliximab during the SARS-CoV-2 pandemic: Preliminary results. *Rev. Esp. Enferm. Dig.* **2022**, *114*, 118–119. [CrossRef] [PubMed]

64. Liefferinckx, C.; Bottieau, J.; Toubeau, J.F.; Thomas, D.; Rahier, J.F.; Louis, E.; Baert, F.; Dewint, P.; Pouillon, L.; Lambrecht, G.; et al. Collecting New Peak and Intermediate Infliximab Levels to Predict Remission in Inflammatory Bowel Diseases. *Inflamm. Bowel Dis.* **2022**, *28*, 208–217. [CrossRef] [PubMed]
65. Bar-Yoseph, H.; Levhar, N.; Selinger, L.; Manor, U.; Yavzori, M.; Picard, O.; Fudim, E.; Kopylov, U.; Eliakim, R.; Ben-Horin, S.; et al. Early drug and anti-infliximab antibody levels for prediction of primary nonresponse to infliximab therapy. *Aliment. Pharmacol. Ther.* **2018**, *47*, 212–218. [CrossRef] [PubMed]
66. Ungar, B.; Engel, T.; Yablecovitch, D.; Lahat, A.; Lang, A.; Avidan, B.; Har-Noy, O.; Carter, D.; Levhar, N.; Selinger, L.; et al. Prospective Observational Evaluation of Time-Dependency of Adalimumab Immunogenicity and Drug Concentrations: The POETIC Study. *Am. J. Gastroenterol.* **2018**, *113*, 890–898. [CrossRef]
67. Ward, M.G.; Thwaites, P.A.; Beswick, L.; Hogg, J.; Rosella, G.; Van Langenberg, D.; Reynolds, J.; Gibson, P.R.; Sparrow, M.P. Intra-patient variability in adalimumab drug levels within and between cycles in Crohn's disease. *Aliment. Pharmacol. Ther.* **2017**, *45*, 1135–1145. [CrossRef]
68. Casteele, N.V.; Baert, F.; Bian, S.; Dreesen, E.; Compernolle, G.; Van Assche, G.; Ferrante, M.; Vermeire, S.; Gils, A. Subcutaneous Absorption Contributes to Observed Interindividual Variability in Adalimumab Serum Concentrations in Crohn's Disease: A Prospective Multicentre Study. *J. Crohn's Colitis* **2019**, *13*, 1248–1256. [CrossRef]
69. Casteele, N.V.; Gils, A. Editorial: Variability in adalimumab trough and peak serum concentrations. *Aliment. Pharmacol. Ther.* **2017**, *45*, 1475–1476. [CrossRef]
70. Ye, B.D.; Leszczyszyn, J.; Dudkowiak, R.; Lahat, A.; Gawdis-Wojnarska, B.; Pukitis, A.; Horynski, M.; Farkas, K.; Kierkuś, J.; Kowalski, M.; et al. Exposure-response relationship of subcutaneous infliximab (CT-P13 SC) in patients with active Crohn's disease and ulcerative colitis: Analysis from a multicenter, randomized controlled pivotal trial. *United Eur. Gastroenterol. Week* **2020**, *8* (Suppl. S1), 385–386. Available online: https://ueg.eu/library/exposure-response-relationship-of-subcutaneous-infliximab-ct-p13-sc-in-patients-with-active-crohns-disease-and-ulcerative-colitis-analysis-from-a-multicenter-randomized-controlled-pivotal-trial/235451 (accessed on 22 August 2022).
71. Dai, Z.H.; Xu, X.T.; Ran, Z.H. Associations Between Obesity and the Effectiveness of Anti-Tumor Necrosis Factor-alpha Agents in Inflammatory Bowel Disease Patients: A Literature Review and Meta-analysis. *Ann. Pharmacother.* **2020**, *54*, 729–741. [CrossRef]
72. Singh, S.; Facciorusso, A.; Singh, A.G.; Vande Casteele, N.; Zarrinpar, A.; Prokop, L.J.; Grunvald, E.L.; Curtis, J.R.; Sandborn, W.J. Obesity and response to anti-tumor necrosis factor-alpha agents in patients with select immune-mediated inflammatory diseases: A systematic review and meta-analysis. *PLoS ONE* **2018**, *13*, e0195123. [CrossRef]
73. Singh, S.; Proudfoot, J.; Xu, R.; Sandborn, W.J. Obesity and Response to Infliximab in Patients with Inflammatory Bowel Diseases: Pooled Analysis of Individual Participant Data from Clinical Trials. *Am. J. Gastroenterol.* **2018**, *113*, 883–889. [CrossRef] [PubMed]
74. Gu, P.; Chhabra, A.; Chittajallu, P.; Chang, C.; Mendez, D.; Gilman, A.; Fudman, D.I.; Xi, Y.; Feagins, L.A. Visceral Adipose Tissue Volumetrics Inform Odds of Treatment Response and Risk of Subsequent Surgery in IBD Patients Starting Antitumor Necrosis Factor Therapy. *Inflamm. Bowel Dis.* **2022**, *28*, 657–666. [CrossRef] [PubMed]
75. Brandse, J.F.; van den Brink, G.R.; Wildenberg, M.E.; van der Kleij, D.; Rispens, T.; Jansen, J.M.; Mathot, R.A.; Ponsioen, C.Y.; Löwenberg, M.; D'Haens, G.R. Loss of Infliximab into Feces Is Associated with Lack of Response to Therapy in Patients with Severe Ulcerative Colitis. *Gastroenterology* **2015**, *149*, 350–355. [CrossRef] [PubMed]
76. Kim, J.; Hayton, W.L.; Robinson, J.M.; Anderson, C.L. Kinetics of FcRn-mediated recycling of IgG and albumin in human: Pathophysiology and therapeutic implications using a simplified mechanism-based model. *Clin. Immunol.* **2007**, *122*, 146–155. [CrossRef] [PubMed]
77. Pyzik, M.; Rath, T.; Lencer, W.I.; Baker, K.; Blumberg, R.S. FcRn: The Architect Behind the Immune and Nonimmune Functions of IgG and Albumin. *J. Immunol.* **2015**, *194*, 4595–4603. [CrossRef] [PubMed]
78. Colombel, J.F.; Sandborn, W.J.; Reinisch, W.; Mantzaris, G.J.; Kornbluth, A.; Rachmilewitz, D.; Lichtiger, S.; D'Haens, G.; Diamond, R.H.; Broussard, D.L.; et al. Infliximab, azathioprine, or combination therapy for Crohn's disease. *N. Engl. J. Med.* **2010**, *362*, 1383–1395. [CrossRef]
79. Colombel, J.F.; Adedokun, O.J.; Gasink, C.; Gao, L.L.; Cornillie, F.J.; D'Haens, G.R.; Rutgeerts, P.J.; Reinisch, W.; Sandborn, W.J.; Hanauer, S.B. Combination Therapy with Infliximab and Azathioprine Improves Infliximab Pharmacokinetic Features and Efficacy: A Post Hoc Analysis. *Clin. Gastroenterol. Hepatol.* **2019**, *17*, 1525–1532. [CrossRef]
80. Kennedy, N.A.; Heap, G.A.; Green, H.D.; Hamilton, B.; Bewshea, C.; Walker, G.J.; Thomas, A.; Nice, R.; Perry, M.H.; Bouri, S.; et al. Predictors of anti-TNF treatment failure in anti-TNF-naive patients with active luminal Crohn's disease: A prospective, multicentre, cohort study. *Lancet Gastroenterol. Hepatol.* **2019**, *4*, 341–353. [CrossRef]
81. Schultheiss, J.P.D.; Mahmoud, R.; Louwers, J.M.; van der Kaaij, M.T.; van Hellemondt, B.P.; van Boeckel, P.G.; Mahmmod, N.; Jharap, B.; Fidder, H.H.; Oldenburg, B. Loss of response to anti-TNFalpha agents depends on treatment duration in patients with inflammatory bowel disease. *Aliment. Pharmacol. Ther.* **2021**, *54*, 1298–1308. [CrossRef]
82. Baert, F.; Noman, M.; Vermeire, S.; Van Assche, G.; Haens, G.D.; Carbonez, A.; Rutgeerts, P. Influence of immunogenicity on the long-term efficacy of infliximab in Crohn's disease. *N. Engl. J. Med.* **2003**, *348*, 601–608. [CrossRef]
83. D'Haens, G.; Reinisch, W.; Schreiber, S.; Cummings, F.; Irving, P.; Ye, B.; Kim, D.; Yoon, S.; Ben-Horin, S. Comparison of combination subcutaneous infliximab and an immunomodulator versus subcutaneous infliximab monotherapy: Post-hoc analysis of a randomised clinical trial. *United Eur. Gastroenterol. Week* **2021**, *9* (Suppl. S1), P0467. Available online: https://programme.ueg.eu/week2021/#/details/presentations/1284 (accessed on 22 August 2022).

84. Ungar, B.; Chowers, Y.; Yavzori, M.; Picard, O.; Fudim, E.; Har-Noy, O.; Kopylov, U.; Eliakim, R.; Ben-Horin, S. The temporal evolution of antidrug antibodies in patients with inflammatory bowel disease treated with infliximab. *Gut* **2014**, *63*, 1258–1264. [CrossRef] [PubMed]
85. Mahmoud, R.; Schultheiss, J.P.D.; Fidder, H.H.; Oldenburg, B. Letter: Loss of response to anti-TNFalpha agents depends on treatment duration in patients with inflammatory bowel disease-authors' reply. *Aliment. Pharmacol. Ther.* **2022**, *55*, 499–500. [CrossRef] [PubMed]
86. Vande Casteele, N.; Gils, A.; Singh, S.; Ohrmund, L.; Hauenstein, S.; Rutgeerts, P.; Vermeire, S. Antibody response to infliximab and its impact on pharmacokinetics can be transient. *Am. J. Gastroenterol.* **2013**, *108*, 962–971. [CrossRef] [PubMed]
87. Wang, S.L.; Ohrmund, L.; Hauenstein, S.; Salbato, J.; Reddy, R.; Monk, P.; Lockton, S.; Ling, N.; Singh, S. Development and validation of a homogeneous mobility shift assay for the measurement of infliximab and antibodies-to-infliximab levels in patient serum. *J. Immunol. Methods* **2012**, *382*, 177–188. [CrossRef]
88. Egea-Pujol, L.; Reddy, R.; Patel, S.; Christie, R.; Salbato, J.; Shah, S.; Hauenstein, S.; Singh, S. Homogenous Mobility Shift Assay (HMSA) Overcomes the Limitations of ELISA and ECLIA Assays for Monitoring Infliximab (IFX), Adalimumab (ADA), and Associated Anti-drug Antibodies in Serum: 1817. *Off. J. Am. Coll. Gastroenterol.* **2013**, *108*, S548. [CrossRef]
89. Nice, R.; Chanchlani, N.; Green, H.; Bewshea, C.; Ahmad, T.; Goodhand, J.R.; McDonald, T.J.; Perry, M.H.; Kennedy, N.A. Validating the positivity thresholds of drug-tolerant anti-infliximab and anti-adalimumab antibody assays. *Aliment. Pharmacol. Ther.* **2021**, *53*, 128–137. [CrossRef]
90. Weisshof, R.; Ungar, B.; Blatt, A.; Dahan, A.; Pressman, S.; Waterman, M.; Kopylov, U.; Ben-Horin, S.; Chowers, Y. Anti-infliximab Antibodies with Neutralizing Capacity in Patients with Inflammatory Bowel Disease: Distinct Clinical Implications Revealed by a Novel Assay. *Inflamm. Bowel Dis.* **2016**, *22*, 1655–1661. [CrossRef]
91. Buurman, D.J.; Maurer, J.M.; Keizer, R.J.; Kosterink, J.G.; Dijkstra, G. Population pharmacokinetics of infliximab in patients with inflammatory bowel disease: Potential implications for dosing in clinical practice. *Aliment. Pharmacol. Ther.* **2015**, *42*, 529–539. [CrossRef]
92. Malissen, B.; Tamoutounour, S.; Henri, S. The origins and functions of dendritic cells and macrophages in the skin. *Nat. Rev. Immunol.* **2014**, *14*, 417–428. [CrossRef]
93. Kim, H.; Alten, R.; Cummings, F.; Danese, S.; D'Haens, G.; Emery, P.; Ghosh, S.; de Saint Joseph, C.G.; Lee, J.; Lindsay, J.O.; et al. Innovative approaches to biologic development on the trail of CT-P13: Biosimilars, value-added medicines, and biobetters. *MAbs* **2021**, *13*, 1868078. [CrossRef] [PubMed]
94. Mohanan, D.; Slutter, B.; Henriksen-Lacey, M.; Jiskoot, W.; Bouwstra, J.A.; Perrie, Y.; Kundig, T.M.; Gander, B.; Johansen, P. Administration routes affect the quality of immune responses: A cross-sectional evaluation of particulate antigen-delivery systems. *J. Control Release* **2010**, *147*, 342–349. [CrossRef]
95. Hamuro, L.; Kijanka, G.; Kinderman, F.; Kropshofer, H.; Bu, D.X.; Zepeda, M.; Jawa, V. Perspectives on Subcutaneous Route of Administration as an Immunogenicity Risk Factor for Therapeutic Proteins. *J. Pharm. Sci.* **2017**, *106*, 2946–2954. [CrossRef] [PubMed]
96. Rutgeerts, P.; Feagan, B.G.; Lichtenstein, G.R.; Mayer, L.F.; Schreiber, S.; Colombel, J.F.; Rachmilewitz, D.; Wolf, D.C.; Olson, A.; Bao, W.; et al. Comparison of scheduled and episodic treatment strategies of infliximab in Crohn's disease. *Gastroenterology* **2004**, *126*, 402–413. [CrossRef]
97. Hanauer, S.B.; Wagner, C.L.; Bala, M.; Mayer, L.; Travers, S.; Diamond, R.H.; Olson, A.; Bao, W.; Rutgeerts, P. Incidence and importance of antibody responses to infliximab after maintenance or episodic treatment in Crohn's disease. *Clin. Gastroenterol. Hepatol.* **2004**, *2*, 542–553. [CrossRef]
98. Schreiber, S.; Ben-Horin, S.; Alten, R.; Westhovens, R.; Peyrin-Biroulet, L.; Danese, S.; Hibi, T.; Takeuchi, K.; Magro, F.; An, Y.; et al. Perspectives on Subcutaneous Infliximab for Rheumatic Diseases and Inflammatory Bowel Disease: Before, During, and After the COVID-19 Era. *Adv. Ther.* **2022**, *39*, 2342–2364. [CrossRef] [PubMed]
99. Bar-Yoseph, H.; Pressman, S.; Blatt, A.; Vainberg, S.G.; Maimon, N.; Starosvetsky, E.; Ungar, B.; Ben-Horin, S.; Shen-Orr, S.S.; Chowers, Y.; et al. Infliximab-Tumor Necrosis Factor Complexes Elicit Formation of Anti-Drug Antibodies. *Gastroenterology* **2019**, *157*, 1338–1351. [CrossRef]
100. Chaigne, B.; Watier, H. Monoclonal antibodies in excess: A simple way to avoid immunogenicity in patients? *J. Allergy Clin. Immunol.* **2015**, *136*, 814–816. [CrossRef]
101. De Almeida, R.; Nakamura, C.N.; de Lima Fontes, M.; Deffune, E.; Felisbino, S.L.; Kaneno, R.; Favaro, W.J.; Billis, A.; Cerri, M.O.; Fusco-Almeida, A.M.; et al. Enhanced immunization techniques to obtain highly specific monoclonal antibodies. *MAbs* **2018**, *10*, 46–54. [CrossRef]
102. Somerfield, J.; Hill-Cawthorne, G.A.; Lin, A.; Zandi, M.S.; McCarthy, C.; Jones, J.L.; Willcox, M.; Shaw, D.; Thompson, S.A.; Compston, A.S.; et al. A novel strategy to reduce the immunogenicity of biological therapies. *J. Immunol.* **2010**, *185*, 763–768. [CrossRef]

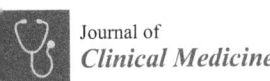

Review

The Role of Low-Dose Oral Methotrexate in Increasing Anti-TNF Drug Levels and Reducing Immunogenicity in IBD

Kathryn Demase [1], Cassandra K. Monitto [1,2], Robert D. Little [1] and Miles P. Sparrow [1,*]

[1] Department of Gastroenterology, Alfred Health and Monash University, Melbourne 3004, Australia
[2] Department of Pharmacy, Alfred Health, Melbourne 3004, Australia
* Correspondence: m.sparrow@alfred.org.au; Tel.: +61-3-9076-2223

Abstract: Concomitant immunomodulation is utilised in combination with anti-TNF therapy for IBD primarily to increase drug levels and prevent anti-drug antibody formation. Whilst thiopurines have traditionally been the immunomodulator of choice in IBD populations, there are concerns regarding the long-term safety of the prolonged use of these agents: particularly an association with lymphoproliferative disorders. Given this, we have explored the existing literature on the use of low-dose oral methotrexate as an alternative immunomodulator for this indication. Although there is a lack of data directly comparing the efficacies of methotrexate and thiopurines as concomitant immunomodulators, the available literature supports the use of methotrexate in improving the pharmacokinetics of anti-TNF agents. Furthermore, low-dose oral methotrexate regimens appear to have comparable efficacies to higher-dose parenteral administration and are better tolerated. We suggest that clinicians should consider the use of low-dose oral methotrexate as an alternative to thiopurines when the primary purpose of concomitant immunomodulation is to improve anti-TNF pharmacokinetics.

Keywords: methotrexate; oral; infliximab; adalimumab; concomitant immunomodulator; pharmacokinetics; inflammatory bowel disease

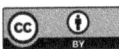

1. Introduction

The role of anti-tumour necrosis factor (anti-TNF) agents within the treatment armamentarium of inflammatory bowel disease (IBD) is well established. Agents such as infliximab (IFX) and adalimumab (ADL) have changed the landscape of medical therapy for both the induction and maintenance of moderate-to-severe ulcerative colitis (UC) and Crohn's disease (CD) [1–6] and now have over 20 years of efficacy and safety data for IBD [7]. Therapeutic drug monitoring (TDM) has become routine in optimising secondary loss of response to anti-TNF therapy in IBD. In particular, TDM of IFX has been shown to improve clinical outcomes and be more cost-effective than empirical dose escalation [8,9]. The data supporting TDM of ADL are, however, less robust [10]. A range of target trough drug levels have been associated with varying depths of clinical, biochemical, and endoscopic remission, as well as perianal fistula healing [11–16].

Combination therapy with immunomodulators such as thiopurines (azathioprine (AZA), mercaptopurine (6-MP)) or methotrexate (MTX) increases anti-TNF drug levels and decreases the formation of anti-drug antibodies (ADAs) [17–19]. The evidence for the benefits of concomitant immunomodulation with ADL is less consistent than that with IFX [20–25]. Thiopurines have traditionally been used as first-line immunomodulators in IBD. Whilst they are effective therapeutic agents both in combination and as monotherapy, their long-term use is associated with serious adverse events (AEs), such as infections, non-melanomatous skin cancers (NMSCs), and lymphoma [26], including hepatosplenic T-cell lymphoma [27]. Although rare, hepatosplenic T-cell lymphoma has high mortality, with a preponderance in young males. Conversely, MTX may have a more tolerable serious side effect profile. It is commonly used in rheumatological conditions both as monotherapy and in combination with anti-TNF agents; however, it is typically reserved for those who are intolerant to thiopurines in IBD [28]. Evidence for its use in IBD is limited to studies of clinical outcomes of parenteral MTX given at varying doses, with few studies addressing the outcomes of using oral MTX to improve anti-TNF pharmacokinetics [29].

This comprehensive literature review examines the current evidence available on the efficacy, safety, and optimal dosing of oral MTX when used as an immunomodulator in combination with anti-TNF therapy for IBD to optimise anti-TNF drug levels and reduce immunogenicity. For when concomitant immunomodulation is used for this purpose, rather than as a second therapeutic agent to treat disease activity, we propose the consideration of low-dose oral ($\leq$12.5 mg/week) MTX, given its favourable safety profile and comparable efficacy.

We conducted a literature search using the PubMed Online database. The search was performed using the following linked search terms: "methotrexate" AND ("anti-TNF" OR "infliximab" OR "adalimumab" OR "golimumab" OR "certolizumab") AND ("inflammatory bowel disease" OR "Crohn's disease" OR "ulcerative colitis") AND ("rheumatoid arthritis" OR "psoriasis" OR "ankylosing spondylitis") AND ("trough level" OR "drug concentration" OR "anti-drug antibody"). The results were restricted to the English language and original research, presenting data on the efficacy of oral low-dose MTX as a concomitant immunomodulator with anti-TNF therapy, published before 1 May 2023. In total, 68 articles were identified, and their titles and abstracts were screened by one reviewer (KD) to ensure their relevance. After screening, seventeen articles were assessed for eligibility, with an additional four articles added from a review of the reference lists of the selected articles. Studies that investigated the general efficacy of concomitant immunomodulation with thiopurines and MTX but failed to stratify their data by type of immunomodulator were excluded. After review, 10 articles were chosen for discussion (Table 1).

Table 1. Summary of original research reporting efficacy of low-dose MTX as a concomitant immunomodulator with anti-TNF therapy.

Study	Design	Anti-TNFs	MTX Dosing, mg/Week	Characteristics	Drug Level, µg/mL	ADA Formation	Clinical Outcomes
Gastroenterology Studies							
Colman (2015) [30]	Retrospective review	IFX ADL CZP	75% used PO MTX 25% used parenteral MTX; 71% used LD-MTX (≤12.5 mg) 29% used HD-MTX (15–25 mg)	73 adult patients with IBD - 74% with CD - Active disease; All on anti-TNF therapy in combination with MTX - 49% on ADL - 40% on IFX - 11% on CZP; Followed for 42 months; Secondary outcomes: - Endoscopic inflammation - Steroid use - Therapy escalation - Addition or escalation of concomitant therapy - Surgery	-	-	No difference in relapse rate between methods of MTX administration - 37% PO vs. 27% parenteral; $p = 0.56$; HD-MTX more likely to maintain remission than LD-MTX; log-rank test $p < 0.01$; No difference in secondary outcomes indicating worsening disease between MTX doses (OR 1.14; 95% CI 0.61–2.13; $p = 0.67$)
Ungar (2017) [31]	Retrospective multi-centre (3) review	ADL	Mix of PO and SC MTX (% not stated); SC dose: 15–25 mg PO dose: 10–15 mg	23 adult patients with IBD - 91% with CD; All developed ADAs with LOR in ADL monotherapy; immunomodulator was added as salvage combination therapy - 14 on thiopurines - 9 on MTX	-	48% of patients had elimination of ADAs - No difference in type of immunomodulator; $p = 0.5$	Patients who had reversal of ADA achieved clinical responses and normalisation of inflammatory markers

Table 1. Cont.

Study	Design	Anti-TNFs	MTX Dosing, mg/Week	Characteristics	Drug Level, μg/mL	ADA Formation	Clinical Outcomes
Chi (2018) [29]	Cross-sectional analysis	IFX	"Primarily low dose oral MTX, mean dose 11.6 mg ± 5.1 mg/week"	223 paediatric and young adult patients with IBD - 83.9% with CD All on IFX - 62.3% as monotherapy - 37.7% as combination therapy Of the combination therapy: - 84.5% used MTX - 15.5% used 6-MP	Higher TLs in combination therapy (15.59 ± 1.20) vs. monotherapy (12.35 ± 0.93); $p = 0.01$ Monotherapy (27.3%) more likely to have subtherapeutic TLs < 3.5 than combination therapy (8.3%): OR 0.13; 95% CI 0.04–0.39; $p < 0.01$ No difference in mean TL between the MTX (15.2) and MP (17.9) groups; $p = 0.41$	Combination therapy (9.5%) was less likely to result in ADAs than monotherapy (20%) (OR 0.3; 95% CI 0.1–0.7; $p < 0.01$) Trend towards higher rates of ADAs in 6-MP (23.08%) vs. MTX (7.04%) use; $p = 0.07$	No difference in clinical or biochemical disease activity between IFX monotherapy and combination therapy
Vasudevan (2019) [32]	Retrospective multi-centre (2) observational study	IFX ADL	PO MTX - 29% used LD-MTX (≤12.5 mg) - 71% used HD-MTX (≥15 mg)	269 adult patients with CD All on anti-TNF therapy and with ≥3 months of combination immunomodulator therapy - 58% on IFX - 42% on ADL - 71% used thiopurines - 29% used MTX	No difference in IFX TLs between thiopurines (5.3) and MTX (5.4); $p = 0.63$ Higher ADL TLs with thiopurines (7.2) vs. MTX (4.3) combination therapy; $p = 0.03$ The thiopurine combination achieved higher rates of therapeutic ADL levels (73%) vs. MTX (18%); $p < 0.01$	–	Higher rates of endoscopic remission in the ADL group with thiopurine combinations (49%) vs. MTX (6%); $p = 0.004$ No differences in remission rate between immunomodulators when used in combination with IFX -65% on thiopurines vs. 54% on MTX; $p = 0.09$ No differences in rate of endoscopic remission between low- and high-dose MTX

Table 1. Cont.

Study	Design	Anti-TNFs	MTX Dosing, mg/Week	Characteristics	Drug Level, μg/mL	ADA Formation	Clinical Outcomes
Borren (2019) [33]	Retrospective review	IFX ADL CZP GOL	PO and SC MTX, 7.5–25 mg 28% used LD-MTX (≤12.5 mg) - 96.8% used PO 72% used HD-MTX (>12.5 mg) - 39% used PO	222 adult patients with IBD - 73.4% with CD All on anti-TNF therapy with varying doses of MTX IFX - 38.1% LD-MTX users - 37.7% HD-MTX users ADL - 44.4% LD-MTX users - 40.9% HD-MTX users CZP - 9.5% LD-MTX users - 7.0% HD-MTX users GOL - 7.9% LD-MTX users - 4.4% HD-MTX users	-	-	No difference in primary composite outcome (IBD-related hospitalisation or surgery, biological change, or steroid initiation) between the LD-MTX (37%) and HD-MTX (47%) groups; $p = 0.15$ Multi-variable analysis showed no difference in individual outcomes for either group
Yarur (2022) COMBO-IBD [19]	Prospective cohort study	IFX	PO MTX - 65.4% used LD-MTX (12.5 mg) - 34.6% used HD-MTX (25 mg)	113 adult patients with IBD - 73% with CD All on IFX - 23% on IFX monotherapy - 23% on MTX in combination - 54% on thiopurines in combination	Higher TLs in the combination MTX group (17.1 [IQR 9.7–23.7]) and thiopurine group (14.5 [IQR 4.5–18.8]) vs. monotherapy (3.8 [IQR 1.8–9.2]); $p = 0.0001$ - Only those on thiopurines combined with 6-TGNs > 145 had higher TLs than in monotherapy Trend towards higher TL in MTX combination therapy than with thiopurines $p = 0.07$	Higher rates of ADAs in monotherapy than in combination therapy (OR 8.6; 95% CI 2.58–29.16) * Not stratified by type of combination therapy	Higher rates of steroid-free deep remission in combination therapy (71.3) vs. monotherapy (46.2); $p = 0.02$ - Use of MTX and thiopurines with 6-TGNs > 145 as combination therapy were both associated with remission

Table 1. Cont.

Study	Design	Anti-TNFs	MTX Dosing, mg/Week	Characteristics	Drug Level, µg/mL	ADA Formation	Clinical Outcomes
Rheumatology Studies							
Maini (1998) [34]	Multi-centre randomised, double-blind placebo-controlled trial	IFX	PO MTX, 7.5 mg	101 adult patients with active RA Randomised into seven groups - IFX 1 mg/kg ± MTX - IFX 3 mg/kg ± MTX - IFX 10 mg/kg ± MTX - Placebo infusion + MTX Followed for 26 weeks	Combination with MTX showed **consistently higher drug levels** 6 weeks after the last infusion in those receiving IFX at 3 mg/kg and at 10 mg/kg IFX 1mg/kg monotherapy resulted in **undetectable TLs** from week 4 vs. stable, detectable TLs in those receiving combination MTX	Rate of ADA formation was inversely proportional to IFX dose MTX combination reduced ADA formation - 53% of IFX 1 mg/kg vs. 15% with MTX - 21% of IFX 3 mg/kg vs. 7% with MTX - 7% of IFX 10 mg/kg vs. 0% with MTX	IFX (1 mg/kg) monotherapy was no better than placebo - MTX combination achieved clinical responses in >60% of the group for a median of 16.5 weeks; $p = 0.006$ vs. IFX (1 mg/kg) monotherapy
Burmester (2013) CONCERTO [35]	Randomised, double blind parallel-armed study	ADL	PO MTX: 2.5 mg 5 mg 10 mg 20 mg	395 adult patients with RA All on ADL Randomised 1:1:1:1 to combination therapy with different MTX doses Followed for 26 weeks	Higher TLs with increasing MTX doses of up to 10 mg/week - Mean TLs of 4.4 (±5.2), 5.7 (±4.9), 6.5 (4.4), 6.9 (3.4) for MTX at 2.5 mg, 5 mg, 10 mg, and 20 mg, respectively	Lower rates of ADAs with increasing MTX doses of up to 10 mg/week - 21%, 13%, 6% and 6% for MTX 2.5 mg, 5 mg, 10 mg, and 20 mg, respectively	Reduced disease activity with increasing MTX doses - Higher proportion of patients meeting the primary endpoint with increasing MTX doses; $p = 0.005$
Ducourau (2020) [36]	Multi-centre randomised trial	ADL	SC MTX, 10 mg	107 adult patients with axial spondylarthritis All on ADL Randomised 1:1 to ADL monotherapy vs. combination with MTX - 51.4% monotherapy - 48.6% combination Followed for 26 weeks	MTX combination therapy was associated with **higher TLs** at all time points; $p < 0.05$ Those with ADAs had lower median TLs (**1.43** [0.00–11.47]) compared to those without ADAs (**8.66** [0.05–18.31]) at week 26; $p < 0.05$	Lower rates of ADAs in MTX combination therapy (25%) vs. ADL monotherapy (47.3%); $p = 0.03$ - MTX combination therapy reduced risk of ADA formation; RR 0.53 (95% CI 0.31–0.91)	Similar rates of clinically inactive disease by week 26 for both groups (40% ADL monotherapy vs. 37%; $p = 0.9$)

102

Table 1. Cont.

Study	Design	Anti-TNFs	MTX Dosing, mg/Week	Characteristics	Drug Level, µg/mL	ADA Formation	Clinical Outcomes
Dermatology Studies							
van der Kraaij (2022) [37]	Randomised control trial	ADL	PO MTX, 10 mg	61 adult patients with psoriasis All on ADL Randomised 1:1 to ADL monotherapy vs. combination with MTX - 49% monotherapy - 51% combination	No difference in median TL between groups; *p* = 0.26 - 5.9 [3.5–8.8] for monotherapy - 6.8 [5.5–9.2] for combination More monotherapy patients failed to reach **therapeutic TLs > 3.2** at week 5 (6.5%) vs. with combination therapy (30%); *p* = 0.02 - This was not significant at week 49; 12.9 vs. 23.3%; *p* = 0.32	Higher rates of ADA formation in monotherapy group (60%) vs. combination therapy group (22.6%); *p* < 0.01 ADAs appeared earlier in monotherapy group vs. combination therapy group - Week 5: 33.3 vs. 3.2%; *p* < 0.01 - Week 49: 46.7 vs. 38.7%; *p* = 0.31	Combination therapy had faster clinical improvement, with 83.9% achieving treatment goals in week 13 vs. 56.7% of monotherapy patients; *p* = 0.03

Abbreviations—Anti-TNF (anti-tumour necrosis factor), IFX (infliximab), ADL (adalimumab), CZP (certolizumab pegol), GOL (golimumab), MTX (methotrexate), PO (oral), SC (subcutaneous), LD (low-dose), HD (high-dose), IBD (inflammatory bowel disease), CD (Crohn's disease), RA (rheumatoid arthritis), LOR (loss of response), TL (trough level), OR (odds ratio), CI (confidence interval), IQR (inter-quartile range), 6-MP (mercaptopurine), 6-TGNs (6-thioguanine nucleotide). * is to indicate a point of interest/qualifying remark relating to the above comment.

2. Pharmacokinetics of Anti-TNFs and the Role of Methotrexate in Increasing Drug Levels and Reducing Immunogenicity

Whilst anti-TNF agents are an effective therapy for IBD, 23–46% of patients treated with standard dosing regimens of IFX or ADL develop secondary loss of response after 12 months [38]. There are multiple proposed pharmacokinetic and pharmacodynamic mechanisms that lead to low drug levels and loss of response. Firstly, clearance of these drugs is increased in active disease. Intestinal inflammation leads to faecal loss of IFX, with higher faecal IFX concentrations found in those with more severe disease and low serum albumin levels [39]. The inverse relationship between baseline albumin levels and anti-TNF clearance [40] may be explained by the interactions between IgG antibodies, such as IFX, or proteins, such as albumin, and the neonatal Fc Receptor (FcRn) [41]. FcRn is found on endothelial cells and plays a role in the recycling and transcytosis of IgG antibodies and serum proteins, preventing them from catabolism and prolonging their half-life. Additionally, elevated C-reactive protein (CRP) levels have been linked to lower IFX trough levels and loss of response in IBD patients [42,43]. The association between these acute phase reactants and reduced drug levels supports the notion that increased anti-TNF clearance correlates with the severity of the disease.

The most investigated mechanism, however, is the immunogenicity of these agents, which elicit ADA formation against the F(ab)2 fragment of the anti-TNF IgG molecule [44]. The presence of ADAs against IFX has been demonstrated to increase drug clearance [40,45,46]. Whilst all biological drugs induce immunogenicity, they do so at varying degrees. This is partly explained by the structural differences amongst anti-TNF agents, whereby lower immunogenicity rates are associated with the degree of humanisation of molecules [18]. A systematic review and meta-analysis by Thomas et al. found a significant difference in incidences of ADAs against IFX compared to ADL. IFX is a chimeric monoclonal antibody (mAb) comprising murine variable and human Fc regions, whilst ADL is a fully humanised mAb. As expected, the incidence of ADAs against ADL was lower than that with IFX (14.1% vs. 25.3%, respectively; $p = 0.03$) [18]. This partly explains the larger body of evidence supporting the use of immunomodulators in combination with IFX compared to other anti-TNF agents.

2.1. Efficacy of Concomitant Immunomodulation in Improving Anti-TNF Levels

Immunomodulators increase the serum concentrations of anti-TNFs. Although the exact mechanism is not well-established, it is presumed that they exert this function by reducing the formation of ADAs. In the SONIC trial, patients with active CD and who received a combination of IFX and AZA had higher IFX levels than those who received IFX monotherapy (3.5 µg/mL vs. 1.6 µg/mL, respectively; $p < 0.001$). These findings were associated with higher corticosteroid-free remission rates in the combination therapy group [47]. Although the advantage of the combination treatment may, in part, be due to an additive immunosuppressive effect of AZA on the underlying disease process, there was also a clear reduction in ADA formation in patients on combination therapy in comparison to monotherapy (0.9% vs. 14.6%, respectively). Post hoc analysis found increasing rates of remission with increasing serum IFX concentrations but no difference between those on combination therapy and those on monotherapy when stratified by drug level [48]. Combination IFX and AZA patients comprised 73.1% of those who achieved the highest quartile of IFX concentrations and only 23.5% of those in the lowest quartile. Furthermore, the addition of immunomodulators can impact outcomes at as early as 4 weeks, which is faster than the onset of their therapeutic efficacy [49]. The benefit of combination therapy has been seen with real-world data from the prospective PANTS UK cohort, which demonstrated that concomitant immunomodulator therapy with thiopurines or MTX prevented ADA formation against IFX and ADL, improved drug levels, and was associated with a higher 54-week clinical remission rate [23].

2.2. Mechanism of Action of Methotrexate in Improving Anti-TNF Pharmacokinetics

MTX is a potent folic acid antagonist with proven efficacy in CD treatment due to its anti-inflammatory and pro-apoptotic properties [50]. However, trials in adult patients with UC found no superiority to the placebo in induction or maintenance of remission [51,52]. MTX exerts its cytotoxic effect by blocking dihydrofolate reductase, interfering with DNA synthesis, and inhibiting de novo purine synthesis. These anti-inflammatory pathways may also enhance the efficacy of biologic agents by reducing TNF and IL-12/23 levels [53], even in the absence of any effect in reducing ADAs. The specific effects on immunological processes that may lead to reductions in ADA formation are complex and not fully understood. A distinct immunomodulatory pathway has been observed in preclinical animal models of immunogenicity and may account for MTX's effects on ADA production. MTX exposure in mice appears to induce T and B cell anergy, thereby blunting their response to antigen stimulation [54,55]. The animals in these studies showed reduced ADA production towards recombinant human proteins when treated with MTX. Furthermore, this response persisted 32 weeks after MTX cessation. Unrelated recombinant human proteins were administered after MTX cessation, and the ADA response was preserved, suggesting that this mechanism is distinct from generalised immunosuppression. Additionally, other immunosuppressive medications, including rapamycin and cyclophosphamide, exhibited no significant effect on the ADA responses, further supporting a unique role of MTX beyond its established immunosuppressive and cytotoxic effects [54]. These "anergic effects" of MTX on T and B cells may explain the mechanism for reducing ADAs that target anti-TNF agents.

3. Efficacy of Methotrexate Compared to Thiopurines as Concomitant Immunomodulators

In contrast to rheumatological conditions, the use of MTX in combination with anti-TNF agents for concomitant immunomodulation in IBD is less common [17]. This may be due to the more limited role MTX plays as a therapeutic agent in adult IBD [56]. Thiopurines, on the other hand, have a robust evidence base for both CD and UC and, as such, are commonly used as monotherapy maintenance agents in many jurisdictions globally. Therefore, when the decision is made to add an anti-TNF agent in patients failing thiopurine monotherapy, most of the patients continue to receive thiopurines for concomitant immunomodulation, with MTX typically reserved for those who either have failed or are intolerant to thiopurines [57]. A preference for thiopurines over MTX is evident across studies that have evaluated the effects of concomitant immunomodulation, with the majority of cohorts showing thiopurine usage rates of 50–70% (Table 1). There may be a trend towards increasing use of MTX as a first-line immunomodulator in the paediatric population due to safety concerns regarding prolonged thiopurine exposure, particularly hepatosplenic T-cell lymphoma. A multi-centre retrospective cohort study found that the proportion of patients who received MTX as their first immunomodulator rose from 14% in 2002 to 60% in 2010 ($p = 0.005$) [57].

3.1. Efficacy of Methotrexate for Concomitant Immunomodulation with Anti-TNFs

A review of the literature pertaining to the efficacy of MTX in regard to anti-TNF pharmacokinetics in both rheumatology and IBD has been summarised in Tables 1 and 2. Overall, MTX has consistently been shown to reduce the formation of ADAs and lead to higher anti-TNF levels. There may be a reduced effect when it is used in combination with ADL compared to with IFX; however, the data on this are mixed [35–37]. Two large, multi-centre randomised control trials that investigated the use of MTX in combination with ADL in rheumatoid arthritis and axial spondylarthritis found it to be effective in reducing rates of ADA formation, increasing trough levels, and achieving clinical responses [35,36]. Conversely, a small, randomised control trial in patients with psoriasis found that there were no differences in the ADL levels in those on monotherapy compared to those receiving concomitant MTX [37]. Despite this, the MTX group did have significantly lower rates of ADA formation and achieved more rapid clinical responses than those on ADL monotherapy. Furthermore, a retrospective observational study of 278 CD patients on IFX or ADL with concomitant immunomodulation with either thiopurines (71%) or MTX (29%) found that those who received thiopurines had higher ADL trough levels compared to those who received MTX [32]. Patients on ADL also had higher rates of endoscopic remission when treated in combination with a thiopurine compared to MTX. These differences were not observed in patients on IFX. Further studies comparing the differential effects of MTX and thiopurines when used in combination with ADL would help clarify these conflicting results.

The data on the effects of concomitant MTX on clinical outcomes in IBD are similarly conflicted. Two randomised control trials found no difference in the rate of treatment failure in those on IFX monotherapy compared to combination therapy with MTX; however, one did show an improvement when used in combination with ADL [58,59]. Conversely, a large prospective cohort study found that the combination of IFX and MTX had higher rates of corticosteroid-free deep remission and was less likely to develop secondary non-response compared to IFX monotherapy [19]. The retrospective data on the effects of varying doses of concomitant MTX on clinical outcomes are also mixed but overall suggest that there is no difference between high- and low-dose regimes [30,32,33].

The efficacy of adding a concomitant immunomodulator (thiopurines or MTX) in eliminating ADAs, improving drug levels, and recapturing clinical responses to anti-TNF therapy is more established. Three retrospective studies have investigated the effects of commencing immunomodulators in patients who had developed immunogenic loss of response to IFX or ADL [31,60,61]. In all three studies, the immunomodulators were associated with reduction and elimination of ADA titres, increases in anti-TNF trough levels, and restored clinical responses. Although only one study reported the differential effects of MTX compared to thiopurines, it found no difference inefficacy between agents on these outcomes [31]. Furthermore, the addition of an immunomodulator was more effective than dose intensification of anti-TNFs alone [61].

Table 2. Summary of original research reporting efficacy of high-dose MTX as a concomitant immunomodulator with anti-TNF therapy for IBD.

Study	Design	Anti-TNF smg/Week	MTX Dosing, PO	Characteristics	Drug Level, μg/mL	ADA Formation	Clinical Outcomes
Vermeire (2007) [28]	Multi-centre (3) prospective cohort study	IFX	SC MTX at 15 mg (12-week induction with 25 mg)	174 adult patients with IBD All commenced IFX (episodic, on-demand regime) - 34% with IFX monotherapy - 37.3% with AZA combination - 28.7% with MTX combination	Higher median IFX levels in combination therapy (6.45) vs. monotherapy (2.42); $p = 0.065$ - No difference between MTX (5.65) and AZA (6.15); $p = 0.27$	Lower rates of ADA formation in combination therapy (46%) vs. monotherapy (73%); $p < 0.001$ MTX (44%, $p = 0.002$) and AZA (48%, $p = 0.004$) had equal efficacies against ADA formation vs. monotherapy No difference in rate of ADA when immunomodulator started at time of IFX vs. preceding 3 months	-
Feagan (2014) COMMIT [58]	Double-blind, placebo-controlled, randomised trial	IFX	SC MTX at 25 mg (escalated from 10 mg to 25 mg over 5 weeks)	126 adult patients with CD All commenced IFX Randomised 1:1 - IFX monotherapy (placebo) - MTX combination	Trend towards higher TLs in MTX group (6.35) vs. monotherapy (3.75); $p = 0.08$	Lower rates of ADA formation in MTX group (4%) vs. monotherapy (20%); $p = 0.01$	No difference in rate of treatment failure at week 50 between MTX (30.6%) and monotherapy (29.8%) groups, (HR, 1.16, 95% CI 0.62–2.17)
Kappelman (2023) [59]	Multi-centre (35), placebo-controlled, randomised trial	IFX ADL	Weight-based PO MTX - 15 mg if >40 kg - 12.5 mg if 30–40 kg - 10 mg if 20–30 kg	297 paediatric (age < 21) patients with CD All commenced either IFX or ADL - 71% IFX - 29% ADL Randomised 1:1 and stratified by anti-TNF - IFX monotherapy (placebo) - MTX combination Followed for 1–3 years	-	No difference in ADA formation with MTX (34%) vs. placebo (47%) group for IFX (RR 0.72, 95% CI 0.49–1.07) No difference for ADL; 15% with MTX vs. 21% with placebo (RR, 0.71 95% CI 0.24–2.07) Those on ADL with ADAs were more likely to have treatment failure (64% vs. 36%, $p = 0.03$) * Serum available for only 70% of patients	MTX use in those on ADL reduced the risk of treatment failure vs. placebo; HR 0.40 (95% CI 0.19–0.81, $p = 0.01$) No significant differences between groups for those on IFX

Abbreviations—Anti-TNF (anti-tumour necrosis factor), IFX (infliximab), ADL (adalimumab), MTX (methotrexate), PO (oral), SC (subcutaneous), IBD (inflammatory bowel disease), CD (Crohn's disease), TL (trough level), HR (hazard ratio), RR (relative risk), CI (confidence interval). * is used to indicate a point of interest/qualifying remark relating to this section.

3.2. Efficacy of Methotrexate Compared to Thiopurines at Augmenting Anti-TNF Pharmacokinetics

In terms of transitioning to the preferential use of MTX for concomitant immunomodulation, the first question that must be answered is whether it is as effective as thiopurines at maintaining anti-TNF trough levels and preventing ADA formation. There have been only two prospective observational studies that have directly compared the efficacies of MTX and thiopurines in combination with anti-TNFs [19,28]. There was no difference in the anti-TNF drug levels between the groups in either study, and MTX was found to be as effective at reducing ADA formation as AZA. The first study was a prospective cohort study of 369 patients with IBD and on maintenance IFX, vedolizumab, or ustekinumab. It investigated the differences in pharmacokinetics between biologic monotherapy and combination therapy with either MTX or thiopurines at varying doses. MTX was given orally, with the majority (65.4%) in low doses of 12.5 mg/week. IFX drug levels were found to be significantly lower in those who received IFX monotherapy (3.8 µg/mL) compared to those on concomitant MTX (17.1 µg/mL, $p = 0.0001$) and thiopurines (14.5 µg/mL, $p = 0.01$), with a trend towards higher levels in the MTX group compared to the thiopurines ($p = 0.07$) [19]. The rates of ADA formation were higher in those on IFX monotherapy compared to combination therapy (OR 8.6; 95% CI 2.59–29.16); however, this was not stratified by type of immunomodulator. The second study followed a cohort of 174 patients with CD across three centres, all of whom were treated with IFX in an episodic on-demand schedule. In total, 37.3% received AZA, 28.7% received MTX, and 34% received no concomitant immunomodulator [28]. MTX was given only to those who had previous thiopurine intolerance. It was administered parenterally at 15 mg/week after a 12-week induction of 25 mg/week. Those researchers found that MTX was as effective at reducing ADA formation as AZA, and both significantly reduced the risk of ADA formation compared to IFX monotherapy. They also showed that there was no significant difference in the rate of ADAs in those who started their concomitant immunomodulators > 3 months prior to commencing IFX compared to those who started the immunomodulators at the time of IFX induction. There was no difference in the median IFX level in those receiving AZA or MTX; this was measured 4 weeks after each infusion (6.15 µg/mL vs. 5.65 µg/mL, respectively; $p = 0.27$) [28].

4. Optimal Methotrexate Dosing for Concomitant Immunomodulation

The optimal dose and route of administration of MTX to optimise anti-TNF levels and prevent ADA formation is yet to be determined. When used as a monotherapy for IBD, MTX has traditionally been given parenterally and in high doses of 15–25 mg weekly [56]. However, high-dose subcutaneous administration may be unnecessary when MTX is used for the purpose of augmenting the pharmacokinetics of anti-TNF agents (Tables 1 and 2).

Oral MTX has been shown to be as effective as parenteral administration in improving clinical outcomes when used in combination with anti-TNFs [30,33], although there is a paucity of data available for direct comparison. A retrospective review of over 200 patients demonstrated no differences in clinical outcomes such as IBD-related hospitalisations or surgery, change in biologic therapy, and steroid initiation between concomitant oral and parenteral MTX [33]. MTX is absorbed in the proximal jejunum to a varying extent between individuals, resulting in a bioavailability ranging from 30 to 90% [62]. This was demonstrated in patients with a range of rheumatological and dermatological conditions and appears to be independent of gastrointestinal disease involvement. Indeed, two small studies of patients with quiescent CD found oral MTX to have a bioavailability of 73–86% compared to subcutaneous administration [63,64]. Evidence around potential reduced absorption in those with proximal small bowel disease is lacking [65].

The saturable, dose-dependent mechanism of MTX absorption means the bioavailability of the oral formulation is higher at lower doses of up to 15 mg [65]. This explains why MTX, at low doses of 10–12.5 mg/week, is sufficient to reduce ADA formation and increase anti-TNF levels in both rheumatology and IBD [19,29,34,35,37], as exemplified in the CON-

CERTO trial [35]. This large randomised double-blind parallel-armed study investigated the effects of oral MTX at 2.5 mg, 5 mg, 10 mg, and 20 mg/week doses in combination with ADL in almost 400 patients with rheumatoid arthritis. There were lower rates of ADAs with increasing doses of MTX of up to 10 mg, with corresponding increases in the mean ADL levels, of up to 6.5 µg/mL, for those on 10 mg/week compared to 4.4 µg/mL in the 2.5 mg/week group. This dose-dependent effect was limited to a ceiling of 10 mg/week, with no difference in ADL levels compared to the 20 mg/week group. Improvement in clinical disease activity also plateaued at an MTX dose of 10 mg/week. These results have been reiterated in IBD cohorts with MTX doses of 10–12.5 mg/week [19,29,33]. A prospective cohort study of patients with IBD on IFX found that concomitant oral MTX improved trough levels to 17.1 µg/mL compared to 3.8 µg/mL in those on IFX monotherapy ($p = 0.001$). The improvement in IFX levels with MTX was numerically higher than that with thiopurines (14.5 µg/mL), although this did not reach significance ($p = 0.07$). The majority of the patients in the MTX group received doses of 12.5 mg/week [19]. Similarly, a cross-sectional study of over 200 paediatric patients found that concomitant low-dose oral MTX increased IFX trough levels to 15.59 µg/mL compared to 12.35 µg/mL in those who received IFX monotherapy ($p = 0.01$) [29].

Role of Therapeutic Drug Monitoring in Guiding Methotrexate Dosing

Although TDM and metabolite monitoring are well-established for anti-TNFs and thiopurines, there is no such role to guide MTX administration. MTX is a prodrug that only inhibits purine synthesis once it has had a number of glutamic acid residues added to it to form MTX polyglutamates [66]. Long-chain MTX-polyglutamates (MTX-PGs) are not effluxed efficiently from cells and therefore are a measure of intra-cellular MTX concentration [67]. A systematic review of the use of MTX-PG monitoring in inflammatory arthropathies has demonstrated that there may be a role for TDM in targeting disease activity but that it was not useful in predicting MTX toxicity or AEs [68]. A small cross-sectional study in a paediatric Crohn's cohort found a trend towards increased short-chain MTX-PGs in those who were in remission compared to those with active disease [67]. Conversely, a similar retrospective study in adult IBD patients found that increased long-chain MTX-PG concentrations were associated with worse clinical disease activity and a higher rate of AEs [69]. Given this paucity of evidence, there is no established role for TDM of MTX via polyglutamate testing.

5. Safety Profile of Methotrexate as a Concomitant Immunomodulator with Anti-TNF Agents

The side effect profile of thiopurines has been well-described, with a range of mild-to-moderate AEs reported [26,70]; however, it is the more serious AEs, including infections, NMSC, and lymphoma, associated with their prolonged use that cause concern. These risks are increased when thiopurines are used in combination with anti-TNF agents [27,71–75].

MTX has a similar mild-to-moderate side effect profile to that of thiopurines. In fact, a retrospective cohort study of almost 800 patients with IBD found that those on MTX were more likely to discontinue treatment due to nausea, fatigue, and hepatotoxicity than those on thiopurines [70]. Meanwhile, patients who took thiopurines had higher rates of pancreatitis and lower leukocyte and neutrophil counts at 1 year. The patients on MTX were older and had higher rates of prior immunomodulator intolerance compared to those on thiopurines. Oral MTX was better tolerated than subcutaneous administration, with significantly less fatigue (3% vs. 10%, respectively; $p = 0.04$) and a trend towards lower discontinuation rates (32% vs. 45%, respectively; $p = 0.07$). The researchers of that study also found that lower doses (<20 mg oral or <15 mg subcutaneous) were better tolerated, with numerically lower discontinuation rates (24% vs. 40%, respectively; $p = 0.19$) compared to higher doses ($\geq$20 mg oral or $\geq$15 mg subcutaneous). Of note is that these lower doses are still higher than is required for concomitant immunomodulation with anti-TNF therapy.

Supplementation with folic acid reduces the incidence of gastrointestinal side effects and hepatotoxicity, improves tolerability, and helps prevent cytopenias [76,77].

More serious but less common AEs of MTX include interstitial lung disease and pleural or pericardial serositis [78,79]. MTX is not, however, associated with lymphoproliferative disorders when used in monotherapy or in combination with anti-TNF agents [80]. Combination immunosuppressive therapy has raised concern around increasing risk of infective complications. Indeed, a population-based French study of over 190,000 IBD patients showed that concomitant thiopurine and anti-TNF therapy increased the risk of serious and opportunistic infections compared to anti-TNF monotherapy [72]. This same risk is not apparent with concomitant MTX. A large retrospective registry study of almost 8000 patients with rheumatoid arthritis reviewed the risk of infections in patients on combination MTX (mean dose of 13.2 mg/week) and anti-TNF therapy compared to monotherapy with either agent [81]. These data followed patients for 15,047 patient-years. Surprisingly, there were no increased rates of infection in those on concomitant MTX and anti-TNF compared to those on anti-TNF monotherapy (37.1/100 person-years, 95% CI [34.9–39.3] vs. 41.8/100 person-years, 95% CI [37.0–43.3], respectively) [81]. Whilst the risk may differ between rheumatoid arthritis and IBD, these data suggest that MTX may have a lower rate of infective complications than thiopurines.

6. Recommendations for the Use of Low-Dose Oral Methotrexate in Combination with Anti-TNF Agents

Given the potential safety benefits and demonstrated pharmacokinetic efficacy, we suggest clinicians consider using low-dose oral MTX as an alternative to thiopurines for concomitant immunomodulation with anti-TNF therapy for IBD. Low-dose oral MTX is particularly suitable when the primary aim of the concomitant immunomodulation is to reduce immunogenicity and increase anti-TNF drug levels rather than as a second therapeutic agent to treat active disease. Other clinical scenarios where low-dose MTX should be considered for concomitant immunomodulation include:

- EBV-naïve patients, especially males (due to the risk of lymphoproliferative disorders);
- Young males (due to the rare but devastating risk of hepatosplenic T-cell lymphoma);
- Thiopurine-intolerant patients;
- Homozygous thiopurine methyltransferase (TMPT)- or Nudix hydrolase-15 (NUDT15)-deficient patients.

Whilst MTX is contraindicated in pregnancy and should be discontinued at least 3 months prior to conception, it has been shown to be safe in males who are planning on fathering a child [82]. MTX should be avoided in those with chronic liver disease, and dose reductions may be required for those with renal impairment.

7. Conclusions

The available evidence suggests that MTX has comparable efficacy to thiopurines in augmenting the pharmacokinetics of anti-TNF agents. It has also been demonstrated to eliminate ADAs, increase trough levels, and recapture clinical responses in those with loss of response and on anti-TNF monotherapy. There are, however, a lack of head-to-head data comparing these two agents as concomitant immunomodulators. Given the heterogeneity of the dosing regimens that have been studied to date, further investigation with more stringent subgroup analyses and consistent MTX doses will help clarify these findings. Overall, low-dose oral MTX (i.e., 10–12.5 mg weekly) is better tolerated and appears to be as effective as higher-dose parenteral administration in improving anti-TNF pharmacokinetics. Furthermore, given a potentially more favourable serious AE profile compared to thiopurines, low-dose oral MTX may be considered as an alternative first-line option for concomitant immunomodulation alongside anti-TNF therapy.

Author Contributions: Conceptualisation, K.D., R.D.L. and M.P.S.; methodology, K.D., R.D.L. and M.P.S.; literature search and screening, K.D.; original draft preparation, K.D. and C.K.M.; review and editing, K.D., C.K.M., R.D.L. and M.P.S.; supervision, R.D.L. and M.P.S. All authors have read and agreed to the published version of the manuscript.

Funding: This research received no external funding.

Conflicts of Interest: R.D.L. has received educational support from Celltrion Healthcare and Janssen and research support from Celltrion Healthcare. M.P.S. has received educational grants or research support from Ferring, Orphan, Gilead, and Celltrion; has received speaker's fees from Janssen, Abbvie, Ferring, Takeda, Pfizer, Shire, and Celltrion; and has served on advisory boards for Janssen, Takeda, Pfizer, Celgene, Abbvie, MSD, Emerge Health, Gilead, BMS, and Celltrion.

References

1. Hanauer, S.B.; Feagan, B.G.; Lichtenstein, G.R.; Mayer, L.F.; Schreiber, S.; Colombel, J.F.; Rachmilewitz, D.; Wolf, D.C.; Olson, A.; Bao, W.; et al. Maintenance infliximab for Crohn's disease: The ACCENT I randomised trial. *Lancet* **2002**, *359*, 1541–1549. [CrossRef]
2. Rutgeerts, P.; Sandborn, W.J.; Feagan, B.G.; Reinisch, W.; Olson, A.; Johanns, J.; Travers, S.; Rachmilewitz, D.; Hanauer, S.B.; Lichtenstein, G.R.; et al. Infliximab for induction and maintenance therapy for ulcerative colitis. *N. Engl. J. Med.* **2005**, *353*, 2462–2476. [CrossRef] [PubMed]
3. Hanauer, S.B.; Sandborn, W.J.; Rutgeerts, P.; Fedorak, R.N.; Lukas, M.; MacIntosh, D.; Panaccione, R.; Wolf, D.; Pollack, P. Human anti-tumor necrosis factor monoclonal antibody (adalimumab) in Crohn's disease: The CLASSIC-I trial. *Gastroenterology* **2006**, *130*, 323–333. [CrossRef] [PubMed]
4. Sandborn, W.J.; Hanauer, S.B.; Rutgeerts, P.; Fedorak, R.N.; Lukas, M.; MacIntosh, D.G.; Panaccione, R.; Wolf, D.; Kent, J.D.; Bittle, B.; et al. Adalimumab for maintenance treatment of Crohn's disease: Results of the CLASSIC II trial. *Gut* **2007**, *56*, 1232–1239. [CrossRef]
5. Colombel, J.F.; Sandborn, W.J.; Rutgeerts, P.; Enns, R.; Hanauer, S.B.; Panaccione, R.; Schreiber, S.; Byczkowski, D.; Li, J.; Kent, J.D.; et al. Adalimumab for maintenance of clinical response and remission in patients with Crohn's disease: The CHARM trial. *Gastroenterology* **2007**, *132*, 52–65. [CrossRef] [PubMed]
6. Sands, B.E.; Anderson, F.H.; Bernstein, C.N.; Chey, W.Y.; Feagan, B.G.; Fedorak, R.N.; Kamm, M.A.; Korzenik, J.R.; Lashner, B.A.; Onken, J.E.; et al. Infliximab maintenance therapy for fistulizing Crohn's disease. *N. Engl. J. Med.* **2004**, *350*, 876–885. [CrossRef]
7. D'Haens, G.R.; van Deventer, S. 25 years of anti-TNF treatment for inflammatory bowel disease: Lessons from the past and a look to the future. *Gut* **2021**, *70*, 1396–1405. [CrossRef]
8. Steenholdt, C.; Brynskov, J.; Thomsen, O.Ø.; Munck, L.K.; Fallingborg, J.; Christensen, L.A.; Pedersen, G.; Kjeldsen, J.; Jacobsen, B.A.; Oxholm, A.S.; et al. Individualised therapy is more cost-effective than dose intensification in patients with Crohn's disease who lose response to anti-TNF treatment: A randomised, controlled trial. *Gut* **2014**, *63*, 919–927. [CrossRef]
9. Adedokun, O.J.; Sandborn, W.J.; Feagan, B.G.; Rutgeerts, P.; Xu, Z.; Marano, C.W.; Johanns, J.; Zhou, H.; Davis, H.M.; Cornillie, F.; et al. Association between serum concentration of infliximab and efficacy in adult patients with ulcerative colitis. *Gastroenterology* **2014**, *147*, 1296–1307.e5. [CrossRef]
10. Gibson, D.J.; Ward, M.G.; Rentsch, C.; Friedman, A.B.; Taylor, K.M.; Sparrow, M.P.; Gibson, P.R. Review article: Determination of the therapeutic range for therapeutic drug monitoring of adalimumab and infliximab in patients with inflammatory bowel disease. *Aliment. Pharmacol. Ther.* **2020**, *51*, 612–628. [CrossRef]
11. Mitrev, N.; Vande Casteele, N.; Seow, C.H.; Andrews, J.M.; Connor, S.J.; Moore, G.T.; Barclay, M.; Begun, J.; Bryant, R.; Chan, W.; et al. Review article: Consensus statements on therapeutic drug monitoring of anti-tumour necrosis factor therapy in inflammatory bowel diseases. *Aliment. Pharmacol. Ther.* **2017**, *46*, 1037–1053. [CrossRef]
12. Ungar, B.; Levy, I.; Yavne, Y.; Yavzori, M.; Picard, O.; Fudim, E.; Loebstein, R.; Chowers, Y.; Eliakim, R.; Kopylov, U.; et al. Optimizing Anti-TNF-α Therapy: Serum Levels of Infliximab and Adalimumab Are Associated with Mucosal Healing in Patients with Inflammatory Bowel Diseases. *Clin. Gastroenterol. Hepatol.* **2016**, *14*, 550–557.e2. [CrossRef] [PubMed]
13. Yarur, A.J.; Kanagala, V.; Stein, D.J.; Czul, F.; Quintero, M.A.; Agrawal, D.; Patel, A.; Best, K.; Fox, C.; Idstein, K.; et al. Higher infliximab trough levels are associated with perianal fistula healing in patients with Crohn's disease. *Aliment. Pharmacol. Ther.* **2017**, *45*, 933–940. [CrossRef] [PubMed]
14. Mitrev, N.; Kariyawasam, V.; Leong, R.W. Editorial: Infliximab trough cut-off for perianal Crohn's disease—another piece of the therapeutic drug monitoring-guided infliximab dosing puzzle. *Aliment. Pharmacol. Ther.* **2017**, *45*, 1279–1280. [CrossRef] [PubMed]
15. Papamichael, K.; Cheifetz, A.S.; Melmed, G.Y.; Irving, P.M.; Vande Casteele, N.; Kozuch, P.L.; Raffals, L.E.; Baidoo, L.; Bressler, B.; Devlin, S.M.; et al. Appropriate Therapeutic Drug Monitoring of Biologic Agents for Patients with Inflammatory Bowel Diseases. *Clin. Gastroenterol. Hepatol.* **2019**, *17*, 1655–1668.e3. [CrossRef] [PubMed]
16. Cheifetz, A.S.; Abreu, M.T.; Afif, W.; Cross, R.K.; Dubinsky, M.C.; Loftus, E.V.; Osterman, M.T.; Saroufim, A.; Siegel, C.A.; Yarur, A.J.; et al. A Comprehensive Literature Review and Expert Consensus Statement on Therapeutic Drug Monitoring of Biologics in Inflammatory Bowel Disease. *Am. J. Gastroenterol.* **2021**, *116*, 2014–2025. [CrossRef]

17. Garcês, S.; Demengeot, J.; Benito-Garcia, E. The immunogenicity of anti-TNF therapy in immune-mediated inflammatory diseases: A systematic review of the literature with a meta-analysis. *Ann. Rheum. Dis.* **2013**, *72*, 1947–1955. [CrossRef] [PubMed]
18. Thomas, S.S.; Borazan, N.; Barroso, N.; Duan, L.; Taroumian, S.; Kretzmann, B.; Bardales, R.; Elashoff, D.; Vangala, S.; Furst, D.E. Comparative Immunogenicity of TNF Inhibitors: Impact on Clinical Efficacy and Tolerability in the Management of Autoimmune Diseases. A Systematic Review and Meta-Analysis. *BioDrugs Clin. Immunother. Biopharm. Gene Ther.* **2015**, *29*, 241–258. [CrossRef]
19. Yarur, A.J.; McGovern, D.; Abreu, M.T.; Cheifetz, A.; Papamichail, K.; Deepak, P.; Bruss, A.; Beniwal-Patel, P.; Dubinsky, M.; Targan, S.R.; et al. Combination Therapy with Immunomodulators Improves the Pharmacokinetics of Infliximab But Not Vedolizumab or Ustekinumab. *Clin. Gastroenterol. Hepatol.* **2022**, *22*, S1542–S3565. [CrossRef]
20. Karmiris, K.; Paintaud, G.; Noman, M.; Magdelaine-Beuzelin, C.; Ferrante, M.; Degenne, D.; Claes, K.; Coopman, T.; Van Schuerbeek, N.; Van Assche, G.; et al. Influence of trough serum levels and immunogenicity on long-term outcome of adalimumab therapy in Crohn's disease. *Gastroenterology* **2009**, *137*, 1628–1640. [CrossRef]
21. Matar, M.; Shamir, R.; Turner, D.; Broide, E.; Weiss, B.; Ledder, O.; Guz-Mark, A.; Rinawi, F.; Cohen, S.; Topf-Olivestone, C.; et al. Combination Therapy of Adalimumab with an Immunomodulator Is Not More Effective Than Adalimumab Monotherapy in Children With Crohn's Disease: A Post Hoc Analysis of the PAILOT Randomized Controlled Trial. *Inflamm. Bowel Dis.* **2020**, *26*, 1627–1635. [CrossRef] [PubMed]
22. Matsumoto, T.; Motoya, S.; Watanabe, K.; Hisamatsu, T.; Nakase, H.; Yoshimura, N.; Ishida, T.; Kato, S.; Nakagawa, T.; Esaki, M.; et al. Adalimumab Monotherapy and a Combination with Azathioprine for Crohn's Disease: A Prospective, Randomized Trial. *J. Crohn's Colitis* **2016**, *10*, 1259–1266. [CrossRef] [PubMed]
23. Kennedy, N.A.; Heap, G.A.; Green, H.D.; Hamilton, B.; Bewshea, C.; Walker, G.J.; Thomas, A.; Nice, R.; Perry, M.H.; Bouri, S.; et al. Predictors of anti-TNF treatment failure in anti-TNF-naive patients with active luminal Crohn's disease: A prospective, multicentre, cohort study. *Lancet. Gastroenterol. Hepatol.* **2019**, *4*, 341–353. [CrossRef]
24. Kopylov, U.; Al-Taweel, T.; Yaghoobi, M.; Nauche, B.; Bitton, A.; Lakatos, P.L.; Ben-Horin, S.; Afif, W.; Seidman, E.G. Adalimumab monotherapy versus combination therapy with immunomodulators in patients with Crohn's disease: A systematic review and meta-analysis. *J. Crohn's Colitis* **2014**, *8*, 1632–1641. [CrossRef]
25. Chalhoub, J.M.; Rimmani, H.H.; Gumaste, V.V.; Sharara, A.I. Systematic Review and Meta-analysis: Adalimumab Monotherapy Versus Combination Therapy with Immunomodulators for Induction and Maintenance of Remission and Response in Patients with Crohn's Disease. *Inflamm. Bowel Dis.* **2017**, *23*, 1316–1327. [CrossRef] [PubMed]
26. Luber, R.P.; Honap, S.; Cunningham, G.; Irving, P.M. Can We Predict the Toxicity and Response to Thiopurines in Inflammatory Bowel Diseases? *Front. Med.* **2019**, *6*, 279. [CrossRef] [PubMed]
27. Kotlyar, D.S.; Osterman, M.T.; Diamond, R.H.; Porter, D.; Blonski, W.C.; Wasik, M.; Sampat, S.; Mendizabal, M.; Lin, M.V.; Lichtenstein, G.R. A systematic review of factors that contribute to hepatosplenic T-cell lymphoma in patients with inflammatory bowel disease. *Clin. Gastroenterol. Hepatol.* **2011**, *9*, 36–41.e1. [CrossRef] [PubMed]
28. Vermeire, S.; Noman, M.; Van Assche, G.; Baert, F.; D'Haens, G.; Rutgeerts, P. Effectiveness of concomitant immunosuppressive therapy in suppressing the formation of antibodies to infliximab in Crohn's disease. *Gut* **2007**, *56*, 1226–1231. [CrossRef]
29. Chi, L.Y.; Zitomersky, N.L.; Liu, E.; Tollefson, S.; Bender-Stern, J.; Naik, S.; Snapper, S.; Bousvaros, A. The Impact of Combination Therapy on Infliximab Levels and Antibodies in Children and Young Adults with Inflammatory Bowel Disease. *Inflamm. Bowel Dis.* **2018**, *24*, 1344–1351. [CrossRef]
30. Colman, R.J.; Rubin, D.T. Optimal doses of methotrexate combined with anti-TNF therapy to maintain clinical remission in inflammatory bowel disease. *J. Crohn's Colitis* **2015**, *9*, 312–317. [CrossRef]
31. Ungar, B.; Kopylov, U.; Engel, T.; Yavzori, M.; Fudim, E.; Picard, O.; Lang, A.; Williet, N.; Paul, S.; Chowers, Y.; et al. Addition of an immunomodulator can reverse antibody formation and loss of response in patients treated with adalimumab. *Aliment. Pharmacol. Ther.* **2017**, *45*, 276–282. [CrossRef]
32. Vasudevan, A.; Raghunath, A.; Anthony, S.; Scanlon, C.; Sparrow, M.P.; Gibson, P.R.; van Langenberg, D.R. Higher Mucosal Healing with Tumor Necrosis Factor Inhibitors in Combination with Thiopurines Compared to Methotrexate in Crohn's Disease. *Dig. Dis. Sci.* **2019**, *64*, 1622–1631. [CrossRef] [PubMed]
33. Borren, N.Z.; Luther, J.; Colizzo, F.P.; Garber, J.G.; Khalili, H.; Ananthakrishnan, A.N. Low-dose Methotrexate has Similar Outcomes to High-dose Methotrexate in Combination with Anti-TNF Therapy in Inflammatory Bowel Diseases. *J. Crohn's Colitis* **2019**, *13*, 990–995. [CrossRef] [PubMed]
34. Maini, R.N.; Breedveld, F.C.; Kalden, J.R.; Smolen, J.S.; Davis, D.; Macfarlane, J.D.; Antoni, C.; Leeb, B.; Elliott, M.J.; Woody, J.N.; et al. Therapeutic efficacy of multiple intravenous infusions of anti-tumor necrosis factor alpha monoclonal antibody combined with low-dose weekly methotrexate in rheumatoid arthritis. *Arthritis Rheumatol.* **1998**, *41*, 1552–1563. [CrossRef]
35. Burmester, G.R.; Kivitz, A.J.; Kupper, H.; Arulmani, U.; Florentinus, S.; Goss, S.L.; Rathmann, S.S.; Fleischmann, R.M. Efficacy and safety of ascending methotrexate dose in combination with adalimumab: The randomised CONCERTO trial. *Ann. Rheum. Dis.* **2015**, *74*, 1037–1044. [CrossRef] [PubMed]
36. Ducourau, E.; Rispens, T.; Samain, M.; Dernis, E.; Le Guilchard, F.; Andras, L.; Perdriger, A.; Lespessailles, E.; Martin, A.; Cormier, G.; et al. Methotrexate effect on immunogenicity and long-term maintenance of adalimumab in axial spondyloarthritis: A multicentric randomised trial. *RMD Open* **2020**, *6*, e001047. [CrossRef]

37. van der Kraaij, G.; Busard, C.; van den Reek, J.; Menting, S.; Musters, A.; Hutten, B.; de Rie, M.; Ouwerkerk, W.; van Bezooijen, S.J.; Prens, E.; et al. Adalimumab with Methotrexate vs. Adalimumab Monotherapy in Psoriasis: First-Year Results of a Single-Blind Randomized Controlled Trial. *J. Investig. Dermatol.* **2022**, *142*, 2375–2383.e6. [CrossRef]
38. Ben-Horin, S.; Chowers, Y. Review article: Loss of response to anti-TNF treatments in Crohn's disease. *Aliment. Pharmacol. Ther.* **2011**, *33*, 987–995. [CrossRef]
39. Brandse, J.F.; van den Brink, G.R.; Wildenberg, M.E.; van der Kleij, D.; Rispens, T.; Jansen, J.M.; Mathôt, R.A.; Ponsioen, C.Y.; Löwenberg, M.; D'Haens, G.R. Loss of Infliximab into Feces Is Associated with Lack of Response to Therapy in Patients with Severe Ulcerative Colitis. *Gastroenterology* **2015**, *149*, 350–355.e2. [CrossRef]
40. Fasanmade, A.A.; Adedokun, O.J.; Ford, J.; Hernandez, D.; Johanns, J.; Hu, C.; Davis, H.M.; Zhou, H. Population pharmacokinetic analysis of infliximab in patients with ulcerative colitis. *Eur. J. Clin. Pharmacol.* **2009**, *65*, 1211–1228. [CrossRef]
41. Kuo, T.T.; Aveson, V.G. Neonatal Fc receptor and IgG-based therapeutics. *mAbs* **2011**, *3*, 422–430. [CrossRef] [PubMed]
42. Roblin, X.; Marotte, H.; Leclerc, M.; Del Tedesco, E.; Phelip, J.M.; Peyrin-Biroulet, L.; Paul, S. Combination of C-reactive protein, infliximab trough levels, and stable but not transient antibodies to infliximab are associated with loss of response to infliximab in inflammatory bowel disease. *J. Crohn's Colitis* **2015**, *9*, 525–531. [CrossRef] [PubMed]
43. Brandse, J.F.; Mathôt, R.A.; van der Kleij, D.; Rispens, T.; Ashruf, Y.; Jansen, J.M.; Rietdijk, S.; Löwenberg, M.; Ponsioen, C.Y.; Singh, S.; et al. Pharmacokinetic Features and Presence of Antidrug Antibodies Associate with Response to Infliximab Induction Therapy in Patients With Moderate to Severe Ulcerative Colitis. *Clin. Gastroenterol. Hepatol.* **2016**, *14*, 251–258.e2. [CrossRef] [PubMed]
44. Ben-Horin, S.; Yavzori, M.; Katz, L.; Kopylov, U.; Picard, O.; Fudim, E.; Coscas, D.; Bar-Meir, S.; Goldstein, I.; Chowers, Y. The immunogenic part of infliximab is the F(ab')2, but measuring antibodies to the intact infliximab molecule is more clinically useful. *Gut* **2011**, *60*, 41–48. [CrossRef] [PubMed]
45. Ternant, D.; Aubourg, A.; Magdelaine-Beuzelin, C.; Degenne, D.; Watier, H.; Picon, L.; Paintaud, G. Infliximab pharmacokinetics in inflammatory bowel disease patients. *Ther. Drug Monit.* **2008**, *30*, 523–529. [CrossRef]
46. Buurman, D.J.; Maurer, J.M.; Keizer, R.J.; Kosterink, J.G.; Dijkstra, G. Population pharmacokinetics of infliximab in patients with inflammatory bowel disease: Potential implications for dosing in clinical practice. *Aliment. Pharmacol. Ther.* **2015**, *42*, 529–539. [CrossRef]
47. Colombel, J.F.; Sandborn, W.J.; Reinisch, W.; Mantzaris, G.J.; Kornbluth, A.; Rachmilewitz, D.; Lichtiger, S.; D'Haens, G.; Diamond, R.H.; Broussard, D.L.; et al. Infliximab, azathioprine, or combination therapy for Crohn's disease. *N. Engl. J. Med.* **2010**, *362*, 1383–1395. [CrossRef]
48. Colombel, J.F.; Adedokun, O.J.; Gasink, C.; Gao, L.L.; Cornillie, F.J.; D'Haens, G.R.; Rutgeerts, P.J.; Reinisch, W.; Sandborn, W.J.; Hanauer, S.B. Combination Therapy with Infliximab and Azathioprine Improves Infliximab Pharmacokinetic Features and Efficacy: A Post Hoc Analysis. *Clin. Gastroenterol. Hepatol.* **2019**, *17*, 1525–1532.e1. [CrossRef]
49. Macaluso, F.S.; Sapienza, C.; Ventimiglia, M.; Renna, S.; Rizzuto, G.; Orlando, R.; Di Pisa, M.; Affronti, M.; Orlando, E.; Cottone, M.; et al. The addition of an immunosuppressant after loss of response to anti-tnfalpha monotherapy in inflammatory bowel disease: A 2-year study. *Inflamm. Bowel Dis.* **2018**, *24*, 394–401. [CrossRef]
50. Nielsen, O.H.; Coskun, M.; Steenholdt, C.; Rogler, G. The role and advances of immunomodulator therapy for inflammatory bowel disease. *Expert Rev. Gastroenterol. Hepatol.* **2015**, *9*, 177–189. [CrossRef]
51. Herfarth, H.; Barnes, E.L.; Valentine, J.F.; Hanson, J.; Higgins, P.D.R.; Isaacs, K.L.; Jackson, S.; Osterman, M.T.; Anton, K.; Ivanova, A.; et al. Methotrexate Is Not Superior to Placebo in Maintaining Steroid-Free Response or Remission in Ulcerative Colitis. *Gastroenterology* **2018**, *155*, 1098–1108.e9. [CrossRef] [PubMed]
52. Chande, N.; Wang, Y.; MacDonald, J.K.; McDonald, J.W. Methotrexate for induction of remission in ulcerative colitis. *Cochrane Database Syst. Rev.* **2014**, *2014*, CD006618. [CrossRef] [PubMed]
53. Bendtzen, K. Is there a need for immunopharmacologic guidance of anti-tumor necrosis factor therapies? *Arthritis Rheumatol.* **2011**, *63*, 867–870. [CrossRef]
54. Garman, R.D.; Munroe, K.; Richards, S.M. Methotrexate reduces antibody responses to recombinant human alpha-galactosidase A therapy in a mouse model of Fabry disease. *Clin. Exp. Immunol.* **2004**, *137*, 496–502. [CrossRef] [PubMed]
55. Joseph, A.; Munroe, K.; Housman, M.; Garman, R.; Richards, S. Immune tolerance induction to enzyme-replacement therapy by co-administration of short-term, low-dose methotrexate in a murine Pompe disease model. *Clin. Exp. Immunol.* **2008**, *152*, 138–146. [CrossRef] [PubMed]
56. Torres, J.; Bonovas, S.; Doherty, G.; Kucharzik, T.; Gisbert, J.P.; Raine, T.; Adamina, M.; Armuzzi, A.; Bachmann, O.; Bager, P.; et al. ECCO Guidelines on Therapeutics in Crohn's Disease: Medical Treatment. *J. Crohn's Colitis* **2020**, *14*, 4–22. [CrossRef]
57. Sunseri, W.; Hyams, J.S.; Lerer, T.; Mack, D.R.; Griffiths, A.M.; Otley, A.R.; Rosh, J.R.; Carvalho, R.; Grossman, A.B.; Cabrera, J.; et al. Retrospective cohort study of methotrexate use in the treatment of pediatric Crohn's disease. *Inflamm. Bowel Dis.* **2014**, *20*, 1341–1345. [CrossRef]
58. Feagan, B.G.; McDonald, J.W.; Panaccione, R.; Enns, R.A.; Bernstein, C.N.; Ponich, T.P.; Bourdages, R.; Macintosh, D.G.; Dallaire, C.; Cohen, A.; et al. Methotrexate in combination with infliximab is no more effective than infliximab alone in patients with Crohn's disease. *Gastroenterology* **2014**, *146*, 681–688.e1. [CrossRef]

59. Kappelman, M.D.; Wohl, D.A.; Herfarth, H.H.; Firestine, A.M.; Adler, J.; Ammoury, R.F.; Aronow, J.E.; Bass, D.M.; Bass, J.A.; Benkov, K.; et al. Comparative Effectiveness of Anti-TNF in Combination with Low-Dose Methotrexate vs Anti-TNF Monotherapy in Pediatric Crohn's Disease: A Pragmatic Randomized Trial. *Gastroenterology* **2023**, *165*, 149–161.e7. [CrossRef]
60. Ben-Horin, S.; Waterman, M.; Kopylov, U.; Yavzori, M.; Picard, O.; Fudim, E.; Awadie, H.; Weiss, B.; Chowers, Y. Addition of an immunomodulator to infliximab therapy eliminates antidrug antibodies in serum and restores clinical response of patients with inflammatory bowel disease. *Clin. Gastroenterol. Hepatol.* **2013**, *11*, 444–447. [CrossRef] [PubMed]
61. Stallhofer, J.; Guse, J.; Kesselmeier, M.; Grunert, P.C.; Lange, K.; Stalmann, R.; Eckardt, V.; Stallmach, A. Immunomodulator comedication promotes the reversal of anti-drug antibody-mediated loss of response to anti-TNF therapy in inflammatory bowel disease. *Int. J. Color. Dis.* **2023**, *38*, 54. [CrossRef]
62. van Roon, E.N.; van de Laar, M.A. Methotrexate bioavailability. *Clin. Exp. Rheumatol.* **2010**, *28*, S27–S32.
63. Wilson, A.; Patel, V.; Chande, N.; Ponich, T.; Urquhart, B.; Asher, L.; Choi, Y.; Tirona, R.; Kim, R.B.; Gregor, J.C. Pharmacokinetic profiles for oral and subcutaneous methotrexate in patients with Crohn's disease. *Aliment. Pharmacol. Ther.* **2013**, *37*, 340–345. [CrossRef]
64. Kurnik, D.; Loebstein, R.; Fishbein, E.; Almog, S.; Halkin, H.; Bar-Meir, S.; Chowers, Y. Bioavailability of oral vs. subcutaneous low-dose methotrexate in patients with Crohn's disease. *Aliment. Pharmacol. Ther.* **2003**, *18*, 57–63. [CrossRef] [PubMed]
65. Cassinotti, A.; Batticciotto, A.; Parravicini, M.; Lombardo, M.; Radice, P.; Cortelezzi, C.C.; Segato, S.; Zanzi, F.; Cappelli, A.; Segato, S. Evidence-based efficacy of methotrexate in adult Crohn's disease in different intestinal and extraintestinal indications. *Ther. Adv. Gastroenterol.* **2022**, *15*. [CrossRef]
66. Goss, S.L.; Klein, C.E.; Jin, Z.; Locke, C.S.; Rodila, R.C.; Kupper, H.; Burmester, G.R.; Awni, W.M. Methotrexate Dose in Patients With Early Rheumatoid Arthritis Impacts Methotrexate Polyglutamate Pharmacokinetics, Adalimumab Pharmacokinetics, and Efficacy: Pharmacokinetic and Exposure-response Analysis of the CONCERTO Trial. *Clin. Ther.* **2018**, *40*, 309–319. [CrossRef] [PubMed]
67. Morrow, R.; Funk, R.; Becker, M.; Sherman, A.; Van Haandel, L.; Hudson, T.; Casini, R.; Shakhnovich, V. Potential Role of Methotrexate Polyglutamates in Therapeutic Drug Monitoring for Pediatric Inflammatory Bowel Disease. *Pharmaceuticals* **2021**, *14*, 463. [CrossRef] [PubMed]
68. Mohamed, H.J.; Sorich, M.J.; Kowalski, S.M.; McKinnon, R.; Proudman, S.M.; Cleland, L.; Wiese, M.D. The role and utility of measuring red blood cell methotrexate polyglutamate concentrations in inflammatory arthropathies—A systematic review. *Eur. J. Clin. Pharmacol.* **2015**, *71*, 411–423. [CrossRef]
69. Brooks, A.J.; Begg, E.J.; Zhang, M.; Frampton, C.M.; Barclay, M.L. Red blood cell methotrexate polyglutamate concentrations in inflammatory bowel disease. *Ther. Drug Monit.* **2007**, *29*, 619–625. [CrossRef]
70. Vasudevan, A.; Parthasarathy, N.; Con, D.; Nicolaides, S.; Apostolov, R.; Chauhan, A.; Bishara, M.; Luber, R.P.; Joshi, N.; Wan, A.; et al. Thiopurines vs methotrexate: Comparing tolerability and discontinuation rates in the treatment of inflammatory bowel disease. *Aliment. Pharmacol. Ther.* **2020**, *52*, 1174–1184. [CrossRef]
71. Singh, S.; Facciorusso, A.; Dulai, P.S.; Jairath, V.; Sandborn, W.J. Comparative Risk of Serious Infections with Biologic and/or Immunosuppressive Therapy in Patients with Inflammatory Bowel Diseases: A Systematic Review and Meta-Analysis. *Clin. Gastroenterol. Hepatol.* **2020**, *18*, 69–81.e3. [CrossRef] [PubMed]
72. Kirchgesner, J.; Lemaitre, M.; Carrat, F.; Zureik, M.; Carbonnel, F.; Dray-Spira, R. Risk of Serious and Opportunistic Infections Associated with Treatment of Inflammatory Bowel Diseases. *Gastroenterology* **2018**, *155*, 337–346.e10. [CrossRef] [PubMed]
73. Peyrin-Biroulet, L.; Khosrotehrani, K.; Carrat, F.; Bouvier, A.M.; Chevaux, J.B.; Simon, T.; Carbonnel, F.; Colombel, J.F.; Dupas, J.L.; Godeberge, P.; et al. Increased risk for nonmelanoma skin cancers in patients who receive thiopurines for inflammatory bowel disease. *Gastroenterology* **2011**, *141*, 1621–1628.e5. [CrossRef] [PubMed]
74. Siegel, C.A.; Marden, S.M.; Persing, S.M.; Larson, R.J.; Sands, B.E. Risk of lymphoma associated with combination anti-tumor necrosis factor and immunomodulator therapy for the treatment of Crohn's disease: A meta-analysis. *Clin. Gastroenterol. Hepatol.* **2009**, *7*, 874–881. [CrossRef]
75. Lemaitre, M.; Kirchgesner, J.; Rudnichi, A.; Carrat, F.; Zureik, M.; Carbonnel, F.; Dray-Spira, R. Association Between Use of Thiopurines or Tumor Necrosis Factor Antagonists Alone or in Combination and Risk of Lymphoma in Patients with Inflammatory Bowel Disease. *JAMA* **2017**, *318*, 1679–1686. [CrossRef]
76. Shea, B.; Swinden, M.V.; Tanjong Ghogomu, E.; Ortiz, Z.; Katchamart, W.; Rader, T.; Bombardier, C.; Wells, G.A.; Tugwell, P. Folic acid and folinic acid for reducing side effects in patients receiving methotrexate for rheumatoid arthritis. *Cochrane Database Syst. Rev.* **2013**, *2013*, CD000951. [CrossRef]
77. Whittle, S.L.; Hughes, R.A. Folate supplementation and methotrexate treatment in rheumatoid arthritis: A review. *Rheumatology* **2004**, *43*, 267–271. [CrossRef]
78. Kremer, J.M.; Alarcón, G.S.; Weinblatt, M.E.; Kaymakcian, M.V.; Macaluso, M.; Cannon, G.W.; Palmer, W.R.; Sundy, J.S.; St Clair, E.W.; Alexander, R.W.; et al. Clinical, laboratory, radiographic, and histopathologic features of methotrexate-associated lung injury in patients with rheumatoid arthritis: A multicenter study with literature review. *Arthritis Rheumatol.* **1997**, *40*, 1829–1837. [CrossRef]
79. Kremer, J. Major Side Effects of Low-Dose Methotrexate. Available online: https://www.uptodate.com/contents/major-side-effects-of-low-dose-methotrexate (accessed on 18 May 2023).

80. Wolfe, F.; Michaud, K. The effect of methotrexate and anti-tumor necrosis factor therapy on the risk of lymphoma in rheumatoid arthritis in 19,562 patients during 89,710 person-years of observation. *Arthritis Rheumatol.* **2007**, *56*, 1433–1439. [CrossRef]
81. Greenberg, J.D.; Reed, G.; Kremer, J.M.; Tindall, E.; Kavanaugh, A.; Zheng, C.; Bishai, W.; Hochberg, M.C. Association of methotrexate and tumour necrosis factor antagonists with risk of infectious outcomes including opportunistic infections in the CORRONA registry. *Ann. Rheum. Dis.* **2010**, *69*, 380–386. [CrossRef]
82. Sammaritano, L.R.; Bermas, B.L.; Chakravarty, E.E.; Chambers, C.; Clowse, M.E.B.; Lockshin, M.D.; Marder, W.; Guyatt, G.; Branch, D.W.; Buyon, J.; et al. 2020 American College of Rheumatology Guideline for the Management of Reproductive Health in Rheumatic and Musculoskeletal Diseases. *Arthritis Rheumatol.* **2020**, *72*, 529–556. [CrossRef] [PubMed]

Disclaimer/Publisher's Note: The statements, opinions and data contained in all publications are solely those of the individual author(s) and contributor(s) and not of MDPI and/or the editor(s). MDPI and/or the editor(s) disclaim responsibility for any injury to people or property resulting from any ideas, methods, instructions or products referred to in the content.

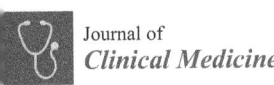

Article

Higher Adalimumab Trough Levels Are Associated with Histologic Remission and Mucosal Healing in Inflammatory Bowel Disease

Rochelle Wong [1], Lihui Qin [2], Yushan Pan [1], Prerna Mahtani [1], Randy Longman [1], Dana Lukin [1], Ellen Scherl [1] and Robert Battat [1,3,*]

[1] Division of Gastroenterology, Department of Medicine, Weill Cornell Medical College, New York, NY 10065, USA
[2] Department of Pathology, Weill Cornell Medical College, New York, NY 10065, USA
[3] Division of Gastroenterology, Centre Hospitalier de l'Universite de Montreal, Montreal, QC H2X 0C1, Canada
* Correspondence: robert.battat@umontreal.ca; Tel.: +1-514-890-8000 (ext. 30787)

Abstract: (1) Many patients with inflammatory bowel disease (IBD) in endoscopic remission have persistent histologic activity, which is associated with worse outcomes. There are limited data on the association between adalimumab drug concentrations and histologic outcomes using validated histologic indices. We aimed to assess the relationship between adalimumab concentrations and the Robarts Histopathology Index (RHI). (2) Patients from a tertiary IBD center from 2013 to 2020 with serum adalimumab (ADA) trough concentrations measured during maintenance therapy ($\geq$14 weeks) and a colonoscopy or flexible sigmoidoscopy with biopsies performed within 90 days of drug level were included. Blinded histologic scoring using the RHI was performed. Primary analysis assessed the relationship between adalimumab drug concentrations and histologic remission using receiver operating characteristic curve analysis. (3) In 36 patients (26 Crohn's Disease, 9 ulcerative colitis, 1 indeterminate), median adalimumab concentrations were higher (17.3 ug/mL, 12.2–24.0) in patients with histologic remission compared to those without (10.3 ug/mL, 6.8–13.9, $p = 0.008$). The optimal ADA concentration identified using the Youden threshold was $\geq$16.3 ug/mL (sensitivity 70%, specificity 90%). Patients with ADA $\geq$ 16.3 ug/mL had higher histologic remission rates (78%) compared to lower ADA concentrations (14%, $p = 0.002$), as well as higher mucosal healing rates (86%) compared to lower levels (12%, $p = 0.001$). Symptoms correlated weakly and non-significantly with both histologic (RHI) scores ($r = 0.25$, $p = 0.2$) and adalimumab concentrations ($r = 0.05$, $p = 0.8$). (4) The current study demonstrated that higher serum adalimumab concentrations ($\geq$16.3 ug/mL) are needed for histologic remission and mucosal healing assessed using the RHI.

Keywords: adalimumab maintenance; therapeutic drug monitoring; mucosal healing

Citation: Wong, R.; Qin, L.; Pan, Y.; Mahtani, P.; Longman, R.; Lukin, D.; Scherl, E.; Battat, R. Higher Adalimumab Trough Levels Are Associated with Histologic Remission and Mucosal Healing in Inflammatory Bowel Disease. *J. Clin. Med.* **2023**, *12*, 6796. https://doi.org/10.3390/jcm12216796

Academic Editors: Konstantinos Papamichael and Jun Kato

Received: 4 August 2023
Revised: 14 October 2023
Accepted: 20 October 2023
Published: 27 October 2023

Copyright: © 2023 by the authors. Licensee MDPI, Basel, Switzerland. This article is an open access article distributed under the terms and conditions of the Creative Commons Attribution (CC BY) license (https://creativecommons.org/licenses/by/4.0/).

1. Introduction

Ulcerative colitis (UC) and Crohn's disease (CD) are chronic inflammatory bowel diseases (IBD) [1,2]. Endoscopic healing in IBD has consistently been associated with reductions in corticosteroid use, hospitalization, and surgery. Thus, endoscopic healing is the recommended primary treatment target for IBD [3–7]. Additionally, improved long-term outcomes are associated with more stringent endoscopic outcomes with a complete absence of disease activity [8–13]. Despite this fact, significant proportions of patients with IBD in endoscopic remission have persistent histologic activity, which is associated with higher rates of symptomatic relapse, corticosteroid use, surgery, and dysplasia [14,15]. Thus, incorporating histology into management is now recommended, and regulatory authorities require the term "mucosal healing" to refer to achieving both endoscopic and histologic remission [16]. Consequently, there has been significant interest in the use of validated histology instruments, such as the Roberts Histopathology Index (RHI), to assess histologic remission [17].

Therapeutic drug monitoring (TDM) has been demonstrated to optimize therapies to maintain efficacy in IBD, in which there are limited existing therapies [18]. Clinical situations during which TDM can be helpful include treatment failure, after successful induction and transition into maintenance therapy, assessing timing for a drug holiday, or during clinical remission when subsequent activity results would change management. Tumor necrosis factor (TNF) antagonist trough and anti-drug antibody concentrations are used in TDM and have been associated with important outcomes in IBD [19]. There are various strategies for providers to utilize TDM that are currently being studied. The standard of care currently involves empiric dose escalation of anti-TNF therapy if the patient does not achieve a response. Reactive TDM, where providers use drug concentration levels and antidrug antibodies to guide decision-making, has been helpful for patients who are suspected or confirmed to have a loss of response to therapy [20]. In contrast, proactive drug monitoring, where the drug is titrated to a target concentration, has been associated with better clinical outcomes, reduced risk of treatment failure, and lower risk of developing antidrug antibodies [21,22].

In both Crohn's disease (CD) and ulcerative colitis (UC), TNF antagonists, such as adalimumab (ADA), are often required to induce and maintain remission. Adalimumab has been found to be effective in achieving and maintaining clinical remission for both CD [23] and UC [24,25] patients, including those who have been treated with prior anti-TNF therapy. Various studies have been published on the optimal therapeutic drug level for adalimumab to achieve clinical, endoscopic, and histologic remission. Levels of 4.8 ug/mL have been associated with clinical remission and >7.5 ug/mL for endoscopic remission [26]. For histologic remission, one study found drug levels >7.8 ug/mL were associated with histologic healing, using standard-of-care pathologist assessment for the absence of microscopic inflammatory infiltrate to define histologic remission but no formal histologic scoring criteria [27]. This initial study suggests higher concentrations may be needed to achieve deeper levels of remission. Another study showed that adalimumab drug concentrations >13.9 ug/mL at week 4 were associated with serological remission at week 24, consistent with emerging literature suggesting that higher concentrations of anti-TNF therapy may be needed to achieve a response [28,29].

However, despite the success of adalimumab therapy to induce and maintain remission, significant proportions of patients experience either primary non-response or secondary loss of response to anti-TNF therapy [30]. There are limited exposure-response data on adalimumab for validated histologic endpoints [31,32]. A recent randomized controlled trial found reduced efficacy of adalimumab relative to vedolizumab to achieve histologic remission defined using the RHI [33]. A potential explanation for suboptimal histologic outcomes with adalimumab may be inadequate drug concentrations. However, data on the relationship between serum adalimumab concentrations and histologic outcomes with validated indices are lacking. The RHI is a responsive indicator of histologic disease and treatment response in UC and CD, [33–35] with similar test characteristics to other histologic indices [36] and validated against endoscopy [37,38]. The RHI has been deemed appropriate to measure histological disease activity in CD [39] and utilized in landmark CD trials.

This study aimed to assess the relationship between serum drug concentrations of adalimumab and a validated histologic disease activity index in patients with IBD using prospectively collected, blinded and objective histologic scores.

2. Materials and Methods

2.1. Study Population

In this retrospective study, patients from a tertiary IBD center from 2013 to 2020 with adalimumab (ADA) trough drug concentrations measured during maintenance therapy ($\geq$14 weeks) and a colonoscopy or flexible sigmoidoscopy with biopsies performed within

90 days of drug level were included. A chart review was performed for demographic data, medication and surgical history, and disease characteristics.

2.2. Data and Outcome Definitions

Serum adalimumab trough concentrations were measured using a homogenous mobility shift assay (Prometheus Laboratories, San Diego, CA, USA). Drug levels were drawn during maintenance therapy for routine drug monitoring, regardless of clinical symptoms or clinical remission. Additional bloodwork was drawn to evaluate for active inflammation if the patient was symptomatically active.

For inclusion criteria, trough levels were defined as drug concentration levels drawn within 7 days prior to the next administration of ADA for patients receiving therapy every 2 weeks, or on the day prior to the next administration for those on weekly injections. However, because the standard practice at our center is to collect serum adalimumab concentrations within 1 day prior to drug administration, the median time of drug concentration measurement prior to the next dose reflected a more stringent trough definition (1.5 days) in this study.

For patients with colonoscopy or flexible sigmoidoscopy performed within 90 days of drug level, histologic scoring using the RHI was performed by a blinded pathologist on the biopsies obtained during ileo-colonoscopy [15,17,34]. Biopsies for CD were taken from endoscopically inflamed segments, or at random if no endoscopic inflammation existed, from at least one segment throughout the ileum and/or colon. Biopsies for UC were also taken from endoscopically inflamed segments, or at random if no endoscopic inflammation existed, from the colon with at least one biopsy from the rectum, given the continuous pattern of inflammation from the rectum in this disease. Additional biopsies were taken from areas that appeared most endoscopically active or affected, such as the presence of ulcers or erythema, in order to accurately assess for inflammation.

Rates of endoscopic remission, defined as the absence of ulcers for CD [3,16] and a Mayo endoscopic score of 0 for UC [3,16] were assessed. Histologic remission, defined as RHI = 0, was also assessed [17,40]. Mucosal healing (MH) was defined as achieving both endoscopic and histologic remission. Rates of clinical (symptomatic) remission were assessed, as defined using a Harvey Bradshaw Index of 4 or less for patients with CD or a partial Mayo score of 2 or less for patients with UC.

2.3. Statistical Analysis

Primary analysis assessed the diagnostic accuracy of adalimumab drug concentrations for histologic remission using receiver operating characteristic curve analysis. Outcome proportions were compared above and below identified optimal (Youden) thresholds using Fisher's exact test. Rates of endoscopic remission and mucosal healing (achieving both endoscopic and histologic remission) were additionally compared using the identified threshold. A p-value < 0.05 was considered significant.

All statistical analyses were performed using STATA SE 15.1 (Statacorp, College Station, TX, USA).

2.4. Ethics

All authors had access to the study data and reviewed and approved the final manuscript. Study protocol and materials were approved by the institutional review board at Weill Cornell Medicine. The study was conducted in accordance with the Declaration of Helsinki and approved by the Institutional Review Board of Weill Cornell Medicine (Protocol code 20-04021893 and date of approval 5 August 2020). All patients provided written informed consent.

3. Results

Thirty-six patients were included (26 CD, 9 UC, 1 indeterminate, Table 1). The median cohort age was 34 years old, and 56% of patients were female. The median ADA drug concentration was 11.1 ug/mL (IQR: 7.0–15.5 ug/mL). The median time from treatment initiation to drug concentration measurement was 103 weeks (IQR 25–75 = 35.6–286). The median time of drug concentration measurement prior to the next dose was 1.5 days. Endoscopic remission was noted in 7/24 (29%) of CD patients and 1/4 (25%) of UC patients. The median RHI score was 8.5 (IQR 25–75 = 0–21.8) and histologic remission was achieved in 10/30 (33%) of patients. Of the 24 patients with both endoscopic and histologic data available, 8 patients (33%) achieved mucosal healing (endo-histologic remission). Median adalimumab concentrations were 12.1 ug/mL in patients with symptomatic remission, 13.9 ug/mL in patients with endoscopic remission, 17.3 ug/mL in patients with histologic remission, and 19.6 ug/mL in patients with complete mucosal healing (endo-histologic remission).

Table 1. Patient Cohort Demographics (n = 36).

Demographics	n(%)
Median Age at Drug Level (years)	34
Gender (female)	20 (0.56)
Type of IBD	
Crohn's Disease	26 (0.72)
Ulcerative Colitis	9 (0.25)
Indeterminate Colitis	1 (0.02)
Adalimumab	
Median Drug Level Concentration (IQR 25–75)	11.1 (7.0–15.5)
Median Dose (mg)	40
Median Frequency (every X weeks)	2
Median Days of Therapy (d)	718
Median Weeks of Therapy (wk)	103
Age at Diagnosis	
Age < or = 16	11 (0.31)
Age 17–40	15 (0.42)
Age > or = 41	8 (0.22)
Unknown	2 (0.06)
Montreal Classification	
Crohn's Disease (n = 26)	
B1—inflamed, non-stricturing, non-penetrating	13 (0.50)
B2—stricturing	6 (0.23)
B3—fistulizing (penetrating)	7 (0.26)
CD: L1 ileal	5 (0.19)
CD: L2 colonic	3 (0.12)
CD: L3 ileocolonic	17 (0.65)
CD: L4 isolated upper GI disease	6 (0.23)
Ulcerative Colitis (n = 9)	
UC: left-sided (rectum to splenic flexure)	5 (0.56)
UC: Extensive (beyond splenic flexure, including ascending/transverse colon)	4 (0.44)
Endoscopy	
CD: Presence of ulcers (lack of remission)	7/24 (0.29)
UC: Mayo Score <2 (presence of remission)	1/4 (0.25)
Histology	
RHI score = 0 (histologic remission)	10/30 (0.33)
Median RHI Score	8.5
Mucosal Healing	
Endohistologic Remission	8/24 (0.33)

Table 1. Cont.

Demographics	n(%)
Medication History	
Previously used mesalamine	28 (0.78)
Previously used sulfasalazine	5 (0.14)
Previously used budesonide	14 (0.39)
Previously used 6-mercaptopurine	14 (0.39)
Previously used methotrexate	5 (0.14)
Previously used azathioprine	6 (0.17)
Prior TNF exposure	13 (0.36)
Prior Vedolizumab exposure	1 (0.03)
Prior steroid (prednisone) use	19 (0.53)
Surgical History	
Previous IBD-related abdominal surgery	12 (0.33)

3.1. Relationship between Adalimumab Concentrations and Histology

Median adalimumab concentrations were higher (17.3 ug/mL, 12.2–24.0) in patients with histologic remission compared to patients without histologic remission (10.3 ug/mL, 6.8–13.9, $p = 0.008$). The area under the curve for ADA concentrations to identify histologic remission was 0.80 (95% CI 0.61–0.99, Figure 1). The optimal ADA concentration identified using the Youden threshold was ≥ 16.3 ug/mL (sensitivity 70%, specificity 90%, positive likelihood ratio 7.0, negative likelihood ratio 0.33). Patients with ADA ≥ 16.3 ug/mL had higher histologic remission rates (78%) compared to patients with lower ADA concentrations (14%, $p= 0.002$, Figure 2).

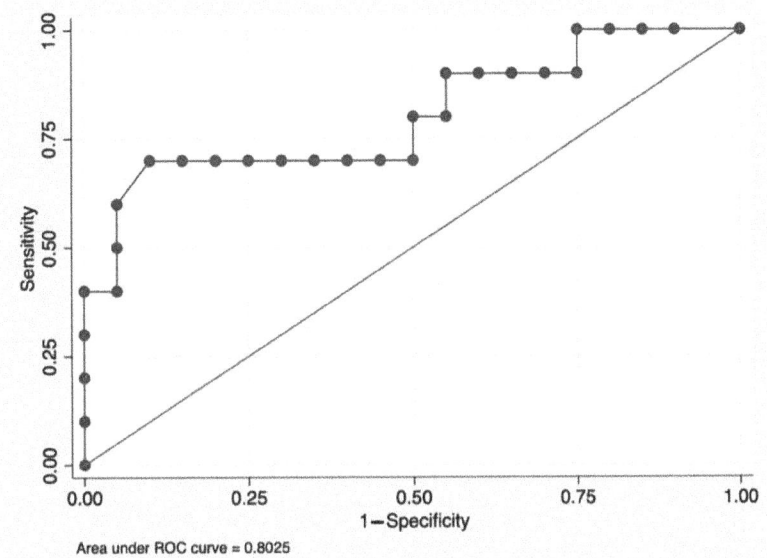

Figure 1. Area Under the Receiver Operator Curve Analysis for Histologic Remission (RHI = 0) and adalimumab drug concentrations.

In quartile analysis of drug concentrations associated with the primary outcome, 17% (1/6) of patients achieved mucosal healing in quartile 1 (0–7 ug/mL), 17% (1/6) of patients achieved mucosal healing in quartile 2 (7–12.3 ug/mL), 14% (1/7) of patients achieved mucosal healing in quartile 3 (12.4–16.3 ug/mL), and 100% (5/5) achieved mucosal healing in quartile 4 (16.4–26.4 ug/mL).

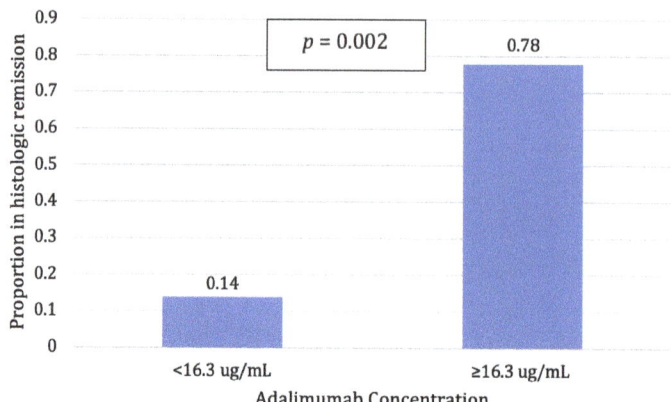

Figure 2. Patients with higher adalimumab (ADA) concentrations achieved statistically significantly higher histologic remission rates than patients with lower ADA concentrations ($p = 0.002$).

3.2. Relationship between Adalimumab Concentrations and Endo-Histologic Outcomes

The median adalimumab concentrations were significantly higher (19.6 ug/mL, 14.6–24.9) in patients with complete mucosal healing (both endoscopic and histologic remission) compared to patients without complete mucosal healing (10.3 ug/mL, 5.9–13.9, $p = 0.009$). Using the previously identified threshold, patients with an adalimumab concentration ≥16.3 ug/mL also had higher rates of complete mucosal healing (86%) compared to patients with lower adalimumab concentrations (12%, $p = 0.001$, Figure 3).

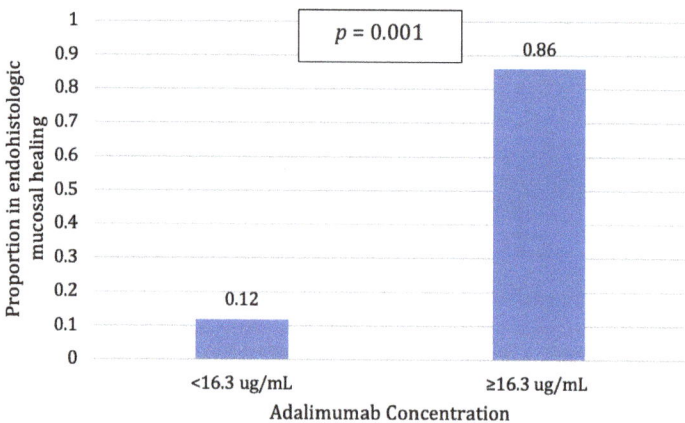

Figure 3. Patients with higher ADA concentrations achieved statistically significantly higher mucosal healing (endohistologic remission) rates than patients with lower ADA concentrations ($p = 0.001$).

Using the previously identified threshold, patients with an adalimumab concentration ≥16.3 ug/mL had higher endoscopic remission (100%) compared to patients with lower adalimumab concentrations (57%, $p = 0.04$). In addition, the median adalimumab concentrations were numerically higher (13.9 ug/mL, 7.7–17.0) in patients with endoscopic remission compared to patients without endoscopic remission (9.1 ug/mL, 6.1–13.0, $p = 0.16$).

3.3. Relationship between Adalimumab Concentrations and Symptomatic Outcomes

The median adalimumab concentrations were similar between patients with (12.1 ug/mL, 5.9–14.5) and without (10.9 ug/mL, 8.9–16.0) symptomatic (clinical) remission. The area under the curve for ADA concentrations to identify symptomatic remission was 0.45 (95%

CI 0.24–0.66). Symptoms correlated weakly and non-significantly with both histologic (RHI) scores (r = 0.25, p = 0.2) and adalimumab concentrations (r = 0.05, p = 0.8).

3.4. Relationship between Adalimumab Concentrations and Composite Outcome of Mucosal Healing and Clinical Remission

The median adalimumab concentrations for patients with both mucosal healing and clinical remission was 18.9 ug/mL, IQR 13.7–22.7, while the median adalimumab concentration for patients without both was 11.2 ug/mL, IQR 7–14.8, p = 0.15. Similar numerical differences existed with a smaller sample size of those with endoscopic, symptomatic, and histologic data. Using the previously identified threshold, patients with an adalimumab concentration ≥16.3 ug/mL trended toward higher mucosal healing and clinical remission (43%) compared to patients with lower adalimumab concentrations (6%, p = 0.06, Figure 4).

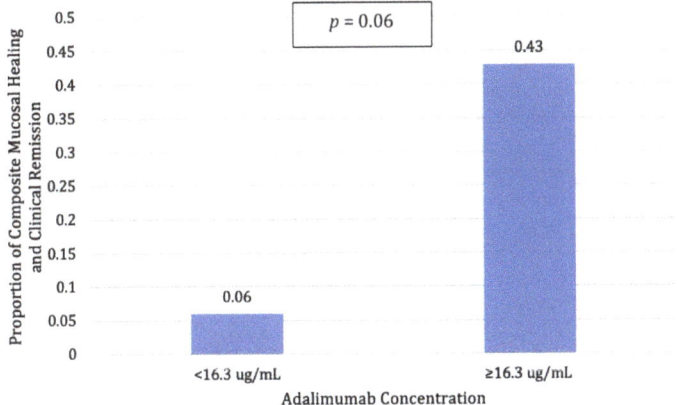

Figure 4. Patients with higher ADA concentrations trended towards improved mucosal healing and clinical remission when compared to patients with lower ADA concentrations (p = 0.06).

4. Discussion

Histologic remission and MH may better predict relapse and long-term outcomes than clinical or endoscopic remission alone [19,30]. Thus, histopathology has been suggested as an adjunctive goal in therapeutic targets in management guidelines [3]. Consequently, understanding the exposure-response relationship between common biologic therapies and these outcomes is important. Adalimumab has been shown to have inferior histologic outcomes to other agents [33]. However, data on the relationship between validated histologic disease activity indices and adalimumab drug concentrations are lacking. The current study was the first to uniquely describe and demonstrate a significant relationship between adalimumab maintenance trough concentrations and histologic outcomes using a validated histologic index.

Therapeutic drug monitoring (TDM), defined as using serum drug concentrations and the presence of anti-drug antibodies to guide management, can be helpful in patients with both a primary non-response or secondary loss of response to biologic therapy [41]. As TDM becomes more incorporated into clinical practice and management, it will be important to clarify the target goal for patients to achieve histologic remission and mucosal healing. The current recommended target adalimumab concentration is 7.5 ug/mL to achieve endoscopic remission [42]. However, this level is best correlated with the lack of endoscopic lesions and may not achieve mucosal healing (endohistologic remission) due to low sensitivity [27]. Our study suggests that a higher than traditional serum ADA target (≥16.3 ug/mL) is needed to achieve histologic remission. Several prior studies have reported on the higher maintenance of adalimumab concentrations, which achieved higher rates of histologic remission and mucosal healing in IBD patients [27,43]. However, the main strength of our study is that it is the first to use a validated histologic scoring tool, as well as a blinded histologic disease activity assessment, in contrast to previous studies that lacked validated histologic scoring tools and utilized retrospectively reviewed pathology [27].

One strength of our study was the use of stringent endoscopic and histologic outcomes. It has been suggested that early proactive monitoring of mucosal inflammation and mucosal healing within 6 months of biologic initiation is associated with a reduction in complications at 24 months, including corticosteroid use, change in biologic, IBD-related hospitalization, or surgery [44]. However, rather than using noninvasive monitoring, such as fecal calprotectin, endoscopic evaluation, or cross-sectional radiographic enterogarphy, our primary outcome was the most stringent of histologic remission, defined as RHI of 0. This has been already strongly associated with patient clinical and endoscopic remission status [40]. An RHI score of 0 ensures complete histologic remission outcomes. Our use of mucosal healing, defined as endo-histologic remission, as an endpoint also better reflects current practice. Although not formally defined as a therapeutic target, histopathology showing active mucosal inflammation on biopsy may increase clinical suspicion for underappreciated endoscopic disease activity, and prompt treatment adjustments or earlier disease activity reassessments.

Limitations of the current study include its retrospective study design, its limited sample size, and a low proportion of patients being in complete endo-histologic remission. However, between-group differences in histologic and MH rates were not only statistically significant but also had strikingly large numerical differences. It is important to note the evolving definitions of mucosal healing [45]. We define mucosal healing in our study to be combined endoscopic and histologic remission, in line with recent Food and Drug Administration (FDA) recommendations. Prior studies have used similar terminology to define only endoscopic remission [46,47]. Our study also defines endoscopic remission for UC as Mayo 0. Mayo 0 shows a lower risk of clinical relapse than Mayo 1, but no differences in risk of hospitalization or IBD surgery [48]. Drug concentration thresholds may differ depending on the outcome of interest. Ungar et al. defined mucosal healing as endoscopic score remission and found that ADA serum levels > 7.1 ug/mL predicted endoscopic MH with 85% specificity, while the current study data suggest a higher ADA level is required to achieve both endoscopic and histologic remission.

Another limitation to consider is that a serum ADA target of 16.3 ug/mL may be difficult to achieve. Proactive therapeutic drug monitoring, which utilizes dose escalation to achieve a threshold concentration regardless of disease activity, may be a strategy to achieve higher adalimumab concentrations appropriately and cost-effectively [49,50]. Testing has more commonly been performed at trough, as the presence of the drug can interfere with the detection of anti-TNF antibodies. The timing of when to measure drug serum concentrations can also be unclear when practicing therapeutic drug monitoring. However, recent data suggest that serum adalimumab concentrations are stable in the first 9 days after injection and can reasonably predict therapeutic trough drug levels, potentially allowing for earlier decision-making based on non-trough adalimumab levels [51,52]. One study by Kato et al. found serum ADA levels are predictive of clinical outcomes regardless of trough timing [53]. This may be helpful for patients on more frequent dosing of adalimumab, while the timing of drug levels may be more important to make for patients requiring longer follow-up. Future studies are needed to investigate the feasibility of this TDM practice.

5. Conclusions

To conclude, this study reports a serum ADA concentration that is higher than traditional targets ($\geq$16.3 ug/mL) is associated with higher rates of histologic remission and mucosal healing.

Author Contributions: Conceptualization, R.W. and R.B.; methodology, R.W. and R.B.; formal analysis, R.B.; investigation, R.W., L.Q. and Y.P.; resources, P.M.; data curation, R.W., Y.P. and P.M.; writing—original draft preparation, R.W. and R.B.; writing—review and editing, R.W., L.Q., Y.P., P.M., R.L., D.L., E.S. and R.B.; supervision, R.B.; project administration, P.M. and R.B. All authors have read and agreed to the published version of the manuscript.

Funding: This work was supported by grants from the NIH R01DK114252-01A1.

Institutional Review Board Statement: Study protocol and materials were approved by the institutional review board at Weill Cornell Medicine (protocol code 20-04021893 and date of approval 5 August 2020).

Informed Consent Statement: All patients provided written informed consent.

Data Availability Statement: Data not publicly available. Data available on request.

Conflicts of Interest: R.L: Consulting for Pfizer. D.L: Consulting for Abbvie, Boehringer Ingelheim, Bristol Meyers Squibb, Eli Lilly, Fresenius Kabi, Janssen, Palatin Technologies, Pfizer, Prometheus Laboratories. Grants: Abbvie, Janssen, Takeda. E.S: Consulting for AbbVie, Crohn's and Colitis Foundation of American (CCFA), Entera Health, Evidera, GI Health Foundation, Janssen, Protagonist Therapeutics, Seres Health, Takeda Pharmaceuticals, Bristol Myers Squibb. Grants: Abbott (Abbvie), AstraZeneca, CCFA, Janssen Research & Development, Johns Hopkins University, National Institute of Diabetes and Digestive and Kidney (NIDDK), National Institute of Health (NIH), New York Crohn's Foundation, Pfizer, UCB, UCSF-CCFA Clinical Research Alliance, Genentech, Seres Therapeutics, Celgene Corporation. Stock shareholder for Gilead. Honoraria for GI Health Foundation and Janssen for non-branded Speaker's bureau. R.B: Speaking/Consulting/Advertising Boards: Prometheus Laboratories, Bristol Myers Squibb, Janssen, Abbvie, Takeda, Pfizer, Eli Lilly. All other authors (R.W., L.Q., Y.P., P.M) have no conflicts to disclose.

References

1. Mekhjian, H.S.; Switz, D.M.; Melnyk, C.S.; Rankin, G.B.; Brooks, R.K. Clinical Features and Natural History of Crohn's Disease. *Gastroenterology* **1979**, *77*, 898–906. [CrossRef] [PubMed]
2. Lichtenstein, G. *The Clinician's Guide to Inflammatory Bowel Disease*; Slack Incorporated: Thorofare, NJ, USA, 2003.
3. Peyrin-Biroulet, L.; Sandborn, W.; Sands, B.E.; Reinisch, W.; Bemelman, W.; Bryant, R.V.; D'Haens, G.; Dotan, I.; Dubinsky, M.; Feagan, B.; et al. Selecting Therapeutic Targets in Inflammatory Bowel Disease (STRIDE): Determining Therapeutic Goals for Treat-to-Target. *Am. J. Gastroenterol.* **2015**, *110*, 1324–1338. [CrossRef]
4. Dulai, P.S.; Levesque, B.G.; Feagan, B.G.; D'Haens, G.; Sandborn, W.J. Assessment of Mucosal Healing in Inflammatory Bowel Disease: Review. *Gastrointest. Endosc.* **2015**, *82*, 246–255. [CrossRef] [PubMed]
5. Shah, S.C.; Colombel, J.-F.; Sands, B.E.; Narula, N. Systematic Review with Meta-Analysis: Mucosal Healing Is Associated with Improved Long-Term Outcomes in Crohn's Disease. *Aliment. Pharmacol. Ther.* **2016**, *43*, 317–333. [CrossRef]
6. Khanna, R.; Bressler, B.; Levesque, B.G.; Zou, G.; Stitt, L.W.; Greenberg, G.R.; Panaccione, R.; Bitton, A.; Paré, P.; Vermeire, S.; et al. Early Combined Immunosuppression for the Management of Crohn's Disease (REACT): A Cluster Randomised Controlled Trial. *Lancet* **2015**, *386*, 1825–1834. [CrossRef]
7. Shah, S.C.; Colombel, J.-F.; Sands, B.E.; Narula, N. Mucosal Healing Is Associated With Improved Long-Term Outcomes of Patients With Ulcerative Colitis: A Systematic Review and Meta-Analysis. *Clin. Gastroenterol. Hepatol.* **2016**, *14*, 1245–1255.e8. [CrossRef]
8. Barreiro-de Acosta, M.; Vallejo, N.; de la Iglesia, D.; Uribarri, L.; Bastón, I.; Ferreiro-Iglesias, R.; Lorenzo, A.; Domínguez-Muñoz, J.E. Evaluation of the Risk of Relapse in Ulcerative Colitis According to the Degree of Mucosal Healing (Mayo 0 vs 1): A Longitudinal Cohort Study. *J. Crohns Colitis* **2016**, *10*, 13–19. [CrossRef]
9. Ikeya, K.; Sugimoto, K.; Kawasaki, S.; Iida, T.; Maruyama, Y.; Watanabe, F.; Hanai, H. Tacrolimus for Remission Induction in Ulcerative Colitis: Mayo Endoscopic Subscore 0 and 1 Predict Long-Term Prognosis. *Dig. Liver Dis.* **2015**, *47*, 365–371. [CrossRef] [PubMed]
10. Manginot, C.; Baumann, C.; Peyrin-Biroulet, L. An Endoscopic Mayo Score of 0 Is Associated with a Lower Risk of Colectomy than a Score of 1 in Ulcerative Colitis. *Gut* **2015**, *64*, 1181–1182. [CrossRef]
11. Meucci, G.; Fasoli, R.; Saibeni, S.; Valpiani, D.; Gullotta, R.; Colombo, E.; D'Incà, R.; Terpin, M.; Lombardi, G. IG-IBD Prognostic Significance of Endoscopic Remission in Patients with Active Ulcerative Colitis Treated with Oral and Topical Mesalazine: A Prospective, Multicenter Study. *Inflamm. Bowel Dis.* **2012**, *18*, 1006–1010. [CrossRef]
12. Nakarai, A.; Kato, J.; Hiraoka, S.; Inokuchi, T.; Takei, D.; Moritou, Y.; Akita, M.; Takahashi, S.; Hori, K.; Harada, K.; et al. Prognosis of Ulcerative Colitis Differs between Patients with Complete and Partial Mucosal Healing, Which Can Be Predicted from the Platelet Count. *World J. Gastroenterol.* **2014**, *20*, 18367–18374. [CrossRef] [PubMed]

13. Yokoyama, K.; Kobayashi, K.; Mukae, M.; Sada, M.; Koizumi, W. Clinical Study of the Relation between Mucosal Healing and Long-Term Outcomes in Ulcerative Colitis. *Gastroenterol. Res. Pract.* **2013**, *2013*, 192794. [CrossRef]
14. Christensen, B.; Hanauer, S.B.; Erlich, J.; Kassim, O.; Gibson, P.R.; Turner, J.R.; Hart, J.; Rubin, D.T. Histologic Normalization Occurs in Ulcerative Colitis and Is Associated With Improved Clinical Outcomes. *Clin. Gastroenterol. Hepatol.* **2017**, *15*, 1557–1564.e1. [CrossRef] [PubMed]
15. Christensen, B.; Erlich, J.; Gibson, P.R.; Turner, J.R.; Hart, J.; Rubin, D.T. Histologic Healing Is More Strongly Associated with Clinical Outcomes in Ileal Crohn's Disease than Endoscopic Healing. *Clin. Gastroenterol. Hepatol.* **2020**, *18*, 2518–2525.e1. [CrossRef]
16. Ma, C.; Sedano, R.; Almradi, A.; Vande Casteele, N.; Parker, C.E.; Guizzetti, L.; Schaeffer, D.F.; Riddell, R.H.; Pai, R.K.; Battat, R.; et al. An International Consensus to Standardize Integration of Histopathology in Ulcerative Colitis Clinical Trials. *Gastroenterology* **2021**, *160*, 2291–2302. [CrossRef]
17. Mosli, M.H.; Feagan, B.G.; Zou, G.; Sandborn, W.J.; D'Haens, G.; Khanna, R.; Shackelton, L.M.; Walker, C.W.; Nelson, S.; Vandervoort, M.K.; et al. Development and Validation of a Histological Index for UC. *Gut* **2017**, *66*, 50–58. [CrossRef] [PubMed]
18. Mitrev, N.; Vande Casteele, N.; Seow, C.H.; Andrews, J.M.; Connor, S.J.; Moore, G.T.; Barclay, M.; Begun, J.; Bryant, R.; Chan, W.; et al. Review Article: Consensus Statements on Therapeutic Drug Monitoring of Anti-Tumour Necrosis Factor Therapy in Inflammatory Bowel Diseases. *Aliment. Pharmacol. Ther.* **2017**, *46*, 1037–1053. [CrossRef]
19. Afif, W.; Leighton, J.A.; Hanauer, S.B.; Loftus, E.V.; Faubion, W.A.; Pardi, D.S.; Tremaine, W.J.; Kane, S.V.; Bruining, D.H.; Cohen, R.D.; et al. Open-Label Study of Adalimumab in Patients with Ulcerative Colitis Including Those with Prior Loss of Response or Intolerance to Infliximab. *Inflamm. Bowel Dis.* **2009**, *15*, 1302–1307. [CrossRef]
20. Yanai, H.; Lichtenstein, L.; Assa, A.; Mazor, Y.; Weiss, B.; Levine, A.; Ron, Y.; Kopylov, U.; Bujanover, Y.; Rosenbach, Y.; et al. Levels of Drug and Antidrug Antibodies Are Associated with Outcome of Interventions after Loss of Response to Infliximab or Adalimumab. *Clin. Gastroenterol. Hepatol.* **2015**, *13*, 522–530.e2. [CrossRef]
21. Papamichael, K.; Chachu, K.A.; Vajravelu, R.K.; Vaughn, B.P.; Ni, J.; Osterman, M.T.; Cheifetz, A.S. Improved Long-Term Outcomes of Patients With Inflammatory Bowel Disease Receiving Proactive Compared with Reactive Monitoring of Serum Concentrations of Infliximab. *Clin. Gastroenterol. Hepatol.* **2017**, *15*, 1580–1588.e3. [CrossRef]
22. Papamichael, K.; Juncadella, A.; Wong, D.; Rakowsky, S.; Sattler, L.A.; Campbell, J.P.; Vaughn, B.P.; Cheifetz, A.S. Proactive Therapeutic Drug Monitoring of Adalimumab Is Associated with Better Long-Term Outcomes Compared with Standard of Care in Patients with Inflammatory Bowel Disease. *J. Crohns Colitis* **2019**, *13*, 976–981. [CrossRef]
23. Townsend, C.M.; Nguyen, T.M.; Cepek, J.; Abbass, M.; Parker, C.E.; MacDonald, J.K.; Khanna, R.; Jairath, V.; Feagan, B.G. Adalimumab for Maintenance of Remission in Crohn's Disease. *Cochrane Database Syst. Rev.* **2020**, *2020*, CD012877. [CrossRef]
24. Sandborn, W.J.; Van Assche, G.; Reinisch, W. Adalimumab in the Treatment of Moderate-to-Severe Ulcerative Colitis: ULTRA 2 Trial Results. *Gastroenterol. Hepatol.* **2013**, *9*, 317–320.
25. Reinisch, W.; Sandborn, W.J.; Hommes, D.W.; D'Haens, G.; Hanauer, S.; Schreiber, S.; Panaccione, R.; Fedorak, R.N.; Tighe, M.B.; Huang, B.; et al. Adalimumab for Induction of Clinical Remission in Moderately to Severely Active Ulcerative Colitis: Results of a Randomised Controlled Trial. *Gut* **2011**, *60*, 780–787. [CrossRef] [PubMed]
26. Hinojosa, J.; Muñoz, F.; Martínez-Romero, G.J. Relationship between Serum Adalimumab Levels and Clinical Outcome in the Treatment of Inflammatory Bowel Disease. *Dig. Dis.* **2019**, *37*, 444–450. [CrossRef] [PubMed]
27. Yarur, A.J.; Jain, A.; Hauenstein, S.I.; Quintero, M.A.; Barkin, J.S.; Deshpande, A.R.; Sussman, D.A.; Singh, S.; Abreu, M.T. Higher Adalimumab Levels Are Associated with Histologic and Endoscopic Remission in Patients with Crohn's Disease and Ulcerative Colitis. *Inflamm. Bowel Dis.* **2016**, *22*, 409–415. [CrossRef] [PubMed]
28. Zittan, E.; Steinhart, A.H.; Goldstein, P.; Milgrom, R.; Gralnek, I.M.; Silverberg, M.S. Post-Induction High Adalimumab Drug Levels Predict Biological Remission at Week 24 in Patients With Crohn's Disease. *Clin. Transl. Gastroenterol.* **2021**, *12*, e00401. [CrossRef]
29. de Souza, L.R.; Magro, D.O.; Teixeira, F.V.; Parra, R.S.; Miranda, E.F.; Féres, O.; Saad-Hossne, R.; Soares Prates Herrerias, G.; Nisihara, R.M.; Coy, C.S.R.; et al. Adalimumab Serum Concentrations, Clinical and Endoscopic Disease Activity in Crohn's Disease: A Cross-Sectional Multicentric Latin American Study. *Pharmaceutics* **2023**, *15*, 586. [CrossRef]
30. Ben-Horin, S.; Kopylov, U.; Chowers, Y. Optimizing Anti-TNF Treatments in Inflammatory Bowel Disease. *Autoimmun. Rev.* **2014**, *13*, 24–30. [CrossRef]
31. Papamichael, K.; Rakowsky, S.; Rivera, C.; Cheifetz, A.S.; Osterman, M.T. Infliximab Trough Concentrations during Maintenance Therapy Are Associated with Endoscopic and Histologic Healing in Ulcerative Colitis. *Aliment. Pharmacol. Ther.* **2018**, *47*, 478–484. [CrossRef]
32. Papamichael, K.; Rakowsky, S.; Rivera, C.; Cheifetz, A.S.; Osterman, M.T. Association Between Serum Infliximab Trough Concentrations During Maintenance Therapy and Biochemical, Endoscopic, and Histologic Remission in Crohn's Disease. *Inflamm. Bowel Dis.* **2018**, *24*, 2266–2271. [CrossRef] [PubMed]
33. Peyrin-Biroulet, L.; Loftus, E.V.; Colombel, J.-F.; Danese, S.; Rogers, R.; Bornstein, J.D.; Chen, J.; Schreiber, S.; Sands, B.E.; Lirio, R.A. Histologic Outcomes With Vedolizumab Versus Adalimumab in Ulcerative Colitis: Results from An Efficacy and Safety Study of Vedolizumab Intravenous Compared to Adalimumab Subcutaneous in Participants with Ulcerative Colitis (VARSITY). *Gastroenterology* **2021**, *161*, 1156–1167.e3. [CrossRef] [PubMed]

34. Löwenberg, M.; Vermeire, S.; Mostafavi, N.; Hoentjen, F.; Franchimont, D.; Bossuyt, P.; Hindryckx, P.; Rispens, T.; de Vries, A.; van der Woude, C.J.; et al. Vedolizumab Induces Endoscopic and Histologic Remission in Patients with Crohn's Disease. *Gastroenterology* **2019**, *157*, 997–1006.e6. [CrossRef] [PubMed]
35. Novak, G.; Parker, C.E.; Pai, R.K.; MacDonald, J.K.; Feagan, B.G.; Sandborn, W.J.; D'Haens, G.; Jairath, V.; Khanna, R. Histologic Scoring Indices for Evaluation of Disease Activity in Crohn's Disease. *Cochrane Database Syst. Rev.* **2017**, *2017*, CD012351. [CrossRef]
36. Solitano, V.; Schaeffer, D.F.; Hogan, M.; Pai, R.K.; Zou, G.; Pai, R.K.; Vande Casteele, N.; Parker, C.E.; Remillard, J.; Christensen, B.; et al. P479 Reliability and Responsiveness of Histologic Disease Activity Indices in Crohn's Disease. *J. Crohn's Colitis* **2023**, *17*, i608–i609. [CrossRef]
37. Shah, J.; Dutta, U.; Das, A.; Sharma, V.; Mandavdhare, H.; Sharma, P.; Kalsi, D.; Popli, P.; Kochhar, R. Relationship between Mayo Endoscopic Score and Histological Scores in Ulcerative Colitis: A Prospective Study. *JGH Open* **2019**, *4*, 382–386. [CrossRef]
38. Reinisch, W.; De Hertogh, G.; Protic, M.; Chan, L.S.; Magro, F.; Pollack, P.; Feagan, B.G.; Harpaz, N.; Pai, R. DOP56 Histologic Disease Activity Correlates with Endoscopic Severity in Patients with Moderate to Severe Crohn's Disease. *J. Crohn's Colitis* **2022**, *16*, i103–i105. [CrossRef]
39. Almradi, A.; Ma, C.; D'Haens, G.R.; Sandborn, W.J.; Parker, C.E.; Guizzetti, L.; Borralho Nunes, P.; De Hertogh, G.; Feakins, R.M.; Khanna, R.; et al. An Expert Consensus to Standardise the Assessment of Histological Disease Activity in Crohn's Disease Clinical Trials. *Aliment. Pharmacol. Ther.* **2021**, *53*, 784–793. [CrossRef]
40. Pai, R.K.; Khanna, R.; D'Haens, G.R.; Sandborn, W.J.; Jeyarajah, J.; Feagan, B.G.; Vande Casteele, N.; Jairath, V. Definitions of Response and Remission for the Robarts Histopathology Index. *Gut* **2019**, *68*, 2101–2102. [CrossRef] [PubMed]
41. Cheifetz, A.S.; Abreu, M.T.; Afif, W.; Cross, R.K.; Dubinsky, M.C.; Loftus, E.V.; Osterman, M.T.; Saroufim, A.; Siegel, C.A.; Yarur, A.J.; et al. A Comprehensive Literature Review and Expert Consensus Statement on Therapeutic Drug Monitoring of Biologics in Inflammatory Bowel Disease. *Am. J. Gastroenterol.* **2021**, *116*, 2014–2025. [CrossRef]
42. Feuerstein, J.D.; Nguyen, G.C.; Kupfer, S.S.; Falck-Ytter, Y.; Singh, S.; Gerson, L.; Hirano, I.; Nguyen, G.C.; Rubenstein, J.H.; Smalley, W.E.; et al. American Gastroenterological Association Institute Guideline on Therapeutic Drug Monitoring in Inflammatory Bowel Disease. *Gastroenterology* **2017**, *153*, 827–834. [CrossRef] [PubMed]
43. Juncadella, A.; Papamichael, K.; Vaughn, B.P.; Cheifetz, A.S. Maintenance Adalimumab Concentrations Are Associated with Biochemical, Endoscopic, and Histologic Remission in Inflammatory Bowel Disease. *Dig. Dis. Sci.* **2018**, *63*, 3067–3073. [CrossRef] [PubMed]
44. Limketkai, B.N.; Singh, S.; Jairath, V.; Sandborn, W.J.; Dulai, P.S. US Practice Patterns and Impact of Monitoring for Mucosal Inflammation After Biologic Initiation in Inflammatory Bowel Disease. *Inflamm. Bowel Dis.* **2019**, *25*, 1828–1837. [CrossRef]
45. Mazzuoli, S.; Guglielmi, F.W.; Antonelli, E.; Salemme, M.; Bassotti, G.; Villanacci, V. Definition and Evaluation of Mucosal Healing in Clinical Practice. *Dig. Liver Dis.* **2013**, *45*, 969–977. [CrossRef] [PubMed]
46. Ungar, B.; Levy, I.; Yavne, Y.; Yavzori, M.; Picard, O.; Fudim, E.; Loebstein, R.; Chowers, Y.; Eliakim, R.; Kopylov, U.; et al. Optimizing Anti-TNF-α Therapy: Serum Levels of Infliximab and Adalimumab Are Associated with Mucosal Healing in Patients with Inflammatory Bowel Diseases. *Clin. Gastroenterol. Hepatol.* **2016**, *14*, 550–557.e2. [CrossRef]
47. Roblin, X.; Marotte, H.; Rinaudo, M.; Tedesco, E.D.; Moreau, A.; Phelip, J.M.; Genin, C.; Peyrin-Biroulet, L.; Paul, S. Association Between Pharmacokinetics of Adalimumab and Mucosal Healing in Patients with Inflammatory Bowel Diseases. *Clin. Gastroenterol. Hepatol.* **2014**, *12*, 80–84.e2. [CrossRef]
48. Viscido, A.; Valvano, M.; Stefanelli, G.; Capannolo, A.; Castellini, C.; Onori, E.; Ciccone, A.; Vernia, F.; Latella, G. Systematic Review and Meta-Analysis: The Advantage of Endoscopic Mayo Score 0 over 1 in Patients with Ulcerative Colitis. *BMC Gastroenterol.* **2022**, *22*, 92. [CrossRef]
49. Papamichael, K.; Dubinsky, M.C.; Cheifetz, A.S. Proactive Therapeutic Drug Monitoring of Adalimumab in Patients with Crohn's Disease. *Gastroenterology* **2023**, *164*, 164–165. [CrossRef]
50. Yao, J.; Jiang, X.; You, J.H.S. Proactive Therapeutic Drug Monitoring of Adalimumab for Pediatric Crohn's Disease Patients: A Cost-Effectiveness Analysis. *J. Gastroenterol. Hepatol.* **2021**, *36*, 2397–2407. [CrossRef] [PubMed]
51. Ward, M.G.; Thwaites, P.A.; Beswick, L.; Hogg, J.; Rosella, G.; Van Langenberg, D.; Reynolds, J.; Gibson, P.R.; Sparrow, M.P. Intra-Patient Variability in Adalimumab Drug Levels within and between Cycles in Crohn's Disease. *Aliment. Pharmacol. Ther.* **2017**, *45*, 1135–1145. [CrossRef]
52. Vande Casteele, N.; Gils, A. Editorial: Variability in Adalimumab Trough and Peak Serum Concentrations. *Aliment. Pharmacol. Ther.* **2017**, *45*, 1475–1476. [CrossRef] [PubMed]
53. Kato, M.; Sugimoto, K.; Ikeya, K.; Takano, R.; Matsuura, A.; Miyazu, T.; Ishida, N.; Tamura, S.; Tani, S.; Yamade, M.; et al. Therapeutic Monitoring of Adalimumab at Non-Trough Levels in Patients with Inflammatory Bowel Disease. *PLoS ONE* **2021**, *16*, e0254548. [CrossRef] [PubMed]

Disclaimer/Publisher's Note: The statements, opinions and data contained in all publications are solely those of the individual author(s) and contributor(s) and not of MDPI and/or the editor(s). MDPI and/or the editor(s) disclaim responsibility for any injury to people or property resulting from any ideas, methods, instructions or products referred to in the content.

Review

Drug Clearance in Patients with Inflammatory Bowel Disease Treated with Biologics

Tina Deyhim, Adam S. Cheifetz and Konstantinos Papamichael *

Center for Inflammatory Bowel Diseases, Division of Gastroenterology, Beth Israel Deaconess Medical Center, Boston, MA 02215, USA; tdeyhim@bidmc.harvard.edu (T.D.); acheifet@bidmc.harvard.edu (A.S.C.)
* Correspondence: kpapamicl@bidmc.harvard.edu

Abstract: Biological therapy is very effective for treating patients with moderate to severe inflammatory bowel disease (IBD). However, up to 40% can have primary non-response, and up to 50% of the patients can experience a loss of response to anti-tumor necrosis factor therapy. These undesirable outcomes can be attributed to either a mechanistic failure or pharmacokinetic (PK) issues characterized by an inadequate drug exposure and a high drug clearance. There are several factors associated with accelerated clearance of biologics including increased body weight, low serum albumin and immunogenicity. Drug clearance has gained a lot of attention recently as cumulative data suggest that there is an association between drug clearance and therapeutic outcomes in patients with IBD. Moreover, clearance is used by model informed precision dosing (MIDP) tools, or PK dashboards, to adjust the dosing for reaching a target drug concentration threshold towards a more personalized application of TDM. However, the role of drug clearance in clinical practice is yet to be determined. This comprehensive review aims to present data regarding the variables affecting the clearance of specific biologics, the association of clearance with therapeutic outcomes and the role of clearance monitoring and MIPD in patients with IBD.

Keywords: clearance; inflammatory bowel disease; therapeutic drug monitoring; anti-TNF therapy; vedolizumab; ustekinumab; mirikizumab; risankizumab; model informed precision dosing; pharmacokinetic dashboard

1. Introduction

Biological therapy is very effective for treating patients with moderate to severe inflammatory bowel diseases (IBD) such as Crohn's disease (CD) and ulcerative colitis (UC). However, up to 40% and 80% of the patients can have primary non-response and primary non-remission to anti-tumor necrosis factor (anti-TNF) therapy, respectively [1]. Moreover, up to half of the patients with IBD may experience secondary loss of response [2]. Therapeutic drug monitoring (TDM) can help to explain these unwanted outcomes attributed either to a mechanistic failure in the presence of adequate drug concentration or pharmacokinetic (PK) issues characterized by an inadequate drug exposure and a high drug clearance [3].

Drug clearance is expressed as the volume of plasma in the vascular compartment that is cleared of drug per unit of time, and it is estimated using Bayesian modeling [3]. Mechanisms underlying the clearance of monoclonal antibodies include intracellular catabolism and endocytosis, increase in target load, protein-losing enteropathy and binding to anti-drug antibodies. There are several factors associated with the above mechanisms that can influence the clearance of biologics including body weight, serum albumin and immunogenicity (Figure 1) [4–46]. In particular, increased body weight, decreased albumin and anti-drug antibodies (ADAs) have been associated with higher clearance for almost all the biologics currently used in IBD (Figure 1).

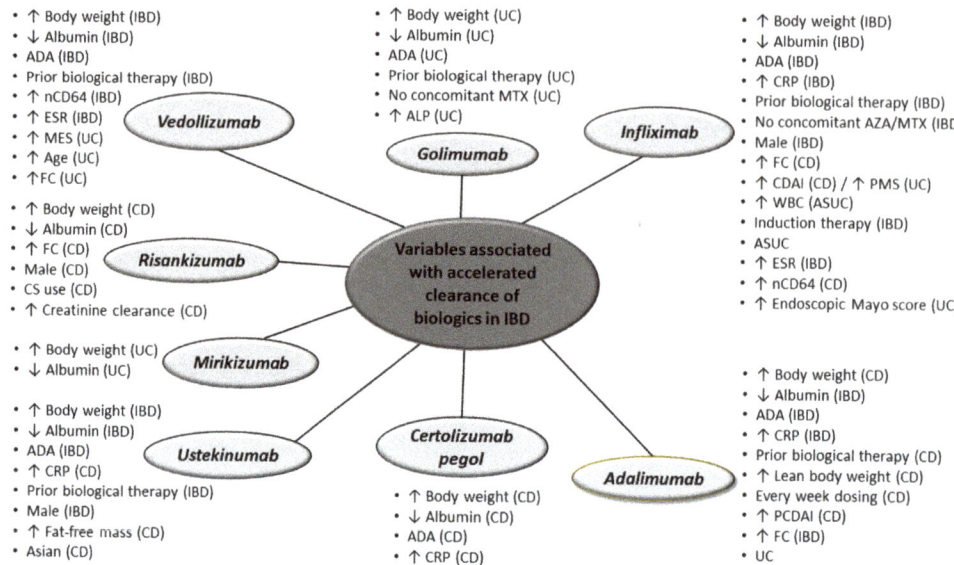

Figure 1. Variables associated with higher clearance of biologics in patients with inflammatory bowel disease. CD: Crohn's disease; IBD: inflammatory bowel disease; UC: ulcerative colitis; ADA; anti-drug antibodies; CRP: C-reactive protein, AZA: azathioprine, MTX: methotrexate, FC: fecal calprotectin, CDAI: Crohn's disease activity index, PMS: partial Mayo score, WBC: white blood count, ESR: erythrocyte sedimentation rate, EOW: every other week, PCDAI: pediatric CDAI, ALP: alkaline phosphatase; nCD64: neutrophil CD64; ↑ higher; ↓ lower.

Drug clearance has gained a lot of attention recently as an increased estimated baseline clearance may identify patients at high risk of underexposure to biologics and PK-related treatment failure. Furthermore, a sudden increase in clearance during therapy can precede the decrease in drug concentrations and may predict a flare prior to the development of symptoms or low drug concentrations. Moreover, cumulative data suggest that there is an association between drug clearance and therapeutic outcomes in patients with IBD (Table 1) [17,21,22,24,32,36,40,47–51].

Table 1. Estimated clearance of biologics associated with therapeutic outcomes in patients with inflammatory bowel disease.

Author (Year)	Study Design	Drug	Population (N)	Estimated Clearance Time Point	Estimated Clearance Threshold, L/Day	Therapeutic Outcome (Time Point)
Battat (2021) [47]	Retrospective	IFX	ASUC (N = 39)	Baseline	≥0.627	Colectomy (6 months)
Vande Casteele (2019) [48]	ACT 1 and 2 RCTs	IFX	UC (N = 484)	Baseline	<0.397	MES ≤ 1 (week 8)
Vande Casteele (2019) [48]	ACT 1 and 2 RCTs	IFX	UC (N = 484)	Baseline	<0.364	MES ≤ 1 (week 30)
Peticollin (2019) [17]	Prospective	IFX	IBD (N = 91)	At time of de-escalation	>0.320	Relapse following treatment de-escalation

Table 1. Cont.

Author (Year)	Study Design	Drug	Population (N)	Estimated Clearance Time Point	Estimated Clearance Threshold, L/Day	Therapeutic Outcome (Time Point)
Whaley (2023) [21]	Prospective	IFX	ASUC * (N = 38)	Day 3 after drug initiation	>0.480	Colectomy
Chung (2023) [24]	Retrospective	IFX	CD (N = 85)	Baseline	<0.230	Remission (5 months)
Chung (2023) [24]	Retrospective	IFX	CD (N = 85)	Baseline	<0.238	Remission (10 months)
Chung (2023) [24]	Retrospective	IFX	CD (N = 85)	Baseline	<0.243	Remission (16 months)
Chung (2023) [24]	Retrospective	IFX	CD (N = 85)	End of induction	<0.230	Remission (5 months)
Chung (2023) [24]	Retrospective	IFX	CD (N = 85)	End of induction	<0.213	Remission (10 months)
Chung (2023) [24]	Retrospective	IFX	CD (N = 85)	End of induction	<0.252	Remission (16 months)
Vermeire (2022) [22]	Prospective	IFX	IBD (N = 276)	Baseline, weeks 2, 6, 14	<0.250	CRP-based clinical remission
Abraham (2023) [49]	Prospective	IFX	IBD (N = 275)	Maintenance	>0.294	Active disease, drug discontinuation
Wright (2023) [50]	Retrospective	ADM	CD (N = 237)	Maintenance #	<0.350	SES-CD < 3
Wright (2023) [50]	Retrospective	ADM	CD (N = 237)	Maintenance #	<0.280	FC < 100 ug/g
Wright (2023) [50]	Retrospective	ADM	CD (N = 237)	Maintenance #	<0.300	CRP-based clinical remission
Lefevre (2022) [32]	PRECiSE 1 and 2 RCTs	CZP	CD (N = 964)	Baseline	>0.500	Drug TC < 36 µg/mL (week 6)
Vande Casteele (2022) [51]	Retrospective	VDZ	IBD (N = 695)	Baseline	<0.170	Clinical remission (week 52)
Vande Casteele (2022) [51]	Retrospective	VDZ	IBD (N = 695)	Baseline	<0.160	Deep remission (week 52)
Osterman (2019) [36]	GEMINI 1 RCT	VDZ	UC (N = 693)	Week 6	<0.140	Clinical response (week 14)
Colman (2022) [40]	Prospective	VDZ	IBD (N = 21)	Baseline	<0.161	FC < 250 mg/g (week 14)

* Pediatric; # The sampling time for adalimumab pharmacokinetics were matched to the study visit assessment, occurring anytime relative to the last dose. IFX: infliximab; ADM: adalimumab; CZP: certolizumab pegol; VDZ: vedolizumab; ASUC: acute severe ulcerative colitis; IBD: inflammatory bowel disease; MES: Mayo endoscopic score; CD: Crohn's disease; UC: ulcerative colitis; FC: fecal calprotectin; CRP: C-reactive protein; SES-CD: Simple Endoscopic Score for Crohn's Disease; RCT: randomized controlled trial; TC: trough concentration.

Finally, clearance is used by model informed precision dosing (MIDP) tools, or PK dashboards, to adjust the dosing for reaching a target drug concentration threshold, typically depending on the desired therapeutic set by the treating physician. However, the role of drug clearance in clinical practice is yet to be determined.

The aim of this comprehensive review is to present data regarding the variables affecting the clearance of specific biologics, the association of clearance with therapeutic outcomes and the role of clearance monitoring and MIPD in patients with IBD.

2. Variables Affecting Clearance of Biologics

2.1. Infliximab

Numerous factors have been shown to accelerate infliximab clearance in patients with IBD. The most frequently identified variables from studies were increased body weight, lower albumin and immunogenicity (Figure 1) [4–20]. Other factors that can lead to high clearance include male gender [5,12,18], induction compared to maintenance therapy [14,21,22], prior biologic therapy [13], an increased Crohn's disease activity index (CDAI) [11], as well as elevated fecal calprotectin [10,11], C-reactive protein (CRP) [14,23,24] and erythrocyte sedimentation rate (ESR) [10]. On the other hand, concomitant immunomodulators (IMMs) (thiopurines/methotrexate) were found to decrease infliximab clearance by around 15% [6,9,17]. This is probably due to the fact that IMM can prevent or suppress immunogenicity as well as decrease the TNF target-antigen burden and consequently the target-mediated elimination of infliximab; although, the mechanisms by which IMM decrease infliximab clearance have not been clearly defined yet [17].

A post hoc analysis of the REACH and ACCENT I randomized controlled trials (RCTs) showed that the clearance was higher in those who developed ADAs or had low baseline albumin [6]. Moreover, concurrent IMM use decreased infliximab clearance by 14% [6]. Data from the Phase I study of maintenance subcutaneous therapy with the infliximab biosimilar CT-P13 in patients with IBD showed that clearance could be increased by 43.2%, 30.1% and 39% by an elevated body weight (from 70 to 120 kg), lower albumin (from 44 to 32 gr/L) and positive ADAs, respectively [13]. The same study showed that patients previously treated with biologics also exhibited a higher drug clearance compared to anti-TNF naïve patients, probably reflecting a more refractory disease and a higher tendency to develop ADAs [13]. A multi-center prospective study including pediatric patients with CD showed that median clearance was higher in ADA-positive compared to ADA-negative patients (0.0111 L/h vs. 0.0094 L/h, $p < 0.001$) [8]. A post hoc analysis of the TAILORIX RCT showed that higher infliximab clearance in patients with CD was associated with increased fecal calprotectin, decreased albumin, increased CDAI and immunogenicity [11]. In a PK analysis of the ACT1 and ACT2, RCTs increased body weight, and lower albumin predicted a higher infliximab clearance in UC. The same study also showed that the mean clearance was 47.1% higher for patients with positive ADAs [12]. A prospective PK study regarding patients with IBD showed that concomitant azathioprine use led to a 15.1% decrease in infliximab clearance [17].

2.2. Adalimumab

Several factors have been shown to accelerate adalimumab clearance in patients with IBD including body weight, lower albumin and immunogenicity. (Figure 1) [26–30]. Other factors associated with increased clearance include prior biologic exposure [50], every week dosing [27], UC [29], elevated CRP [29,30] and higher fecal calprotectin [29].

A post hoc analysis of the SERENE CD and UC RCTs identified increased body weight, lower baseline albumin and immunogenicity as variables associated with higher drug clearance [29]. Other factors associated with accelerated adalimumab clearance were UC and elevated baseline fecal calprotectin and CRP levels. The PK analysis of the IMAgINE-1 RCT showed that increased body weight, higher baseline CRP and lower baseline albumin levels were associated with a greater clearance of adalimumab in pediatric CD [30]. In a prospective multicenter study, positive ADAs increased the clearance of a typical patient with CD from 0.330 L/d to 0.525 L/d [26]. Similarly, another study showed a four-fold increase in adalimumab clearance in the presence of ADAs in patients with CD [27].

2.3. Certolizumab Pegol

Variables associated with a higher clearance of certolizumab pegol in patients with CD include increased body weight, lower albumin, immunogenicity and elevated CRP (Figure 1) [31,32].

In a certolizumab pegol PK modeling study, body weight (46.8–100.5 kg) increased the median clearance from 82 to 120%; albumin (32–48 g/L) decreased drug clearance from 123 to 85%; CRP (0.5–54.0 mg/L) increased the median clearance from 83 to 113%; and positive ADAs increased the median clearance by 142–174% [31]. A PK analysis on phase 2 and 3 certolizumab pegol clinical trials demonstrated that the predicted baseline certolizumab pegol clearance of ≥0.5 L/d was associated with a higher probability of a sub-therapeutic drug concentration at week 6 [32]. The same study using the PRECiSE 1 and 2 RCTs datasets identified a baseline certolizumab pegol clearance associated with composite remission (CDAI ≤ 150 and fecal calprotectin concentration ≤ 250 µg/g) at both week 6 [odds ratio (OR): 0.92; 95% confidence interval (CI): 0.87–0.96] and week 26 (OR: 0.93; 95%CI 0.88–0.97) [32].

2.4. Golimumab

Limited data show that the factors associated with a higher golimumab clearance in patients with UC include increased body weight, lower albumin, immunogenicity, previous biological therapy and a lack of concomitant methotrexate use (Figure 1) [33,34].

A population PK model developed on pooled data from studies regarding adults (NCT00487539 and NCT00488631) and children with moderate-to-severe UC (NCT 01900574), as well as children with polyarticular juvenile idiopathic arthritis (NCT01230827), showed that golimumab clearance increased with body weight and immunogenicity, while the clearance decreased with higher baseline albumin and concomitant methotrexate. Patients receiving methotrexate had a 17% lower clearance compared to those on golimumab monotherapy, and positive ADAs were associated with a 21% higher drug clearance [34]. In the same line, in a PK study of 56 patients with moderate-to-severe UC, golimumab clearance was 31% higher when ADAs were detected [33].

2.5. Vedolizumab

Several factors have been identified to accelerate vedolizumab clearance in patients with IBD; the most important ones being increased body weight, lower albumin and immunogenicity (Figure 1) [35–40]. Other factors that can lead to a high clearance include prior biological therapy [36,38,39], older age [36], and higher endoscopic Mayo score [35], as well as elevated fecal calprotectin [36,39], CRP [39] and ESR [40].

The prospective multicenter LOVE-CD (NCT02646683) study showed that vedolizumab clearance was higher in patients with CD with lower serum albumin concentrations (+26%, from 41 g/L to 28 g/L), presence of ADAs (+89% compared to no ADAs) and previous exposure to other biologic therapies (+25% compared to no biologic naïve patients) [38]. A PK study of the GEMINI 1 RCT demonstrated that the vedolizumab clearance was higher in patients with UC with a history of prior anti-TNF treatment, lower serum albumin and higher fecal calprotectin [36].

2.6. Ustekinumab

Several factors have been identified to accelerate the ustekinumab clearance in patients with IBD including increased body weight, lower albumin and immunogenicity (Figure 1) [41–44]. Other factors that can lead to a high clearance include prior exposure to biologics [42,43], increasing fat-free mass [43], male gender [42,44], Asian race [42] and higher CRP levels [42].

Data from four phase IIb/III ustekinumab clinical trials (C0743T26, CNTO1275CRD3001, CNTO1275CRD3002, CNTO1275CRD3003) demonstrated that increased body weight, elevated CRP, decreased albumin, TNF antagonist failure status (11% higher in failed patients), immunogenicity (increased by 13% in positive ADA status), sex (17% higher in males) and race (14% higher in Asian compared to non-Asian races) were associated with a higher clearance in CD [42]. In a PK analysis of UNIFI (NCT02407236), clearance increased non-linearly with body weight in patients with UC [44]. Moreover, a higher ustekinumab clearance was associated with lower albumin, male sex and immunogenicity [44].

2.7. Risankizumab

A PK analysis from a phase I study in healthy participants (NCT05305222) and phase II and III studies in CD (NCT02031276, ADVANCE, MOTIVATE and FORTIFY) identified increased body weight, decreased albumin, increased fecal calprotectin, corticosteroid use, increased creatinine clearance and male gender as variables associated with higher risakinumab clearance (Figure 1) [45]. Neutralizing antibodies and ADAs were not identified as significant covariates for risankizumab clearance [45].

2.8. Mirikizumab

A PK analysis of three RCTs (NCT02589665, NCT03518086, NCT03524092), including 1362 patients with UC, identified increased body weight and decreased albumin as factors associated with higher mirikizumab clearance (Figure 1) [46].

3. Association of Clearance with Therapeutic Outcomes

There is cumulating evidence suggesting that a higher clearance is associated with sub-therapeutic drug concentrations and unwanted therapeutic outcomes in patients with IBD, while a lower drug clearance is associated with clinical, biomarker, endoscopic and deep remission (Table 1).

Regarding infliximab, a PK analysis of the ACT 1 and two RCTs found a linear relationship between the baseline infliximab clearance and week 8 Mayo endoscopic scores (MES) ($p < 0.001$). Based on a receiver operating characteristic (ROC) curve analysis, a threshold of <0.397 L/d was associated with week 8 MES of ≤ 1 with a sensitivity (SN), specificity (SP), positive predictive value and area under the curve (AUC) of 75%, 48%, 68% and 0.64, respectively [48]. A prospective study of 31 children with IBD showed that patients who achieved deep remission at week 24 had a lower infliximab clearance at week 6 (0.202 L/d vs. 0.269 L/d, $p = 0.020$) and week 12 (0.215 L/d vs. 0.243 L/day, $p = 0.022$) compared to patients not achieving deep remission [52]. In a retrospective study of patients with acute severe UC, the median baseline calculated clearance was higher in patients requiring a colectomy at 6 months than in patients without a colectomy (0.733 vs. 0.569 L/d; $p = 0.005$). An infliximab clearance threshold of 0.627 L/d identified patients who required a colectomy with 80% SN and 82.8% SP (AUC: 0.80) [47]. A multivariable analysis identified the baseline infliximab clearance as the only factor associated with colectomy [47]. A retrospective study of 36 patients with corticosteroid-refractory acute UC showed that the infliximab clearance increased over time in those requiring a colectomy [14]. A prospective study by Peticollin et al. aiming to explore the link between PK parameters and the probability of relapse after de-escalation of infliximab therapy in patients with IBD showed that a drug clearance higher than 0.320 L/d at the time of infliximab de-escalation was associated with a shorter time to relapse [17].

There are only limited data regarding the association of adalimumab clearance with clinical outcomes in patients with IBD (Table 1). A recent retrospective cohort study including patients with CD showed that the median clearance was lower in patients achieving endoscopic remission as compared to those with persistent active endoscopic disease (0.247 L/d vs. 0.326 L/d, $p < 0.01$) [50]. Of note, there was no significant difference in the median adalimumab concentration between patients with endoscopic remission compared to those without (9.3 μg/mL vs. 11.7 μg/mL), implying that drug clearance may be a more superior PK measure than drug concentration to predict outcomes and a better reflection of inflammatory burden than drug concentration. While highly correlated with one another, clearance performed better than drug concentration alone with respect to all investigated outcomes based on the higher AUC in the ROC curve analysis [50].

Regarding the association of vedolizumab clearance with clinical outcomes in patients with IBD, the ERELATE study showed that baseline vedolizumab clearance thresholds of <0.17 L/d and <0.16 L/d were associated with clinical and deep remission at week 52, respectively [51]. The same study showed that clearance in the lower quartiles was associated with higher rates of favorable therapeutic outcomes, including clinical and deep remission assessed either at week 14 or week 52 [51]. In a propensity-score-based case-matching analysis using data from the GEMINI 1, the RCT clinical response and remission rates at week 14 were 26.6% and 5.9%, respectively, in the highest vedolizumab clearance quartile (0.23 to <0.55 L/d) compared to 65.5% and 35.7, respectively, in the lowest vedolizumab clearance concentration quartile (0.03 to <0.14 L/d) at week 6 [36]. In a prospective multicenter study in children with IBD, starting with a vedolizumab baseline clearance of less than 0.161 L/d predicted a fecal calprotectin remission (<250 µg/g) at the end of the induction [40].

Currently, there are no data available regarding the association of ustekinumab, mirikzumab or risankizumab clearance with therapeutic outcomes in patients with IBD.

4. Clearance Monitoring and Model Informed Precision Dosing

The optimal dose of a biologic is not the same for every patient with IBD due to the high interindividual variability in the monoclonal antibodies' PK, and one size does not fit all [3]. Clinical decisions based only on TDM are rather empirical as they are based on analog flowcharts or decision trees that refer more to a trial-and-error treatment optimization, underestimating the true value of TDM [53]. One of the most important aspects of PK is clearance. Clearance precedes changes in drug concentrations and can be an early predictor of disease relapse or development of immunogenicity. A recent study showed that a combination of infliximab concentration and clearance was a better predictor of CRP-based clinical remission compared to either one alone [54]. Another study showed that clearance may be even better than drug concentrations for predicting favorable therapeutic outcomes in patients with CD treated with adalimumab [50].

Baseline clearance, although imprecise as it is estimated only based on patients' clinical and demographic data, can be used to identify patients at high risk of underexposure requiring early proactive TDM and an intensified induction regimen [55]. Drug clearance during biologic therapy is more accurately estimated as drug concentrations are taken into account and can be used by an MIPD tool towards a more personalized implementation of TDM, allowing patient-specific dosing forecasts to accurately achieve a predefined drug concentration target [55]. Of note, clearance monitoring and MIPD do not require TDM at a trough but can operate with intermediate drug concentrations. This allows for more flexibility in the sampling and an extended window of opportunity to adjust dosing. This is particularly important for reactive TDM, as patients are symptomatic and cannot wait until the next drug administration for a clinical decision to be made. A recent study showed an excellent correlation of forecasted infliximab trough concentrations from mid-cycle blood samples with measured trough specimens [56].

MIPD typically uses Bayesian modeling to estimate clearance based on population PK modeling and patient data and a software tool to predict the optimal dosing for achieving a target drug concentration. Preliminary data from retrospective and prospective studies both in adult and pediatric patients with IBD treated with infliximab support the concept of MIPD-based proactive TDM for maintaining therapeutic drug concentrations, showing the benefits of reduced immunogenicity, higher response rates, drug durability and fewer complications [52,57–63]. Most importantly, the PRECISION RCT (NCT02453776) demonstrated that a PK dashboard-based proactive TDM of infliximab was superior to standard dosing for sustaining remission during maintenance therapy [64].

The real-world impact of infliximab precision-guided dosing on management of patients with IBD was demonstrated by a recent study of 275 patients and 37 providers, where in 58% of cases, providers modified the treatment plans based on the results of the MIDP, including dose modifications (41%) and drug discontinuation (8%). Moreover, all providers reported that MIPD was beneficial in guiding treatment decisions and added more value to their practice than routine TDM [49]. A physiologically based pharmacokinetic model was recently used to predict the PK of anti-TNF agents in pregnant women, fetuses and infants to inform dosing decisions for infliximab, adalimumab and golimumab in pregnancy and vaccination regimens for infants [65]. However, wide utilization of MIPD in clinical practice is hindered by its limited availability, high cost, undetermined optimal TDM sampling based also on the assay used, the lack of clearly defined targets for drug concentrations among different IBD phenotypes and the complexity of bedside implementation. Preliminary data suggest that an MIPD tool can be embedded within the electronic health record, guiding clinical decisions in real time for pediatric patients with CD treated with infliximab or adalimumab [10,66].

5. Conclusions

Cumulative data suggest that clearance monitoring of biologics can predict therapeutic outcomes in IBD. Preliminary data also demonstrate the importance of clearance when estimated by MIPD tools for providing dosing recommendations towards treatment optimization. However, more prospective studies are needed to establish the role of MIPD of biologics in IBD and to investigate the efficacy of a novel therapeutic strategy that includes the combination of MIPD-based proactive TDM and pharmacodynamics monitoring. The ongoing RCTs TITRATE (NCT03937609), MODIFI (NCT04982172), REMODEL-CD (NCT05660746) and OPTIMIZE (NCT04835506) will shed more light on the role of MIPD of infliximab in IBD. Future perspectives regarding the use of MIPD include the incorporation of additional factors such as visceral adipose tissue, human leukocyte antigen haplotypes or drug concentration at the site of inflammation that could increase the accuracy of the estimated clearance and the dosing predictions.

Author Contributions: T.D. and K.P.: manuscript drafting, reviewing and editing. A.S.C.: manuscript reviewing and editing. All authors have read and agreed to the published version of the manuscript.

Funding: This research received no external funding.

Institutional Review Board Statement: Not applicable.

Informed Consent Statement: Not applicable.

Data Availability Statement: Not applicable.

Conflicts of Interest: K.P. received lecture/speaker fees from Physicians Education Resource LLC and Grifols; scientific advisory board fees from ProciseDx Inc and Scipher Medicine Corporation; and serves as a consultant for Prometheus Laboratories Inc. A.S.C. served as a consultant and/or advisory board member for Janssen, Abbvie, Protagonist, Spherix, Artizan, Food is Good, Clario, Pfizer, Fresenius Kabi, Artugen, ProciseDx, Prometheus, Equillium, Samsung, Arena, Bacainn, Bristol Myers Squibb, Takeda; unbranded speaker for BMS and Abbvie. T.D declares no conflicts of interest.

References

1. Papamichael, K.; Gils, A.; Rutgeerts, P.; Levesque, B.G.; Vermeire, S.; Sandborn, W.J.; Casteele, V. Role for therapeutic drug monitoring during induction therapy with TNF antagonists in IBD: Evolution in the definition and management of primary nonresponse. *Inflamm. Bowel Dis.* **2015**, *21*, 182–197. [CrossRef]
2. Miligkos, M.; Papamichael, K.; Vande Casteele, N.; Mantzaris, G.M.; Gils, A.; Levesque, B.G.; Zintzaras, E. Efficacy and safety profile of anti-tumor necrosis factor-α versus anti-integrin agents for the treatment of Crohn's disease: A network meta-analysis of indirect comparisons. *Clin. Ther.* **2016**, *38*, 1342–1358. [CrossRef]
3. Kantasiripitak, W.; Wang, Z.; Spriet, I.; Ferrante, M.; Dreesen, E. Recent advances in clearance monitoring of monoclonal antibodies in patients with inflammatory bowel diseases. *Exp. Rev. Clin. Pharmacol.* **2021**, *14*, 1455–1466. [CrossRef]
4. Edlund, H.; Steenholdt, C.; Ainsworth, M.A.; Goebgen, E.; Brynskov, J.; Thomsen, O.; WHuisinga, W.; Kloft, C. Magnitude of increased infliximab clearance imposed by anti-infliximab antibodies in Crohn's disease is determined by their concentration. *AAPS J.* **2017**, *19*, 223–233. [CrossRef]
5. Fasanmade, A.A.; Adedokun, O.J.; Ford, J.; Hernandez, D.; Johanns, J.; Hu, C.; Davis, H.M.; Zhou, H. Population pharmacokinetic analysis of infliximab in patients with ulcerative colitis. *Eur. J. Clin. Pharmacol.* **2009**, *65*, 1211–1228. [CrossRef]
6. Fasanmade, A.A.; Adedokun, O.J.; Blank, M.; Zhou, H.; Davis, H.M. Pharmacokinetic Properties of infliximab in children and adults with Crohn's disease: A retrospective analysis of data from 2 phase III clinical trials. *Clin. Ther.* **2011**, *33*, 946–964. [CrossRef]
7. Fasanmade, A.A.; Adedokun, O.J.; Olson, A.; Strauss, R.; Davis, H.M. Serum albumin concentration: A predictive factor of infliximab pharmacokinetics and clinical response in patients with ulcerative colitis. *Int. J. Clin. Pharmacol. Ther.* **2010**, *48*, 297–308. [CrossRef]

8. Colman, R.J.; Xiong, Y.; Mizuno, T.; Hyams, J.S.; Noe, J.D.; Boyle, B.; D'Haens, G.R.; van Limbergen, J.; Chun, K.; Yang, J.; et al. Antibodies-to-infliximab accelerate clearance while dose intensification reverses immunogenicity and recaptures clinical response in paediatric Crohn's disease. *Aliment. Pharmacol. Ther.* **2022**, *55*, 593–603. [CrossRef]
9. Grisic, A.M.; Eser, A.; Huisinga, W.; Reinisch, W.; Kloft, C. Quantitative relationship between infliximab exposure and inhibition of C-reactive protein synthesis to support inflammatory bowel disease management. *Br. J. Clin. Pharmacol.* **2021**, *87*, 2374–2384. [CrossRef]
10. Xiong, Y.; Mizuno, T.; Colman, R.; Hyams, J.; Noe, J.D.; Boyle, B.; Tsai, Y.T.; Dong, M.; Jackson, K.; Punt, N.; et al. Real-World infliximab pharmacokinetic study informs an electronic health record-embedded dashboard to guide precision dosing in children with Crohn's disease. *Clin. Pharmacol. Ther.* **2021**, *109*, 1639–1647. [CrossRef]
11. Dreesen, E.; Berends, S.; Laharie, D.; D'Haens, G.; Vermeire, S.; Gils, A.; Mathôt, R. Modelling of the relationship between infliximab exposure, faecal calprotectin and endoscopic remission in patients with Crohn's disease. *Br. J. Clin. Pharmacol.* **2021**, *87*, 106–118. [CrossRef]
12. Adedokun, O.J.; Xu, Z.; Padgett, L.; Blank, M.; Johanns, J.; Griffiths, A.; Ford, J.; Zhou, H.; Guzzo, C.; Davis, H.M.; et al. Pharmacokinetics of infliximab in children with moderate-to-severe ulcerative colitis: Results from a randomized, multicenter, open-label, phase 3 study. *Inflamm. Bowel Dis.* **2013**, *19*, 2753–2762. [CrossRef]
13. Hanzel, J.; Bukkems, L.H.; Gecse, K.B.; D'Haens, G.R.; Mathôt, R.A. Population pharmacokinetics of subcutaneous infliximab CT-P13 in Crohn's disease and ulcerative colitis. *Aliment. Pharmacol. Ther.* **2021**, *54*, 1309–1319. [CrossRef]
14. Kevans, D.; Murthy, S.; Mould, D.R.; Silverberg, M.S. Accelerated clearance of infliximab is associated with treatment failure in patients with corticosteroid-refractory acute ulcerative colitis. *J. Crohn's Colitis* **2018**, *12*, 662–669. [CrossRef]
15. Matsuoka, K.; Hamada, S.; Shimizu, M.; Nanki, K.; Mizuno, S.; Kiyohara, H.; Arai, M.; Sugimoto, S.; Iwao, Y.; Ogata, H.; et al. Factors contributing to the systemic clearance of infliximab with long-term administration in Japanese patients with Crohn's disease: Analysis using population pharmacokinetics. *Int. J. Clin. Pharmacol. Ther.* **2020**, *58*, 89. [CrossRef]
16. Petitcollin, A.; Leuret, O.; Tron, C.; Lemaitre, F.; Verdier, M.C.; Paintaud, G.; Bouguen, G.; Willot, S.; Bellissant, E.; Ternant, D. Modeling immunization to infliximab in children with Crohn's disease using population pharmacokinetics: A pilot study. *Inflamm. Bowel Dis.* **2018**, *24*, 1745–1754. [CrossRef]
17. Petitcollin, A.; Brochard, C.; Siproudhis, L. Pharmacokinetic parameters of infliximab influence the rate of relapse after de-escalation in adults with inflammatory bowel diseases. *Clin. Pharmacol. Ther.* **2019**, *106*, 605–615. [CrossRef]
18. Buurman, D.J.; Maurer, J.M.; Keizer, R.J.; Kosterink, J.G.W.; Dijkstra, G. Population pharmacokinetics of infliximab in patients with inflammatory bowel disease: Potential implications for dosing in clinical practice. *Aliment. Pharmacol. Ther.* **2015**, *42*, 529–539. [CrossRef]
19. Brandse, J.F.; Mould, D.; Smeekes, O.; Ashruf, Y.; Kuin, S.; Strik, A.; van den Brink, G.R.; D'Haens, G.R. A real-life population pharmacokinetic study reveals factors associated with clearance and immunogenicity of infliximab in inflammatory bowel disease. *Inflamm. Bowel Dis.* **2017**, *23*, 650–660. [CrossRef]
20. Schreiber, S.; Ben-Horin, S.; Leszczyszyn, J.; Dudkowiak, R.; Lahat, A.; Gawdis-Wojnarska, B.; Pukitis, A.; Horynski, M.; Farkas, K.; Kierkus, J.; et al. Randomized controlled trial: Subcutaneous vs intravenous infliximab CT-P13 maintenance in inflammatory bowel disease. *Gastroenterology* **2021**, *160*, 2340–2353. [CrossRef]
21. Whaley, K.G.; Xiong, Y.; Karns, R.; Hyams, J.S.; Kugathasan, S.; Boyle, B.M.; Walters, T.D.; Kelsen, J.; LeLeiko, N.; Shapiro, J.; et al. Multicenter cohort study of infliximab pharmacokinetics and therapy response in pediatric acute severe ulcerative colitis. *Clin. Gastroenterol. Hepatol.* **2023**, *21*, 1338–1347. [CrossRef] [PubMed]
22. Vermeire, S.; D'Haens, G.; Laharie, D.; Dreesen, E.; Rabizadeh, S.; Jain, A.; Spencer, E.A.; Panetta, J.C.; Dubinsky, M.; Dervieux, T. Infliximab clearance pre-therapy and during induction predicts long term disease control in inflammatory bowel disease. *Gastroenterology* **2022**, *162*, S45–S46. [CrossRef]
23. Le Tilly, O.; Bejan-Angoulvant, T.; Paintaud, G.; Ternant, D. Letter to Dreesen et al. on their article "Modelling of the Relationship Between Infliximab Exposure, Faecal Calprotectin, and Endoscopic Remission in Patients with Crohn's Disease"—A comprehensive review of infliximab population pharmacokinetic modelling publications. *Br. J. Clin. Pharmacol.* **2021**, *87*, 1594–1595. [CrossRef] [PubMed]
24. Chung, A.; Carroll, M.; Almeida, P.; Petrova, A.; Isaac, D.; Mould, D.; Wine, E.; Huynh, H. Early infliximab clearance predicts remission in children with Crohn's disease. *Dig. Dis. Sci.* **2023**, *68*, 1995–2005. [CrossRef]
25. Bauman, L.E.; Xiong, Y.; Mizuno, T.; Minar, P.; Fukuda, T.; Dong, M.; Rosen, M.J.; Vinks, A.A. Improved population pharmacokinetic model for predicting optimized infliximab exposure in pediatric inflammatory bowel disease. *Inflamm. Bowel Dis.* **2020**, *26*, 429–439. [CrossRef] [PubMed]
26. Vande Casteele, N.; Baert, F.; Bian, S.; Dreesen, E.; Compernolle, G.; Van Assche, G.; Ferrante, M.; Vermeire, S.; Gils, A. Subcutaneous absorption contributes to observed interindividual variability in adalimumab serum concentrations in Crohn's disease: A prospective multicentre study. *J. Crohn's Colitis* **2019**, *13*, 1248–1256. [CrossRef]
27. Berends, S.E.; Strik, A.S.; Van Selm, J.C.; Löwenberg, M.; Ponsioen, C.Y.; D'Haens, G.R.; Mathôt, R.A. Explaining interpatient variability in adalimumab pharmacokinetics in patients with Crohn's disease. *Ther. Drug Monit.* **2018**, *40*, 202–211. [CrossRef]
28. Ternant, D.; Karmiris, K.; Vermeire, S.; Desvignes, C.; Azzopardi, N.; Bejan-Angoulvant, T.; Van Assche, G.; Paintaud, G. Pharmacokinetics of adalimumab in Crohn's disease. *Eur. J. Clin. Pharmacol.* **2015**, *71*, 1155–1157. [CrossRef]

29. Ponce-Bobadilla, A.V.; Stodtmann, S.; Chen, M.J.; Winzenborg, I.; Mensing, S.; Blaes, J.; Haslberger, T.; Laplanche, L.; Dreher, I.; Mostafa, N.M. Assessing the impact of immunogenicity and improving prediction of trough concentrations: Population pharmacokinetic modeling of adalimumab in patients with Crohn's disease and ulcerative colitis. *Clin. Pharmacokinet.* **2023**, *62*, 623–634. [CrossRef]
30. Sharma, S.; Eckert, D.; Hyams, J.S.; Mensing, S.; Thakkar, R.B.; Robinson, A.M.; Rosh, J.R.; Ruemmele, F.M.; Awni, W.M. Pharmacokinetics and exposure–efficacy relationship of adalimumab in pediatric patients with moderate to severe Crohn's disease: Results from a randomized, multicenter, phase-3 study. *Inflamm. Bowel Dis.* **2015**, *21*, 783–792. [CrossRef]
31. Vande Casteele, N.; Mould, D.R.; Coarse, J.; Hasan, I.; Gils, A.; Feagan, B.; Sandborn, W.J. Accounting for pharmacokinetic variability of certolizumab pegol in patients with Crohn's disease. *Clin. Pharmacokinet.* **2017**, *56*, 1513–1523. [CrossRef] [PubMed]
32. Lefevre, P.L.C.; Dulai, P.S.; Wang, Z.; Guizzetti, L.; Feagan, B.G.; Pop, A.; Yassine, M.; Shackelton, L.M.; Jairath, V.; Sandborn, W.J.; et al. A clinical prediction model to determine probability of response to certolizumab pegol for Crohn's disease. *BioDrugs.* **2022**, *36*, 85–93. [CrossRef]
33. Dreesen, E.; Kantasiripitak, W.; Detrez, I.; Stefanović, S.; Vermeire, S.; Ferrante, M.; Bouillon, T.; Drobne, D.; Gils, A. A Population pharmacokinetic and exposure–response model of golimumab for targeting endoscopic remission in patients with ulcerative colitis. *Inflamm. Bowel Dis.* **2020**, *26*, 570–580. [CrossRef]
34. Xu, Y.; Adedokun, O.J.; Chan, D.; Hu, C.; Xu, Z.; Strauss, R.S.; Hyams, J.S.; Turner, D.; Zhou, H. Population pharmacokinetics and exposure-response modeling analyses of golimumab in children with moderately to severely active ulcerative colitis. *J. Clin. Pharmacol.* **2019**, *59*, 590–604. [CrossRef]
35. Rosario, M.; Dirks, N.L.; Gastonguay, M.R.; Fasanmade, A.A.; Wyant, T.; Parikh, A.; Sandborn, W.J.; Feagan, B.G.; Reinisch, W.; Fox, I. Population pharmacokinetics-pharmacodynamics of vedolizumab in patients with ulcerative colitis and Crohn's disease. *Aliment. Pharmacol. Ther.* **2015**, *42*, 188–202. [CrossRef] [PubMed]
36. Osterman, M.T.; Rosario, M.; Lasch, K.; Barocas, M.; Wilbur, J.D.; Dirks, N.L.; Gastonguay, M.R. Vedolizumab exposure levels and clinical outcomes in ulcerative colitis: Determining the potential for dose optimisation. *Aliment. Pharmacol. Ther.* **2019**, *49*, 408–418. [CrossRef] [PubMed]
37. Okamoto, H.; Dirks, N.L.; Rosario, M.; Hori, T.; Hibi, T. Population pharmacokinetics of vedolizumab in Asian and non-Asian patients with ulcerative colitis and Crohn's disease. *Intest. Res.* **2021**, *19*, 95–105. [CrossRef]
38. Hanzel, J.; Dreesen, E.; Vermeire, S.; Löwenberg, M.; Hoentjen, F.; Bossuyt, P.; Clasquin, E.; Baert, F.J.; D'Haens, G.R.; Mathôt, R. Pharmacokinetic-pharmacodynamic model of vedolizumab for targeting endoscopic remission in patients with Crohn disease: Post-hoc analysis of the LOVE-CD study. *Inflamm. Bowel Dis.* **2022**, *28*, 689–699. [CrossRef]
39. Colman, R.J.; Mizuno, T.; Fukushima, K.; Haslam, D.B.; Hyams, J.S.; Boyle, B.; Noe, J.D.; D'Haens, G.R.; Van Limbergen, J.; Chun, K.; et al. Real world population pharmacokinetic study in children and young adults with inflammatory bowel disease discovers novel blood and stool microbial predictors of vedolizumab clearance. *Aliment. Pharmacol. Ther.* **2023**, *57*, 524–539. [CrossRef]
40. Colman, R.; Mizuno, T.; Hyams, J.; Noe, J.; Boyle, B.; Denson, L.; Vinks, A.; Minar, P. Real-world vedolizumab pharmacokinetic study in children identifies two novel biomarkers of drug clearance. *Gastroenterology* **2022**, *162*, S100. [CrossRef]
41. Wang, Z.; Verstockt, B.; Sabino, J.; Vermeire, S.; Ferrante, M.; Declerck, P.; Dreesen, E. Population pharmacokinetic-pharmacodynamic model-based exploration of alternative ustekinumab dosage regimens for patients with Crohn's disease. *Br. J. Clin. Pharmacol.* **2022**, *88*, 323–335. [CrossRef] [PubMed]
42. Adedokun, O.J.; Xu, Z.; Gasink, C.; Kowalski, K.; Sandborn, W.J.; Feagan, B. Population pharmacokinetics and exposure–response analyses of ustekinumab in patients with moderately to severely active Crohn's disease. *Clin. Ther.* **2022**, *44*, 1336–1355. [CrossRef]
43. Aguiar Zdovc, J.; Hanžel, J.; Kurent, T.; Sever, N.; Koželj, M.; Smrekar, N.; Novak, G.; Štabuc, B.; Dreesen, E.; Thomas, D.; et al. Ustekinumab dosing individualization in crohn's disease guided by a population pharmacokinetic–pharmacodynamic model. *Pharmaceutics* **2021**, *13*, 1587. [CrossRef] [PubMed]
44. Xu, Y.; Hu, C.; Chen, Y.; Miao, X.; Adedokun, O.J.; Xu, Z.; Sharma, A.; Zhou, H. Population pharmacokinetics and exposure-response modeling analyses of ustekinumab in adults with moderately to severely active ulcerative colitis. *J. Clin. Pharmacol.* **2020**, *60*, 889–902. [CrossRef] [PubMed]
45. Suleiman, A.A.; Goebel, A.; Bhatnagar, S.; D'Cunha, R.; Liu, W.; Pang, Y. Population pharmacokinetic and exposure–response analyses for efficacy and safety of risankizumab in patients with active Crohn's disease. *Clin. Pharmacol. Ther.* **2023**, *113*, 839–850. [CrossRef]
46. Chua, L.; Friedrich, S.; Zhang, X.C. Mirikizumab pharmacokinetics in patients with moderately to severely active ulcerative colitis: Results from phase III LUCENT Studies. *Clin. Pharmacokinet.* **2023**, *62*, 1479–1491. [CrossRef]
47. Battat, R.; Hemperly, A.; Truong, S.; Whitmire, N.; Boland, B.S.; Dulai, P.S.; Holmer, A.K.; Nguyen, N.H.; Singh, S.; Vande Casteele, N.; et al. Baseline clearance of infliximab is associated with requirement for colectomy in patients with acute severe ulcerative colitis. *Clin. Gastroenterol. Hepatol.* **2021**, *19*, 511–518. [CrossRef]
48. Vande Casteele, N.; Jeyarajah, J.; Jairath, V.; Feagan, B.G.; Sandborn, W.J. Infliximab exposure-response relationship and thresholds associated with endoscopic healing in patients with ulcerative colitis. *Clin. Gastroenterol. Hepatol.* **2019**, *17*, 1814–1821. [CrossRef]
49. Abraham, B.P.; Ziring, D.A.; Dervieux, T.; Han, P.A.; Shim, A.; Battat, R. Real-world impact of infliximab precision-guided dosing on management of patients with IBD. *Am. J. Manag. Care* **2023**, *29*, S227–S235. [CrossRef]

50. Wright, E.K.; Chaparro, M.; Gionchetti, P.; Hamilton, A.L.; Schulberg, J.; Gisbert, J.P.; Valerii, M.C.; Rizzello, F.; De Cruz, P.; Panetta, J.C.; et al. Adalimumab clearance, rather than trough level, may have greatest relevance to crohn's disease therapeutic outcomes assessed clinically and endoscopically. *J. Crohn's Colitis* 2023, jjad140, *Online ahead of print*. [CrossRef]
51. Vande Casteele, N.; Sandborn, W.J.; Feagan, B.G. Real-world multicentre observational study including population pharmacokinetic modelling to evaluate the exposure–response relationship of vedolizumab in inflammatory bowel disease: ERELATE Study. *Aliment. Pharmacol. Ther.* 2022, *56*, 463–476. [CrossRef]
52. Kantasiripitak, W.; Wicha, S.G.; Thomas, D.; Hoffman, I.; Ferrante, M.; Vermeire, S.; Karen van Hoeve, K.; Dreesen, E. A model-based tool for guiding infliximab induction dosing to maximise long-term deep remission in children with inflammatory bowel diseases. *J. Crohn's Colitis* 2023, jjad009. [CrossRef]
53. Wang, Z.; Dreesen, E. Therapeutic drug monitoring of anti-tumor necrosis factor agents: Lessons learned and remaining issues. *Curr. Opin. Pharmacol.* 2020, *55*, 53–59. [CrossRef] [PubMed]
54. Dubinsky, M.C.; Rabizadeh, S.; Panetta, J.C.; Spencer, E.A.; Everts-van der Wind, A.; Dervieux, T. The combination of predictive factors of pharmacokinetic origin associates with enhanced disease control during treatment of pediatric Crohn's disease with infliximab. *Pharmaceutics* 2023, *15*, 2408. [CrossRef] [PubMed]
55. Kantasiripitak, W.; Outtier, A.; Wicha, S.G.; Kensert, K.; Wang, Z.; Sabino, J.; Vermeire, S.; Thomas, D.; Ferrante, M.; Dreesen, E. Multi-model averaging improves the performance of model-guided infliximab dosing in patients with inflammatory bowel diseases. *CPT Pharmacomet. Syst. Pharmacol.* 2022, *11*, 1045–1059. [CrossRef]
56. Primas, C.; Reinisch, W.; Panetta, J.C.; Eser, A.; Mould, D.R.; Dervieux, T. Model informed precision dosing tool forecasts trough infliximab and associates with disease status and tumor necrosis factor-alpha levels of inflammatory bowel diseases. *J. Clin. Med.* 2022, *11*, 3316. [CrossRef]
57. Dubinsky, M.C.; Phan, B.L.; Singh, N.; Rabizadeh, S.; Mould, D.R. Pharmacokinetic dashboard-recommended dosing is different than standard of care dosing in infliximab-treated pediatric IBD patients. *AAPS J.* 2017, *19*, 215–222. [CrossRef] [PubMed]
58. Eser, A.; Primas, C.; Reinisch, S.; Vogelsang, H.; Novacek, G.; Mould, D.R.; Reinisch, W. Prediction of individual serum infliximab concentrations in inflammatory bowel disease by a Bayesian dashboard system. *J. Clin. Pharmacol.* 2018, *58*, 790–802. [CrossRef]
59. Dubinsky, M.C.; Mendiolaza, M.L.; Phan, B.L.; Moran, H.R.; Tse, S.S.; Mould, D.R. Dashboard-driven accelerated infliximab induction dosing increases infliximab durability and reduces immunogenicity. *Inflamm. Bowel Dis.* 2022, *28*, 1375–1385. [CrossRef]
60. Santacana Juncosa, E.; Rodríguez-Alonso, L.; Padullés Zamora, A.; Guardiola, J.; Rodríguez-Moranta, F.; Nilsson, K.S.; Minguet, J.B.; Rego, F.M.; Codina, H.C.; Zamora, N.P. Bayes-based dosing of infliximab in inflammatory bowel diseases: Short-term efficacy. *Br. J. Clin. Pharmacol.* 2021, *87*, 494–505. [CrossRef]
61. Papamichael, K.; Cheifetz, A.S. Optimizing therapeutic drug monitoring in inflammatory bowel disease: A focus on therapeutic monoclonal antibodies. *Expert Opin. Drug Metab. Toxicol.* 2021, *17*, 1423–1431. [CrossRef]
62. Serrano-Díaz, L.; Iniesta-Navalón, C.; Gómez-Espín, R.; Nicolás-de Prado, I.; Bernal-Morell, E.; Rentero-Redondo, L. Impact of proactive therapeutic drug monitoring of infliximab during the induction phase in IBD patients. A Bayesian Approach. *Rev. Esp. Enferm. Dig.* 2023, *115*, 435–443. [CrossRef] [PubMed]
63. Díaz, L.S.; Navalón, C.I.; Espín, R.G.; Nicolás-de Prado, I.; Bernal-Morell, E.; Rentero-Redondo, L. Impact of proactive of infliximab monitoring using the Bayesian approach in the maintenance phase in patients with inflammatory bowel disease. *Gastroenterol. Hepatol.* 2023, *46*, 504–511. [CrossRef] [PubMed]
64. Strik, A.S.; Löwenberg, M.; Mould, D.R.; Berends, S.E.; Ponsioen, C.I.; van den Brande, J.M.H.; Jansen, J.M.; Hoekman, D.R.; Brandse, J.F.; Duijvestein, M.; et al. Efficacy of dashboard driven dosing of infliximab in inflammatory bowel disease patients; a randomized controlled trial. *Scand. J. Gastroenterol.* 2021, *56*, 145–154. [CrossRef] [PubMed]
65. Chen, J.; Lin, R.; Guo, G.; Wu, W.; Ke, M.; Ke, C.; Huang, P.; Lin, C. Physiologically-based pharmacokinetic modeling of anti-tumor necrosis factor agents for inflammatory bowel disease patients to predict the withdrawal time in pregnancy and vaccine time in infants. *Clin. Pharmacol. Ther.* 2023, *Online ahead of print*. [CrossRef]
66. Colman, R.J.; Samuels, A.; Mizuno, T.; Punt, N.; Vinks, A.A.; Minar, P. Model-informed precision dosing for biologics is now available at the bedside for patients with inflammatory bowel disease. *Inflamm. Bowel Dis.* 2023, *29*, 1342–1346. [CrossRef] [PubMed]

Disclaimer/Publisher's Note: The statements, opinions and data contained in all publications are solely those of the individual author(s) and contributor(s) and not of MDPI and/or the editor(s). MDPI and/or the editor(s) disclaim responsibility for any injury to people or property resulting from any ideas, methods, instructions or products referred to in the content.

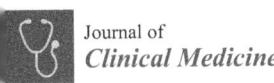

Article

Promising Tools to Facilitate the Implementation of TDM of Biologics in Clinical Practice

Rani Soenen [1,2,3], Christophe Stove [4], Alessio Capobianco [2], Hanne De Schutter [2], Marie Dobbelaere [2], Tahmina Mahjor [2], Merel Follens [2], Jo Lambert [1,2,*] and Lynda Grine [1,2]

1 Department of Dermatology, Ghent University Hospital, 9000 Ghent, Belgium; rani.soenen@uzgent.be (R.S.); lynda.grine@gmail.com (L.G.)
2 Dermatology Research Unit, University Ghent, 9000 Ghent, Belgium; alessio.capobianco@ugent.be (A.C.); hanne.deschutter@ugent.be (H.D.S.); marie.dobbelaere@ugent.be (M.D.); tahmina.mahjor@ugent.be (T.M.); merel.follens@ugent.be (M.F.)
3 Department of Pharmaceutical and Pharmacological Sciences, KU Leuven, 3000 Leuven, Belgium
4 Department of Bioanalysis, Ghent University Hospital, 9000 Ghent, Belgium; christophe.stove@ugent.be
* Correspondence: jo.lambert@uzgent.be

Abstract: Therapeutic drug monitoring (TDM) of biologics—encompassing the measurement of (trough) concentrations and anti-drug antibodies—is emerging as a valuable tool for clinical decision making. While this strategy needs further validation, attention on its implementation into the clinic is warranted. Rapid testing and easy sampling are key to its implementation. Here, we aimed to evaluate the feasibility and volunteers' perception of home microsampling for quantification of adalimumab (ADM) concentrations in psoriasis patients. In addition, we compared lateral flow testing (LFT) with enzyme-linked immunosorbent assay (ELISA). Patients participating in the SUPRA-A study (clinicaltrials.gov NCT04028713) were asked to participate in a substudy where volumetric absorptive microsampling (VAMS) was performed at home. At three time points, whole blood and corresponding serum samples were collected for ADM measurement using an in-house ELISA. In addition, the patients' perspective on microsampling was evaluated via a questionnaire. LFT-obtained ADM concentrations agreed very well with ELISA results (Pearson's correlation = 0.95 and R^2 = 0.89). ADM concentrations determined in both capillary (via finger prick) and corresponding venous blood VAMS samples correlated strongly with serum concentrations (Pearson's correlation = 0.87). Our preliminary data (n = 7) on rapid testing and home-based microsampling are considered promising with regard to TDM implementation for adalimumab, warranting further research.

Keywords: psoriasis; biologics; therapeutic drug monitoring; lateral flow testing; microsampling

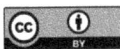

1. Introduction

The management of patients with moderate-to-severe psoriasis has changed dramatically over the past years and has greatly benefited from the use of biologics, monoclonal antibodies targeting specific components of the immune system [1]. The first class of biologics comprises anti-tumor necrosis factor (anti-TNF) agents, including infliximab, adalimumab (ADM), etanercept and golimumab, which remain widely used in psoriasis, in addition to psoriatic arthritis and inflammatory bowel disease [2]. Although the efficacy is superior compared to conventional systemic treatments such as methotrexate [3], real-world evidence on effectiveness revealed primary and secondary non-responders [4–6]. Primary non-responders are considered patients who do not respond or insufficiently respond to the biologic, whereas secondary non-responders include patients who responded well initially, yet lose clinical response over time. A variety of reasons exist for these observations, but the exact mechanisms remain to be unraveled [7].

One explanation entails drug exposure, which is usually measured through the trough (i.e., right before the next drug administration) concentrations in serum or plasma. To this end, a therapeutic window may be defined, making it possible to categorize patients as 'underexposed' or 'overexposed' (Figure 1).

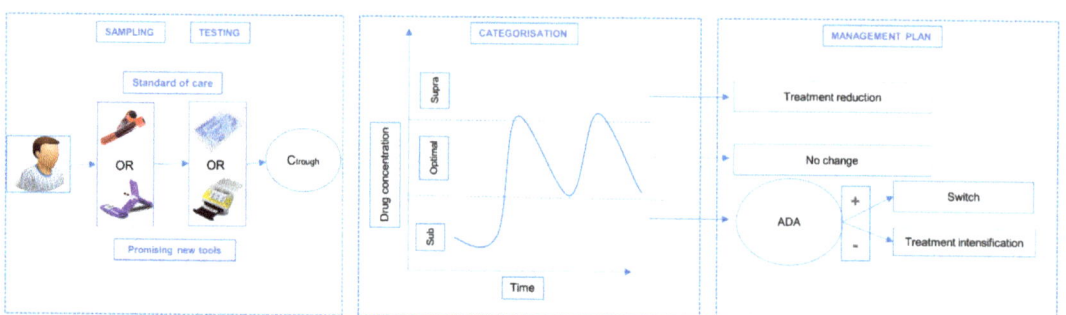

Figure 1. Concept of therapeutic drug monitoring. Therapeutic drug monitoring as proposed in the SUPRA-A trial: blood from the patient is sampled at trough as either whole blood (venipuncture or finger prick). Adalimumab (ADM) concentrations can then be quantified by ELISA or lateral flow testing (LFT). Based on the therapeutic window of ADM (dotted horizontal lines in graph) [8,9], the patients' trough levels can be categorized into three categories: supratherapeutic (above upper threshold of window), optimal (within window), or subtherapeutic (below lower threshold of window). Depending on the categorization, a management plan is set up by the physician and the dose administration can be adapted. In case of subtherapeutic levels, additional testing of immunogenicity may be required to detect anti-drug antibodies (ADA). If ADA-negative, a dose increase (intensification) may be needed. If ADAs are present, a treatment switch is recommended. Figure adapted from Research Foundation—Flanders (FWO) grant proposal (T003218N). Abbreviations: ADA—Anti-Drug Antibodies; Ctrough—serum trough concentration (i.e., drug concentration right before the next drug administration.

The use of the concept of a therapeutic window, and corresponding adaptation of a dosing regimen to ensure that the concentrations of a drug lie within this window, is coined 'therapeutic drug monitoring' (TDM). TDM already found its way in the field of treatment of inflammatory bowel disease with anti-TNF agents [10]. Here, windows have been defined for infliximab, vedolizumab, golimumab, and ADM [8,9,11]. Interestingly, the definition of such windows heavily depend on several factors, including the timing of sampling (induction versus maintenance phase), the quantification assay but also the clinical outcome and of course the disease [10]. To illustrate the latter, Juncadella et al. evaluated ADM concentrations in light of several objective therapeutic outcomes: ADM levels of 11.8, 12.0, and 12.2 µg/mL were associated with biochemical, endoscopic or histological remission in patients with Crohn's disease; respectively [11]. For ulcerative colitis, levels of 10.5, 16.2, and 16.2 µg/mL of ADM were defined as threshold for the respective outcomes. Endoscopic and histological remission required minimum levels of 12 and 12.2 µg/mL of ADM, respectively. Similar observations were made for infliximab [12]. In 2015, we defined a window for ADM in psoriasis of 3.51–7.0 mg/L associating with an optimal clinical effect, which was later confirmed by Wilkinson and colleagues in a larger cohort [8,9]. Currently, the use of TDM in patients with overexposure to ADM (supratherapeutic levels) is being investigated in the SUPRA-A trial (recruitment ongoing; clinicaltrials.gov NCT04028713) [13].

However, for TDM to be implemented in clinical practice, several criteria need to be met: first, a therapeutic window or target concentration should be defined based on a dose–response relationship, linking measurable drug concentrations (typically in serum) to a clinical therapeutic efficacy. In addition, serum concentrations should be available rapidly, in case of clinical flares, in order to propose dose adjustments, and, even more, should be obtained with relative ease for patient, clinician and lab. Currently, TDM of biologics is generally performed in serum as the sample matrix, requiring sampling to be done by a healthcare professional and the patient to leave their home. Not only is this time-consuming for the patient, but during the initial COVID-19 pandemic lockdown, nearly impossible [14]. Hence, alternative sampling methods that can be executed in the comfort of the patients' homes have become more relevant. Sampling via dried blood spots (DBS) has long been a standard method of microsampling, with various studies supporting its feasibility in different patient populations [15–19]. It has numerous advantages, including the collection of microvolumes of equal to or less than 20 µL, which is more suitable for reduced blood flow or when handling infants. Moreover, storage and transfer of DBS does not require freezing, making it suitable for various settings (including patient homes or remote locations). Another asset is the simplicity of collection, omitting centrifugation or wet volume transfers and thus biohazardous handling. Lastly, its costs are much lower regarding transport and storage, making it an attractive option for large trials or—when needed regularly—in patient management.

Despite being a relatively robust sampling method for routine drug monitoring, the implementation of dried blood microsampling is hampered by a few issues. First, since whole blood is used as a source, the presence of haematocrit impacts the viscosity of the sample and thus its spreading on filter paper. This may pose an issue as, for a given volume applied on filter paper, blood with a high haematocrit will yield smaller-sized DBS than blood with a low haematocrit. Consequently, when using a partial-punch approach, the blood volume contained within this punch -and hence also the concentration derived for a compound- will differ. This is also referred to as the haematocrit effect [20,21].

Second, the volume of blood that is collected is not easily controlled. However, recently several devices have been developed that allow volumetric collection of blood from a finger prick [20,21]. One of these newer technologies is called volumetric absorptive microsampling (VAMS), in which a polymeric tip wicks up a fixed volume of blood (e.g., 10, 20 or 30 microliters), irrespective of the hematocrit [20,22]. The use of VAMS for various drugs has been tested and was found to be a reliable sampling method, also for the determination of larger proteins such as monoclonal antibodies [16,23].

After sample collection, the sample still needs to be assessed. Until now, in clinical laboratory settings, the measurement of biologics is predominantly performed by means of enzyme-linked immunosorbent assay (ELISA). ELISAs are antigen-specific, provide quantifiable results, and can easily be implemented in clinical laboratories (in essence only requiring an absorbance microplate reader). On a downside, the execution is rather time-consuming (impacting the turn-over time) and it is rather suitable for high-throughput measurement; i.e., to be cost-effective, multiple samples need to be analyzed simultaneously. Only if sufficient patients in a short time window need to be sampled, ELISA is cost-efficient, which may induce long waiting times to meet the serum sample number. To this end, alternative assays were developed, such as 'rapid' testing via lateral flow testing (LFT) assays. LFT has gained massive use amongst the general public since the COVID-19 pandemic [24]. In the field of TDM, LFT for the measurement of ADM and anti-ADM antibodies has been developed as well [25]. However, the use of such assays has remained limited to the clinical setting, due to the requirement of serum or plasma as a matrix and a specific reader.

Although recent advances in the microsampling and rapid testing field allow for several limitations to be tackled, this is yet to be shown for TDM of ADM in the psoriasis population. Here, we report on a preliminary evaluation of the use of rapid testing and home sampling by patients participating in a study assessing non-inferiority of a TDM-based dose reduction strategy for ADM in psoriasis (Soenen et al.; unpublished). In this study, two promising tools to facilitate TDM, self-sampling at home and rapid testing, were evaluated.

2. Materials and Methods

2.1. Study Design and Data Collection

Subjects were recruited from the SUPRA-A trial (NCT04028713) with ethical approval from the Ethics Committee of Ghent University Hospital in Belgium (EudraCT 2019-001918-42). All participating subjects provided written informed consent. The study was conducted in accordance with the Declaration of Helsinki. At the time of writing, the study had not been completed yet.

In short, patients with confirmed supratherapeutic ADM concentration were randomized 1:1 to a control or intervention arm, the latter implying a lengthening of the dose interval (once every 3 weeks instead of bi-weekly). If the therapeutic response remained stable in the intervention arm, the dose reduction could be extended to every 4 weeks. All patients were asked to participate in a substudy in which the use of VAMS was evaluated as an alternative sampling technique for quantification of ADM.

Study data were collected and managed using REDCap (Research Electronic Data Capture) hosted at Ghent University Hospital [26,27].

2.2. Sample Collection, Transportation, Preparation and Storage

On day 0, patients received a short training by an instructed nurse as well as written instructions on home sampling (Supplementary Figure S1). The first sampling was performed under supervision of the trained nurse in the hospital. Afterwards, patients were asked to self-sample at 9 pre-defined time points (day 3, 5, 7, 14, 21, 28, 35, 42, and 49) using a VAMS device, marketed as Mitra® (Neoteryx LLC, Torrance, CA, USA). In short, the device consists of a plastic handler with an absorbent polymeric tip attached to it, which absorbs a precise volume of blood (20 µL), after a finger prick was performed with a 1.8 mm safety lancet (Novolab, Ergolance Blue 25G, Geraardsbergen, Belgium). For each time point, patients received a home sampling kit containing the following materials to perform home sampling (in duplicate, if needed): lancet, sampling cartridge, cotton ball, adhesive bandage and a prepaid shipping envelope with desiccant. At each time point, 2 VAMS samples were collected by the patients (biological replicates). The VAMS samples were sent by postal service under ambient conditions to the Dermatology Research Unit of Ghent University Hospital for processing. Upon receipt, the tips were first visually inspected for absorption efficiency [28]; i.e., if white spots were still visible we assumed less than 20 µL was absorbed and this was noted for each individual sample. Next, the VAMS tips were transferred to 1.5 mL Eppendorfs with a forceps and 480 µL superblock PBS buffer (ThermoFisher; Waltham, MA, USA) was added. Following an incubation of 1 h at 21 °C at 300 RPM (Eppendorf ThermoMixer C, Hamburg, Germany), each vial was shortly vortexed and tips were removed with cleaned forceps. Extracts were stored at −20 °C until analysis. Overall, extraction was done within 4 days after sampling (ranging from 1 day until 10 days).

In addition, at 3 predefined time points (day 0, day 14 and day 28 or day 0, day 21 and day 42, depending on the randomization arm), whole blood and serum were collected simultaneously, allowing comparison of the different matrices, i.e., capillary VAMS samples (obtained following finger prick), venous VAMS samples and serum (gold standard) samples. Venous VAMS samples were obtained by a trained nurse by touching the surface of ethylenediaminetetraacetic acid (EDTA)-anticoagulated venous whole blood with a VAMS tip. The serum was centrifuged for 10 min at $252 \times g$ at room temperature (Eppendorf centrifuge 5804, Germany), after an incubation time of maximum 24 h. Serum was preserved at minimally −20 °C for a median time of 185 days until analysis. An overview of the sampling time points is depicted in Figure 2.

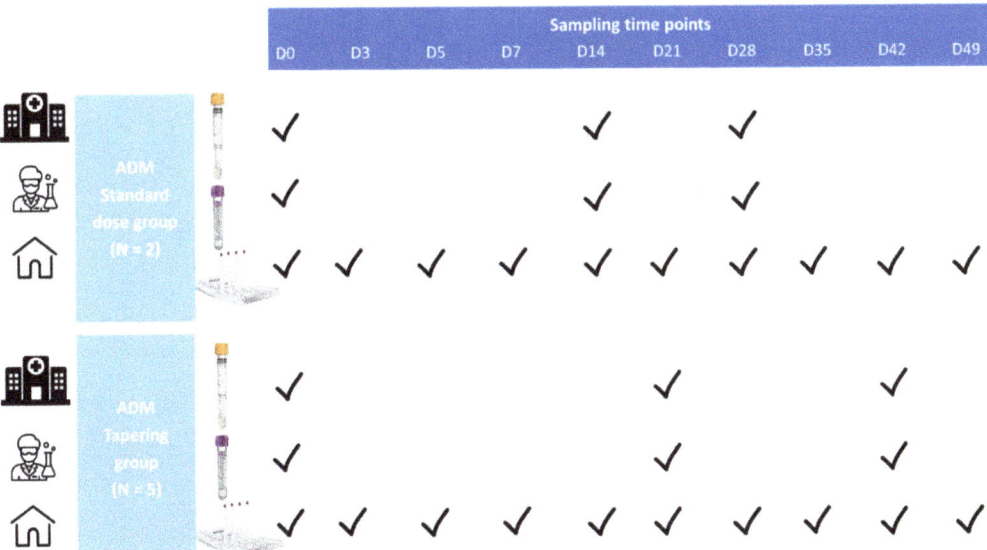

Figure 2. Overview of sampling time points in the substudy of the SUPRA-A trial. Patients were asked to self-sample at 10 predefined time points (day 0 (after training and under supervision of nurse), 3, 5, 7, 14, 21, 28, 35, 42, and 49) using a VAMS device, marketed as Mitra® (Neoteryx LLC, Torrance, CA, USA). At day 0, day 14 and day 28 or day 0, day 21 and day 42 whole blood and serum were collected simultaneously, allowing comparison of the different matrices, i.e., capillary VAMS, venous VAMS and serum (gold standard) samples. Abbreviations: D—Day; N—Number of patients.

2.3. Extraction Efficiency of Adalimumab in Volumetric Absorptive Microsamples

The extraction efficiency of ADM from VAMS tips was evaluated by spiking the blood of healthy volunteers with known ADM concentrations, 0–1–5–10 and 20 µg/mL. After drying for a minimum of 24 h, VAMS tips were extracted and extracts were stored at −20 °C until analysis.

2.4. Quantification of Adalimumab Concentrations
2.4.1. Rapid Testing with Lateral Flow Technique

ADM serum levels were measured using RIDA®QUICK ADM Monitoring lateral flow assay (R-Biopharm AG, Darmstadt, Germany), according to the manufacturer's instructions. In short, after a 5 min pre-incubation of 1:500 diluted sample with "Solution A" and "Solution B" and 15 min developing time on the lateral flow strip, the lateral flow strips were read using a portable reader (RIDA®- QUICK SCAN II, R-Biopharm AG, Darmstadt, Germany). The RIDA®QUICK ADM Monitoring allows quantification of ADM in the 0.5–25.0 µg/mL range [29].

2.4.2. Traditional Detection with ELISA

ADM concentrations in capillary VAMS samples, venous VAMS samples and serum were determined using an in-house developed ADM ELISA with a lower limit of quantification of 0.1 µg/mL [30]. Briefly, MA-ADM28B8 (4 µg/mL) was coated to 96-well plates at 4 °C for 72 h. Serum and VAMS extracts were diluted to a final dilution of 1:2000 in PTAE buffer (phosphate-buffered saline (PBS) + 0.1% bovine serum albumin (BSA) + 0.002% Tween 80 + EDTA), applied on the plate and incubated overnight at 4 °C. The next day, horseradish peroxidase (HRP)-conjugated MA-ADM40D8 was applied for the detection of bound ADM and incubated for 2 h at room temperature. Plates were washed and developed using o-phenylenediamine and H_2O_2 in citrate buffer and the reaction was stopped with H_2SO_4 (4 M). The absorbance was then measured at 492 nm with an ELx808 Absorbance Microplate Reader (BioTek Instrumens Inc., Winooski, VT, USA).

2.5. Statistical Analysis

Correlations and agreements between the results obtained by LFT and ELISA were assessed using the Pearson r correlation coefficient, simple linear regression, and Bland–Altman analysis. A two-tailed p-value < 0.05 was considered significant. All statistics were carried out using the statistical programs Graphpad Prism 8.3.0 (Graphpad software, San Diego, CA, USA) and IBM SPSS Statistics 25 (IBM SPSS, Costa Mesa, CA, USA).

3. Results

3.1. Demographics of Study Cohort

Until present, the SUPRA-A trial recruited a total of 10 patients, of whom 6 were randomized (1:1) in the intervention arm. With the exception of one patient, all patients were male. The cohort had a mean age of 54.2 years, with a mean disease duration of 30.5 years. Treatment duration with ADM ranged from 3.9 years to 12.8 years, with a mean psoriasis area and severity index (PASI) at start of therapy of 8.2. Before randomization, all patients were screened with ELISA for supratherapeutic ADM serum trough concentrations (>8 µg/mL). Patients were randomized if on two out of three time points, supratherapeutic trough levels were measured. Overall, patients had a mean ADM concentration of 9.6 µg/mL during screening, ranging from 7.6 to 13.1 µg/mL.

Seven participants agreed to be included in the substudy for microsampling. All patients were highly educated Caucasian men with an average age of 50.3 years. The range of ADM serum trough concentrations obtained in the screening of this subcohort was the same as the one mentioned above, with a mean of 9.7 µg/mL; five participants were randomized to the intervention group.

3.2. Rapid Testing of Adalimumab Is Feasible and Valuable in Clinical Setting

A total of 15 samples were collected from 10 patients on week 0 and from 5 patients on week 13. One patient in the control arm had dropped out before the sampling of week 13, hence the missing time point. Lateral flow testing was performed independently by two researchers and showed a mean coefficient of variation (CV) of 7.6% (median: 6.4%; range: 0.0–25.1%), which is slightly lower than the interassay precision reported by the manufacturer [29]. The ADM concentrations in these serum samples ranged from 2.9 to 16.2 µg/mL (Table S1). Based on simple linear regression, a significant concentration-dependent variation of the LFT measurements was observed (Figure 3a).

Next, LFT-obtained ADM concentrations (the mean of replicate measurements for both assessments was used) were compared to ELISA-based quantification. The results showed a good agreement with the reference assay, as indicated by a correlation coefficient R^2 of 0.89 (Figure 3b), which is somewhat lower than the correlation coefficient ($R^2 = 0.95$) previously reported by the manufacturer [29]. The Bland–Altman analysis yielded a mean bias of −0.03 µg/mL, indicating the absence of a significant systematic bias between LFT and ELISA (Figure 3c). Noteworthy, the span covered by the upper and lower limits of agreement (LoA) (−1.98–1.93 µg/mL) is rather big, given the relative narrow therapeutic window of ADM, i.e., 3.51–7.0 µg/mL. This may influence clinical decision-making as categorization of patients as sub- or supratherapeutic may differ, depending on the method of analysis used. However, relatively limited number of samples were included at this point in time—future inclusion of more patients will help to further substantiate this finding.

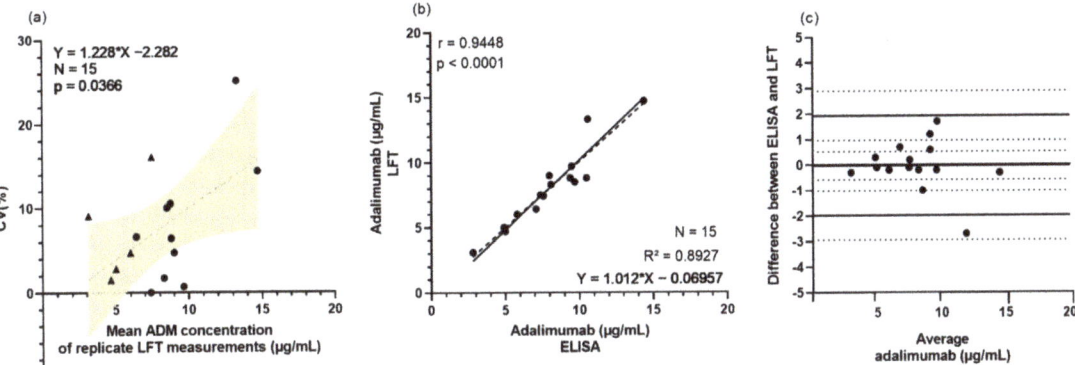

Figure 3. Comparison between LFT and ELISA for quantification of ADM in patient samples from SUPRA-A trial. Serum was collected during ADM maintenance therapy from patients participating in the SUPRA-A trial and drug concentrations were quantified in parallel by two detection methods in duplicate, LFT and ELISA. (**a**) Pearson correlation between the CV (%) and the mean ADM concentrations (µg/mL) measured with LFT by 2 independent researchers. Week 0 and week 13 values are represented by circles and triangles, respectively. The grey range indicates the 95% CI of the best-fit line (simple linear regression). (**b**) Pearson correlation between ADM serum concentrations measured with LFT (Y-axis) and in-house sandwich ELISA (X-axis). (**c**) Bland–Altman plot for ADM quantification by LFT and with in-house sandwich ELISA. Mean bias and limits of agreement are represented by full lines, 95% CI by dotted lines. Abbreviations: ADM—adalimumab; CI—confidence interval; CV—Coefficient of variation; ELISA—enzyme-linked immunosorbent assay; LFT—lateral flow test; N—number of samples.

3.3. VAMS Is Suitable for Extraction of Adalimumab

For validation of the VAMS extraction protocol, the extraction efficiency of ADM from VAMS tips was evaluated by spiking the blood of healthy volunteers with known ADM concentrations, ranging from 0 to 20 µg/mL. Extracts were measured 5 times on different days with an in-house ADM ELISA and a mean extraction efficiency was obtained of 114.4% (SD 13.9%, CV 12.2%).

3.4. Feasibility of Home Sampling by Non-Experienced Patients Using VAMS

Until present, seven patients were included, resulting in 136 capillary VAMS samples (68 replicates; 4 missing), 40 venous VAMS samples (20 replicates; 2 missing) and 19 serum samples (2 missing) which were eligible for ADM quantification. Ten capillary VAMS samples were excluded from analysis after visual inspection due to undersampling (7.4%).

First, the quality of the patient sampling technique was assessed by comparing biological replicates of capillary VAMS. The difference between the replicates was determined (n = 65) and the CV was calculated. The CV obtained for capillary VAMS samples was 13.5%, which was slightly, though significantly higher than the CV of 7.5% observed for venous VAMS samples (Chi2-test, α = 0.05). The latter were prepared by a trained nurse, dipping the VAMS tips in EDTA-anticoagulated venous whole blood. Overall, a very good correlation was observed between biological replicates of the capillary VAMS samples, with no concentration- or time-dependent variation in the imprecision of home sampling (Figure 4a–c).

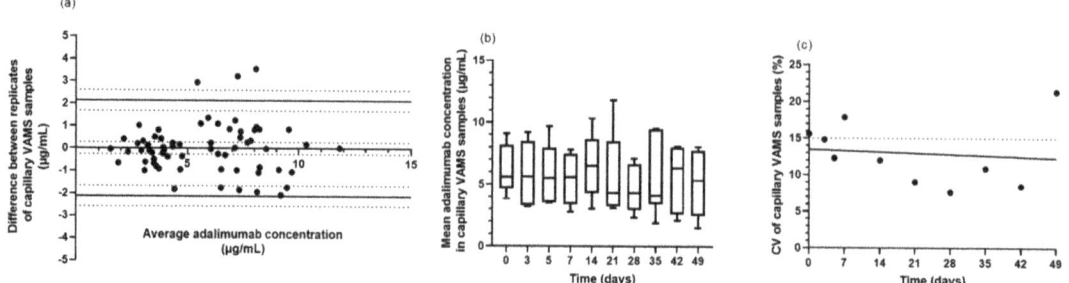

Figure 4. Patients' performance on microsampling (capillary VAMS). Participants self-sampled VAMS twice in a row, these replicates being taken at 10 time points between day 0 and day 49. ADM was measured in capillary VAMS extracts with an in-house ELISA. (**a**) Bland–Altman plot for ADM quantification in capillary VAMS (n = 65). Mean bias and limits of agreement are represented by full lines, 95% CI by dotted lines. (**b**) Boxplots of mean ADM concentrations in capillary VAMS samples, taken at time points between day 0 and day 49. (**c**) CV (%) of replicates from capillary VAMS samples at the sampling time points between day 0 and day 49. The CV (%) threshold of 15% and the best fit curve (simple linear regression) are indicated by a dotted and full line, respectively. Abbreviations: ADM—adalimumab; CI—confidence interval; CV—Coefficient of variation; ELISA—enzyme-linked immunosorbent assay; N—number of samples; VAMS—volumetric absorptive microsampling.

Next, we evaluated how quantification of ADM obtained with VAMS would compare to simultaneously collected serum (gold standard). Hereto, we first compared ADM concentrations obtained from venous VAMS samples (Figure 5a,b) with those obtained from the corresponding serum samples. A good correlation between ADM concentrations in venous VAMS samples [7.32 ± 2.78; 6.92 (5.24–8.63)] and in serum [8.56 ± 2.7; 8.4 (7.3–10.5)] was observed, with a Pearson correlation of 0.87 [mean ± SD; median (IQR), µg/mL].

Then, we examined the concordance of the results obtained from capillary VAMS samples (obtained by patient self-sampling) and simultaneously collected venous VAMS samples. Figure 5c depicts a Pearson correlation of r = 0.91. From the Bland–Altman analysis, a mean significant bias of 1.30 µg/mL was apparent, with 95% CI 0.72–1.87 (Figure 5d; p = 0.0002). This implies that ADM concentrations in venous VAMS samples are overall slightly higher than in capillary VAMS samples, collected at the same time point. This capillary venous difference illustrates the need for the application of a capillary-venous correction factor. Based on our cohort, a capillary-venous correction factor of 1.28 was found.

Finally, we compared ADM concentrations obtained from capillary VAMS samples with those obtained from the corresponding serum samples. As shown in Figure 5 (panel e,f), a good correlation between ADM concentrations in capillary VAMS samples [5.67 ± 2.47; 5.48 (3.52–7.61)] and in serum [8.56 ± 2.7; 8.4 (7.3–10.5)] was observed, with a Pearson correlation of 0.87 [mean ± SD; median (IQR), µg/mL]. A significant mean bias of 2.7 µg/mL (95% CI: 1.96, 3.35) was found by Bland–Altman analysis (p < 0.0001), implying that lower concentrations are obtained from VAMS samples, compared to the corresponding serum samples, which can be expected, as ADM resides in the serum/plasma fraction of blood. By multiplying the ADM concentration from capillary VAMS samples with the capillary-venous and blood-serum correction factors of, respectively, 1.28 and 1.22, the calculated ADM serum concentration was determined (Figure 6). As depicted in Figure 6c, this may be an overcorrection due to the small sample size of this cohort.

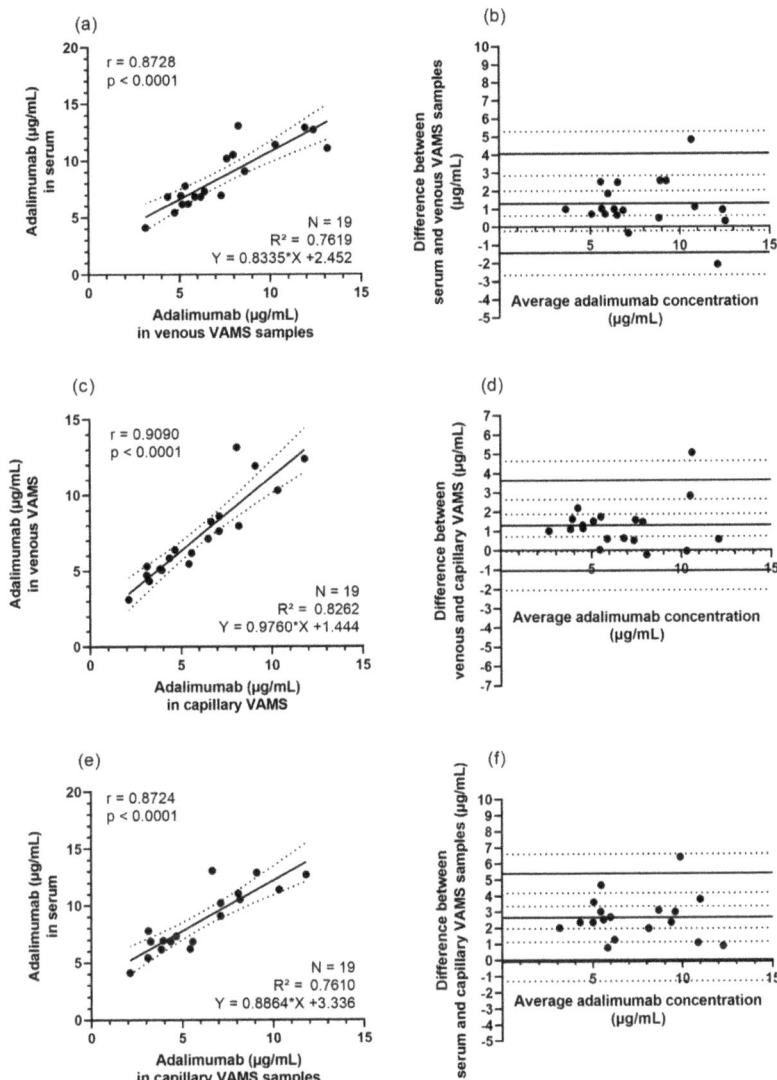

Figure 5. Concordance between capillary VAMS samples, venous VAMS samples and serum (gold standard). (**a**) Pearson correlation of ADM concentrations obtained from venous VAMS samples prepared by nurse (X-axis) and serum (Y-axis). (**b**) Bland–Altman comparison of ADM concentrations in venous VAMS samples and serum. Mean bias and limits of agreement are represented by full lines, 95% CI by dotted lines. (**c**) Pearson correlation of ADM concentrations obtained from mean venous VAMS samples, prepared by a trained nurse (Y-axis) and mean capillary VAMS samples, collected by the patients (X-axis). (**d**) Bland–Altman comparison of ADM concentrations in samples obtained by nurse versus patients. Mean bias and limits of agreement are represented by full lines, 95% CI by dotted lines. (**e**) Pearson correlation of ADM concentrations obtained from capillary VAMS samples collected by patients (X-axis) and serum (Y-axis). (**f**) Bland–Altman comparison of ADM concentrations in capillary VAMS samples and serum. Mean bias and limits of agreement are represented by full lines, 95% CI by dotted lines. Abbreviations: ADM—adalimumab; CI—confidence interval; N—number of samples; VAMS—volumetric absorptive microsampling.

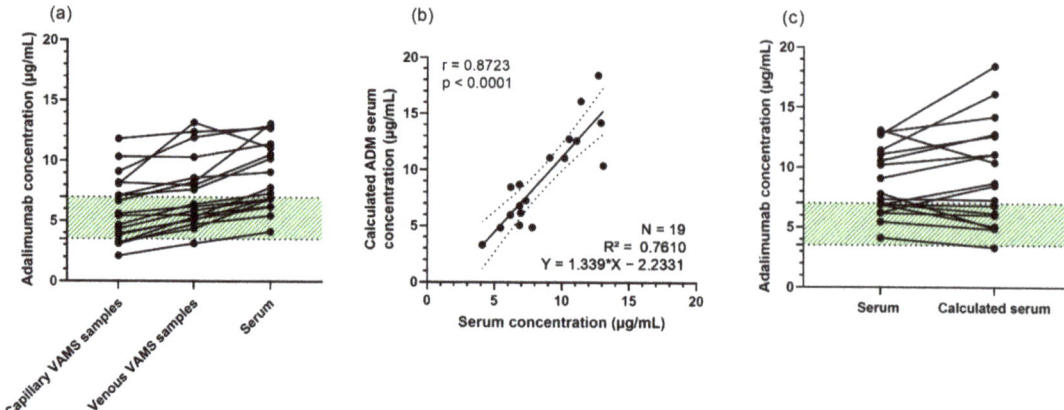

Figure 6. Concordance between capillary VAMS samples, venous VAMS samples and calculated serum (based on a blood-serum and capillary-venous correction factor). (**a**) ADM (µg/mL) in the three matrices, capillary VAMS samples, venous VAMS samples and serum. Green range represents the therapeutic window of ADM (3.51–7.0 µg/mL [8,9]) (**b**) Pearson correlation of ADM concentrations obtained from serum samples (X-axis) and calculated ADM serum concentrations based on a blood-serum correction factor of 1.22 and a capillary correction factor of 1.28 (Y-axis). (**c**) ADM (µg/mL) in serum (gold standard) and calculated ADM serum concentration, based on a blood-serum correction factor of 1.22 and a capillary-venous correction factor of 1.28. Green range represents the therapeutic window of ADM (3.51–7.0 µg/mL [8,9]). Abbreviations: ADM—adalimumab; CI—confidence interval; N—number of samples; VAMS—volumetric absorptive microsampling.

3.5. Patient Experience with VAMS

All participants completed the substudy according to the protocol, which by itself was already considered to be a success regarding acceptance of VAMS as a collection technique. All samples, shipped by regular mail, were received within an acceptable time frame (on average 5 days, range [3–8]).

Next, we used a questionnaire to evaluate the patients' perception on self-sampling at home based on Van Uytfanghe et al. and Mbughuni et al., with minor adaptations [28,31]. The questionnaire consisted of 10 main questions and gauged about the clarity of instructions, experience, performance, user-friendliness, acceptability/pain and preference.

All patients (n = 7) completed the survey. Five out of seven participants (71.4%) had a higher degree (bachelor or master). Except one, none of the respondents had experience with performing VAMS before. All patients judged the clarity of the instructions to be clear or very clear and evaluated the performance as very or rather user-friendly and feasible (Figure 7a). None of the patients felt the need to consult for additional information (data not shown). All patients self-sampled, except for one participant, who stated their partner was a nurse who performed the finger prick (Figure 7b). On a scale of 1 (not painful at all) to 10 (very painful), participants scored 3 or less, with 60% rating it a zero (Figure 7c). Moreover, with the exception of one patient, all patients scored finger prick sampling as less painful compared to a conventional blood draw (Figure 7d). With a higher degree of flexibility/autonomy and no transportation to the clinic, this translates to the vast majority (85.7%) preferring this type of sampling over a conventional blood draw (Figure 7d,e).

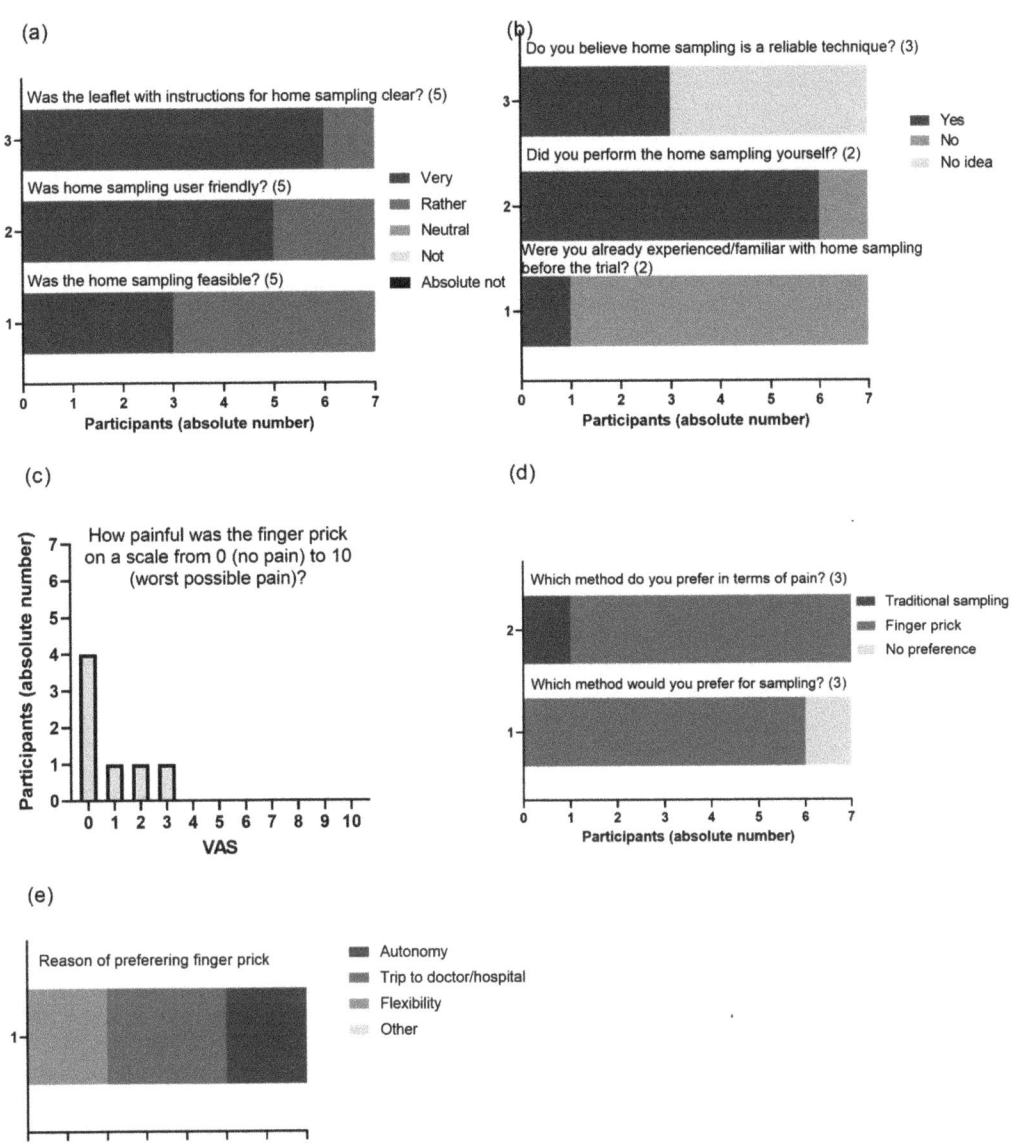

Figure 7. Microsampling was found to be easily executed by patients and preferred over venous sampling. After completing the substudy for microsampling, participants were sent an electronic survey to inquire into their experience. Patients scored questions on execution (**a**) and execution experience (**b**). Pain was quantified (**c**,**d**) and compared to traditional sampling (**d**,**e**). n = 7 The number between brackets in panel (**a**,**b**,**d**) indicates the number of possible answers.

For VAMS to be adopted by patients in the context of TDM in psoriasis, we inquired into patients' acceptance. All participants scored the technique as user-friendly for use at home (Figure 7a). In addition, all patients agreed that it would be feasible to perform this regularly. When asked about an acceptable frequency to use VAMS, a monthly basis had the most votes (data not shown). Although patients were positive about this sampling technique, more than half of the patients was uncertain about the reliability of the sampling technique (Figure 7b), reflecting the gap of knowledge.

4. Discussion

Although the use of TDM in psoriasis is still not standard practice, parallel research into enabling tools is required to facilitate implementation. As Figure 1 illustrates, TDM requires various steps, and especially the first step, encompassing sampling, will pose most challenges regarding implementation. Easy and feasible sampling is a great challenge, with a healthcare professional being required for a traditional blood draw. Furthermore, serum preparation from whole blood requires the sample to be handled in a laboratory setting.

Here, we investigated the home-based use of VAMS by psoriasis patients treated with ADM for drug quantification. We focused on both the technical performance and the patient's user experience. From a technical perspective, our extraction protocol showed a satisfactory extraction efficiency, with adequate reproducibility. As TDM is based on narrow therapeutic windows, a robust extraction is essential to ensure appropriate interpretation and treatment management plan. Patients' performance assessed by replicates was deemed acceptable, with a CV of 13.5%. As no long-term data were collected, at this point no conclusions can be drawn related to 'performance fatigue'. Performance compared to a trained nurse also showed satisfactory results with a slightly, though significantly higher CV than the CV derived under controlled circumstances for sampling, 7.5%. Based on this, it could be estimated that home sampling accounted for 11.2% of the total imprecision of the method.

In addition, a good correlation between the three matrices, capillary VAMS samples, venous VAMS samples and serum was obtained. At this point it is too early to make definitive statements on whether capillary samples can yield data that can reliably steer dose adaptations (this will become clear in the ongoing trial and was beyond the scope of the current pilot study). However, the data so far indicate that 2 kinds of corrections are required to predict serum concentrations based on capillary blood concentrations: a capillary-venous correction of 1.28, and a blood-serum correction of 1.22. The latter is obvious, as ADM resides in the serum fraction of blood, and 20 µL of (dried) blood only contains ~12 µL of serum (in the case of ~40% haematocrit blood). However, more data are needed to validate these correction factors and verify these on independent sample sets. In future, these data will provide further insight into the suitability of VAMS as an adequate substitute for conventional sampling for ADM TDM.

Besides the technical suitability of microsampling for TDM of ADM in psoriasis patients, it is also important to acknowledge the patients' perception, as they are the end users. Based on our questionnaire, it can be concluded that the patients were overall positive about home-based microsampling. Even more, participants in this pilot study preferred this type of sampling over a conventional blood draw, but this needs to be confirmed in a larger cohort. This is in agreement with results obtained by Morgan et al., who showed that 81% of the participants preferred VAMS collection, and is in line with the preference for VAMS in the cohort studied by Verougstraete et al. [23,32]. Essential to implementation, we also investigated the time it took for a sample to reach our laboratory. Based on our limited data, the time window was deemed acceptable for psoriasis management with ADM. Most biologics are administered from twice a month to every 3 months—rendering an average of 5 transport days (range: 3–8 days) acceptable for the physician to adapt the management plan.

In this paper, we did not address the impact of storage conditions on extraction efficiency. However, we refer to Bloem et al. where a similar technique has been investigated for several storage conditions [17]. In addition, Li et al. obtained very encouraging drug recovery data after short and long term storage for biotherapeutics daclizumab and trastuzumab [33]. Ideally, when patients require a change in management plan, results should become available relatively fast, making long-term storage impact irrelevant. The impact of parameters such as temperature and humidity should be investigated in real world settings for conclusive evidence. To lower the threshold of using VAMS within the patient community and empower patients to monitor their drug concentrations, in the future, microsampling kits could become available at the pharmacy, or could be provided by the treating physician upon treatment with biologics.

After sampling, trough drug concentrations are traditionally measured by ELISA, requiring laboratory equipment (e.g., a shaker and dedicated reader) and are time-consuming. An additional disadvantage of ELISA is the ratio of performance time to sample size. As ELISA is standard-dependent, a single sample run is considered wasteful. To this end, the (complementary) use of immunochromatographic lateral flow testing allows for a more satisfactory ratio of performance time to sample size. The LFT assay investigated here was demonstrated to be applicable in clinical practice, with a turnover time of less than 30 min after serum preparation. Although it was compared to only one ELISA kit for ADM quantification [25,34], our data show acceptable results for clinical applicability. As the therapeutic window of ADM is relatively narrow [8,9], interpretation of results should be done taking into account the type of assay. In the limited dataset from this study, a good agreement was found between LFT and ELISA, suggesting that no adaptation of the therapeutic window would be required when implementing this LFT assay—obviously, more samples are required to further substantiate this finding. The current LFT assay was performed on serum samples, and its compatibility with VAMS remains to be elucidated. Ultimately, a combination of both tools would truly enable rapid and easy monitoring.

Limitations of this pilot study inherently include the small sample size for both microsampling and rapid testing. In addition, we did not address various conditions to assess the impact on both tools. For instance, we currently lack data on storage conditions and how ADM concentrations in VAMS samples are affected. All LFT measurements were executed by trained lab personnel. As all measurements were performed in an academic hospital setting, extrapolation to private practices is limited. It should also be noted that the used LFT cassettes are not compatible with all LFT-readers.

Strengths of this study reside in the affinity with real world evidence as SUPRA-A is considered a pragmatic trial, in addition to the use of public postal services for sample transport. Furthermore, participants had access to adequate educational material to execute microsampling. Lastly, in addition to laboratory evaluations, we also considered and investigated the study participants as end users—rendering this study comprehensive.

5. Conclusions

Microsampling for ADM TDM in the context of psoriasis treatment is a valuable alternative to traditional blood sampling, enabling patient-centric TDM. VAMS, as applied here, can be performed by non-experienced patients at home, potentially allowing to reach a greater patient community. In addition, rapid testing by LFT of ADM allows the dermatologist to rapidly obtain results that may impact a patient's treatment plan.

The results presented here provide preliminary evidence, revealing that LFT and microsampling are promising tools to facilitate TDM of ADM in clinical practice. Though the data is from a limited sample size, both tools pose interesting fields of further investigation for TDM in psoriasis.

Supplementary Materials: The following supporting information can be downloaded at: https://www.mdpi.com/article/10.3390/jcm11113011/s1, Figure S1: Written instruction (in Dutch) for patients for home sampling by use of VAMS after finger prick; Table S1: Lateral Flow Testing results of adalimumab concentrations in SUPRA-A trial participants.

Author Contributions: Conceptualization, J.L. and L.G.; Data curation, R.S.; Formal analysis, A.C., H.D.S., M.D., T.M. and R.S.; Funding acquisition, J.L. and L.G.; Investigation, A.C., M.D., T.M. and R.S.; Methodology, C.S., H.D.S., L.G. and R.S.; Project administration, R.S.; Resources, J.L.; Supervision, C.S., J.L. and L.G.; Visualization, R.S.; Writing—original draft, L.G. and R.S.; Writing—review and editing, C.S., M.F., J.L., L.G. and R.S. All authors have read and agreed to the published version of the manuscript.

Funding: This research was funded by the Research Foundation—Flanders (FWO), Belgium (T003218N).

Institutional Review Board Statement: The study was conducted in accordance with the Declaration of Helsinki and approved by the Institutional Review Board (or Ethics Committee) of Ghent University Hospital (EudraCT 2019-001918-42; 22 April 2020).

Informed Consent Statement: Informed consent was obtained from all subjects involved in the study.

Data Availability Statement: The data presented in this study can be found at https://osf.io/2bk7u hosted at Open Science Framework and access can be obtained upon request.

Acknowledgments: We would like to express our gratitude to all patients willing to participate in this study. Special gratitude goes out to Brigitte Blanquart as a dedicated study nurse. In addition, we want to thank Neoteryx and R-Biopharm for the fruitful discussions.

Conflicts of Interest: Lambert has received grants (not personal but for scientific research account University Ghent) from Janssen, AbbVie, and Pfizer; had paid consultancies (not personal but for scientific research account University Ghent) from Abbvie, Almirall, Argenx, BMS, Janssen Cilag, Pfizer, Leo Pharma, Novartis and UCB; and carried out clinical trials for Janssen-Cilag, Merck Serono, Amgen, Pfizer, AbbVie, Celgene, Regeneron and Novartis. Lynda Grine received paid speaker fees from UCB, AbbVie and R-Biopharm. The other authors state no disclosures.

References

1. Brownstone, N.D.; Hong, J.; Mosca, M.; Hadeler, E.; Liao, W.; Bhutani, T.; Koo, J. Biologic treatments of psoriasis: An update for the clinician. *Biol. Targets Ther.* **2021**, *15*, 39–51. [CrossRef]
2. Smolen, J.S.; Aletaha, D.; McInnes, I.B. Rheumatoid arthritis. *Lancet* **2016**, *388*, 2023–2038. [CrossRef]
3. Schmitt, J.; Rosumeck, S.; Thomaschewski, G.; Sporbeck, B.; Haufe, E.; Nast, A. Efficacy and safety of systemic treatments for moderate-to-severe psoriasis: Meta-analysis of randomized controlled trials. *Br. J. Dermatol.* **2014**, *170*, 274–303. [CrossRef] [PubMed]
4. Keystone, E.C.; Rampakakis, E.; Movahedi, M.; Cesta, A.; Stutz, M.; Sampalis, J.S.; Nantel, F.; Maslova, K.; Bombardier, C. Toward Defining Primary and Secondary Nonresponse in Rheumatoid Arthritis Patients Treated with Anti-TNF: Results from the BioTRAC and OBRI Registries. *J. Rheumatol.* **2020**, *47*, 510–527. [CrossRef]
5. Bracke, S.; Lambert, J. Viewpoint on handling anti-TNF failure in psoriasis. *Arch. Dermatol. Res.* **2013**, *305*, 945–950. [CrossRef] [PubMed]
6. De la Brassinne, M.; Ghislain, P.-D.; Lambert, J.L.W.; Lambert, J.; Segaert, S.; Willaert, F. Recommendations for managing a suboptimal response to biologics for moderate-to-severe psoriasis: A Belgian perspective. *J. Dermatolog. Treat.* **2016**, *27*, 128–133. [CrossRef] [PubMed]
7. Edson-Heredia, E.; Sterling, K.L.; Alatorre, C.I.; Cuyun Carter, G.; Paczkowski, R.; Zarotsky, V.; Maeda-Chubachi, T. Heterogeneity of Response to Biologic Treatment: Perspective for Psoriasis. *J. Invest. Dermatol.* **2014**, *134*, 18–23. [CrossRef] [PubMed]
8. Menting, S.P.; Coussens, E.; Pouw, M.F.; van den Reek, J.M.P.A.P.A.; Temmerman, L.; Boonen, H.; De Jong, E.M.G.J.G.J.; Spuls, P.I.; Lambert, J. Developing a Therapeutic Range of Adalimumab Serum Concentrations in Management of Psoriasis. *JAMA Dermatology* **2015**, *151*, 616. [CrossRef]
9. Wilkinson, N.; Tsakok, T.; Dand, N.; Bloem, K.; Duckworth, M.; Baudry, D.; Pushpa-Rajah, A.; Griffiths, C.E.E.M.; Reynolds, N.J.; Barker, J.; et al. Defining the Therapeutic Range for Adalimumab and Predicting Response in Psoriasis: A Multicenter Prospective Observational Cohort Study. *J. Investig. Dermatol.* **2019**, *139*, 115–123. [CrossRef]
10. Papamichael, K.; Cheifetz, A.S. Therapeutic Drug Monitoring in IBD: The New Standard-of-Care for Anti-TNF Therapy. *Am. J. Gastroenterol.* **2017**, *112*, 673–676. [CrossRef]
11. Juncadella, A.; Papamichael, K.; Vaughn, B.P.; Cheifetz, A.S. Maintenance Adalimumab Concentrations Are Associated with Biochemical, Endoscopic, and Histologic Remission in Inflammatory Bowel Disease. *Dig. Dis. Sci.* **2018**, *63*, 3067–3073. [CrossRef] [PubMed]
12. Vande Casteele, N.; Feagan, B.G.; Wolf, D.C.; Pop, A.; Yassine, M.; Horst, S.N.; Ritter, T.E.; Sandborn, W.J. Therapeutic Drug Monitoring of Tumor Necrosis Factor Antagonists in Crohn Disease: A Theoretical Construct to Apply Pharmacokinetics and Guidelines to Clinical Practice. *Inflamm. Bowel Dis.* **2021**, *27*, 1346–1355. [CrossRef] [PubMed]
13. Lambert, J.; Grine, L.; Soenen, R. Dose Tapering Study of Adalimumab in Psoriasis—Full Text View. Available online: https://clinicaltrials.gov/ct2/show/NCT04028713 (accessed on 24 January 2022).
14. Harahap, Y.; Diptasaadya, R.; Purwanto, D.J. Volumetric absorptive microsampling as a sampling alternative in clinical trials and therapeutic drug monitoring during the covid-19 pandemic: A review. *Drug Des. Dev. Ther.* **2020**, *14*, 5757–5771. [CrossRef] [PubMed]

15. Kneepkens, E.L.; Pouw, M.F.; Wolbink, G.J.; Schaap, T.; Nurmohamed, M.T.; de Vries, A.; Rispens, T.; Bloem, K. Dried blood spots from finger prick facilitate therapeutic drug monitoring of adalimumab and anti-adalimumab in patients with inflammatory diseases. *Br. J. Clin. Pharmacol.* **2017**, *83*, 2474–2484. [CrossRef] [PubMed]
16. Mingas, P.D.; Zdovc, J.; Grabnar, I.; Vovk, T. The Evolving Role of Microsampling in Therapeutic Drug Monitoring of Monoclonal Antibodies in Inflammatory Diseases. *Molecules* **2021**, *26*, 1787. [CrossRef]
17. Bloem, K.; Schaap, T.; Boshuizen, R.; Kneepkens, E.L.; Wolbink, G.J.; de Vries, A.; Rispens, T. Capillary blood microsampling to determine serum biopharmaceutical concentration: Mitra® microsampler vs dried blood spot. *Bioanalysis* **2018**, *10*, 815–823. [CrossRef]
18. Delahaye, L.; Veenhof, H.; Koch, B.C.P.; Alffenaar, J.-W.C.; Linden, R.; Stove, C. Alternative Sampling Devices to Collect Dried Blood Microsamples. *Ther. Drug Monit.* **2021**, *43*, 310–321. [CrossRef]
19. Martial, L.C.; Aarnoutse, R.E.; Schreuder, M.F.; Henriet, S.S.; Brüggemann, R.J.M.; Joore, M.A. Cost Evaluation of Dried Blood Spot Home Sampling as Compared to Conventional Sampling for Therapeutic Drug Monitoring in Children. *PLoS ONE* **2016**, *11*, e0167433. [CrossRef]
20. De Kesel, P.M.M.; Sadones, N.; Capiau, S.; Lambert, W.E.; Stove, C.P. Hemato-critical issues in quantitative analysis of dried blood spots: Challenges and solutions. *Bioanalysis* **2013**, *5*, 2023–2041. [CrossRef]
21. Velghe, S.; Delahaye, L.; Stove, C.P. Is the hematocrit still an issue in quantitative dried blood spot analysis? *J. Pharm. Biomed. Anal.* **2019**, *163*, 188–196. [CrossRef]
22. Spooner, N.; Denniff, P.; Michielsen, L.; De Vries, R.; Ji, Q.C.; Arnold, M.E.; Woods, K.; Woolf, E.J.; Xu, Y.; Boutet, V.; et al. A device for dried blood microsampling in quantitative bioanalysis: Overcoming the issues associated blood hematocrit. *Bioanalysis* **2015**, *7*, 653–659. [CrossRef]
23. Verougstraete, N.; Lapauw, B.; Van Aken, S.; Delanghe, J.; Stove, C.; Stove, V. Volumetric absorptive microsampling at home as an alternative tool for the monitoring of HbA1c in diabetes patients. *Clin. Chem. Lab. Med.* **2017**, *55*, 462–469. [CrossRef] [PubMed]
24. Montesinos, I.; Gruson, D.; Kabamba, B.; Dahma, H.; Van den Wijngaert, S.; Reza, S.; Carbone, V.; Vandenberg, O.; Gulbis, B.; Wolff, F.; et al. Evaluation of two automated and three rapid lateral flow immunoassays for the detection of anti-SARS-CoV-2 antibodies. *J. Clin. Virol.* **2020**, *128*, 104413. [CrossRef]
25. Verstockt, B.; Moors, G.; Bian, S.; Van Stappen, T.; Van Assche, G.; Vermeire, S.; Gils, A.; Ferrante, M. Influence of early adalimumab serum levels on immunogenicity and long-term outcome of anti-TNF naive Crohn's disease patients: The usefulness of rapid testing. *Aliment. Pharmacol. Ther.* **2018**, *48*, 731–739. [CrossRef]
26. Harris, P.A.; Taylor, R.; Minor, B.L.; Elliott, V.; Fernandez, M.; O'Neal, L.; McLeod, L.; Delacqua, G.; Delacqua, F.; Kirby, J.; et al. The REDCap consortium: Building an international community of software platform partners. *J. Biomed. Inform.* **2019**, *95*, 103208. [CrossRef]
27. Harris, P.A.; Taylor, R.; Thielke, R.; Payne, J.; Gonzalez, N.; Conde, J.G. Research electronic data capture (REDCap)—A metadata-driven methodology and workflow process for providing translational research informatics support. *J. Biomed. Inform.* **2009**, *42*, 377–381. [CrossRef] [PubMed]
28. Van Uytfanghe, K.; Heughebaert, L.; Stove, C.P. Self-sampling at home using volumetric absorptive microsampling: Coupling analytical evaluation to volunteers' perception in the context of a large scale study. *Clin. Chem. Lab. Med.* **2021**, *59*, e185–e187. [CrossRef]
29. Castillo, C. GN3043_RIDA QUICK_ADM Monitoring_2018-06-28_EN. Available online: https://clinical.r-biopharm.com/wp-content/uploads/2018/08/gn3043_rida_quick_adm-monitoring_2018-06-28_en.pdf (accessed on 24 January 2022).
30. Bian, S.; Van Stappen, T.; Baert, F.; Compernolle, G.; Brouwers, E.; Tops, S.; de Vries, A.; Rispens, T.; Lammertyn, J.; Vermeire, S.; et al. Generation and characterization of a unique panel of anti-adalimumab specific antibodies and their application in therapeutic drug monitoring assays. *J. Pharm. Biomed. Anal.* **2016**, *125*, 62–67. [CrossRef] [PubMed]
31. Mbughuni, M.M.; Stevens, M.A.; Langman, L.J.; Kudva, Y.C.; Sanchez, W.; Dean, P.G.; Jannetto, P.J. Volumetric Microsampling of Capillary Blood Spot vs Whole Blood Sampling for Therapeutic Drug Monitoring of Tacrolimus and Cyclosporin A: Accuracy and Patient Satisfaction. *J. Appl. Lab. Med.* **2020**, *5*, 516–530. [CrossRef]
32. Morgan, P.E. Microsampling Devices for Routine Therapeutic Drug Monitoring-Are We There Yet? *Ther. Drug Monit.* **2021**, *43*, 322–334. [CrossRef]
33. Li, H.; Myzithras, M.; Bolella, E.; Leonard, A.; Ahlberg, J. Whole blood stability evaluation of monoclonal antibody therapeutics using volumetric absorptive microsampling. *Bioanalysis* **2021**, *13*, 621–629. [CrossRef] [PubMed]
34. Rocha, C.; Afonso, J.; Lago, P.; Arroja, B.; Vieira, A.I.; Dias, C.C.; Magro, F. Accuracy of the new rapid test for monitoring adalimumab levels. *Therap. Adv. Gastroenterol.* **2019**, *12*, 1756284819828238. [CrossRef] [PubMed]

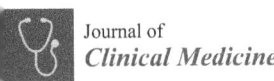

Article

Model Informed Precision Dosing Tool Forecasts Trough Infliximab and Associates with Disease Status and Tumor Necrosis Factor-Alpha Levels of Inflammatory Bowel Diseases

Christian Primas [1], Walter Reinisch [1,*], John C. Panetta [2], Alexander Eser [1], Diane R. Mould [3] and Thierry Dervieux [4,*]

1 Division of Gastroenterology & Hepatology, Medical University of Vienna, A-1090 Vienna, Austria; christian.primas@meduniwien.ac.at (C.P.); dr.eser@gmx.at (A.E.)
2 St. Jude Children's Research Hospital, Memphis, TN 38105, USA; carl.panetta@stjude.org
3 Projection Research LLC, Fort Myers, FL 33901, USA; drmould@pri-home.net
4 Prometheus Laboratories, San Diego, CA 92121, USA
* Correspondence: walter.reinisch@meduniwien.ac.at (W.R.); tdervieux@prometheuslabs.com (T.D.)

Abstract: Background: Substantial inter-and intra-individual variability of Infliximab (IFX) pharmacokinetics necessitates tailored dosing approaches. Here, we evaluated the performances of a Model Informed Precision Dosing (MIPD) Tool in forecasting trough Infliximab (IFX) levels in association with disease status and circulating TNF-α in patients with Inflammatory Bowel Diseases (IBD). Methods: Consented patients undergoing every 8-week maintenance therapy with IFX were enrolled. Midcycle specimens were collected, IFX, antibodies to IFX, albumin were determined and analyzed with weight using nonlinear mixed effect models coupled with Bayesian data assimilation to forecast trough levels. Accuracy of forecasted as compared to observed trough IFX levels were evaluated using Demings's regression. Association between IFX levels, CRP-based clinical remission and TNF-α levels were analyzed using logistic regression and linear mixed effect models. Results: In 41 patients receiving IFX (median dose = 5.3 mg/Kg), median IFX levels decreased from 13.0 to 3.9 µg/mL from mid to end of cycle time points, respectively. Midcycle IFX levels forecasted trough with Deming's slope = 0.90 and R2 = 0.87. Observed end cycle and forecasted trough levels above 5 µg/mL associated with CRP-based clinical remission (OR = 7.2 CI95%: 1.7–30.2; OR = 21.0 CI95%: 3.4–127.9, respectively) ($p < 0.01$). Median TNF-α levels increased from 4.6 to 8.0 pg/mL from mid to end of cycle time points, respectively ($p < 0.01$). CRP and TNF-α levels associated independently and additively to decreased IFX levels ($p < 0.01$). Conclusions: These data establish the value of our MIPD tool in forecasting trough IFX levels in patients with IBD. Serum TNF-α and CRP are reflective of inflammatory burden which impacts exposure.

Keywords: Infliximab; therapeutic drug monitoring; model informed precision dosing; inflammatory bowel disease

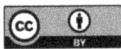

1. Introduction

Therapeutic drug monitoring (TDM) assists gastroenterologists with the management of Inflammatory Bowel Diseases (IBD; Crohn's Disease [CD] and Ulcerative Colitis [UC]) by clinical pharmacokinetic (PK) assessment of Infliximab (IFX) and antibodies to Infliximab (ATI) levels to detect underexposure and to prevent negative outcomes. The American Gastroenterological association has endorsed the TDM of IFX, and maintenance IFX trough threshold of 5 µg/mL was proposed as an effective minimum target level that can maximize TNF-α neutralization capabilities of the drug to promote inflammatory control of the underlying disease [1,2]. Reactively, in the face of uncontrolled disease, TDM can be implemented to inform on the value of dose intensification in the presence of inadequate exposure and accelerated clearance of the drug, while proactively, sustained maintenance of IFX levels to promote drug tolerance can help avoid the re-emergence of inflammation and flare post induction [3,4].

In recent years, modern and sophisticated Model Informed Precision Dosing (MIPD) tools that employ clinical PK have emerged to guide IFX dosing [5], and both retrospective and prospective clinical utility studies support the value of such dosing optimization to improve outcome [6,7]. Ideally, the optimization of IFX dose during maintenance should be proactively based on the identification of patients likely to present with underexposure at the end of infusion cycle, and as such, the collection of specimens during the elimination phase of IFX to forecast trough levels may inform clinicians of impending risk for underexposure that could be addressed by dose intensification.

Inflammatory burden remains a key determinant of IFX exposure; circulating C-reactive Protein (CRP) and fecal calprotectin are commonly measured to assist clinicians to assess underlying inflammation. However, despite the fact that IFX and anti-TNF blockers have been used in IBD and other immune mediated diseases for decades, the association between antigenic TNF-α and IFX PK is very limited, although high levels of TNF-α at baseline or during treatment serves as a sink for IFX thereby promoting underexposure, inadequate disease control, as reported previously in IBD [8] and rheumatoid arthritis [9].

The study establishing the validity of MIPD in forecasting trough concentration and associating with disease control is needed before implementation in clinical practice and the clinical laboratory setting. In this report, we establish the performance characteristics of MIDP in forecasting trough IFX levels and in associating these levels with disease control. We also evaluated the changes in antigenic TNF-α levels during infusion cycle and the impact on IFX exposure.

2. Materials and Methods

2.1. Patients and Laboratory Measurements

Consented patients with IBD (CD and UC) undergoing every 8-week maintenance therapy with IFX were enrolled at a single site. Two specimens were collected within one maintenance cycle, a first specimen collected mid-cycle at least 20 days after infusion, and a second specimen collected towards the end of cycle. Serum was isolated from the clot immediately after specimen collection and stored at $-20\ °C$ until analysis. IFX levels (assay range 0.8–34 µg/mL) and Antibodies to Infliximab (ATI) (cutoff > 3.1 U/mL for positive status) were determined from serum using drug tolerant homogenous mobility shift assay as described previously [10] (Prometheus Laboratories, San Diego, CA, USA). Serum albumin (g/L) and CRP (mg/L) were measured using standard immunoassay techniques (IMMAGE®800 Protein Chemistry Analyzer, Beckman Coulter, Brea, CA, USA) while antigenic TNF-α levels (following one freeze thaw cycle) were measured using high sensitivity immunoassays (Singulex Erenna Assay, MilliporeSigma, Burlington, MA, USA) and expressed as pg/mL [11]. Disease activity was assessed using Harvey-Bradshaw Index and partial Mayo score for CD and UC patients, respectively. Outcome variable consisted of clinical and biochemical remission (HBI and Partial Mayo below 5 and 2 points, respectively, with CRP level below 3 mg/L).

2.2. Model Informed Precision Dosing Tool

Individual PK parameters were estimated using a combinations of nonlinear mixed effect models (Monolix 2020R1, Lixoft, Paris, France) coupled with R functions (version 4.0) translated from MatLab (R2021a) and prior information from previously reported population pharmacokinetics model [7] independently of the patients enrolled in the study. The model employed two compartment pharmacokinetics with random effects on clearance (Cl), volume of distribution (central, [V1] and peripheral [V2]) and intercompartment clearance (Q). Covariates consisted of weight (on Cl, V1, Q and V2), Albumin (on Cl) and positive ATI status (on Cl). All parameters were fixed as described [7], with the exception that the proportional residual error model was set at 0.10. For each subject, mid-cycle IFX levels, ATI status, albumin and weight were used to estimate the conditional distribution of the individual parameters, which represents the uncertainty of the individual parameters given the observations collected above, and the prior information [7]. Conditional distributions of the model parameters (clearance (Cl), central volume of distribution (V1), intercompartmental clearance (Q), and peripheral volume of distribution (V2)) were generated for each patient using Markov Chain Monte Carlo simulations (Metropolis Hastings algorithm), and sampling (n = 100) from those distributions were used to estimate the median forecasted end of cycle, median trough levels (immediately before infusion, 56 days post infusion) and median probability to achieve trough levels above 5 and 10 µg/mL. Prediction intervals (80% corresponding to the 10th and 90th percentile of the estimates levels) were also calculated. All observations below the limit of quantitation of the IFX assay (0.8 µg/mL) were censored.

2.3. Statistical Analysis

Performances of the MIPD in forecasting end of cycle IFX levels using mid-cycle determination was assessed using Deming regression, regression coefficient and Kappa statistics (at 5 µg/mL cutoff). Area under the Receiver Operating Characteristic curve (AUC ROC) and logistic regression were used to evaluate the association of individual parameters with outcome measure. Group comparisons were tested using Kruskal Wallis ANOVA while longitudinal changes in CRP and TNF-α levels in relation to IFX exposure were evaluated using linear mixed effect models.

3. Results

A total of 41 patients with IBD (31 with CD and 10 with UC) undergoing every 8-week maintenance therapy with IFX (median dose = 5.9 mg/Kg [interquartile range, IQR:5.3–6.2]) were enrolled. Mid-cycle specimens were collected 28-day (median) post infusion (interquartile range [IQR]: 26–30-days), while end of cycle were collected 52-days (median) post infusion (IQR: 44–56-days). Patient characteristics and laboratory measures are presented in Table 1, 44% (18/41) patients presented with inactive disease (biochemical and clinical remission). Montreal classification criteria is provided in Table 2. Median individual PK parameter estimated using mid-cycle determination yielded 0.300 L/day CL (IQR 0.240–0.424), with 3.36 (IQR: 3.03–3.70) and 1.56 L (IQR: 1.37–1.77) for V1 and V2, respectively. Median Q was 0.134 L/day (IQR: 0.108–0.153). There was no significant difference in IFX Clearance between the group of patients who received concomitant immunomodulators (median 0.323 L/day, IQR: 0.295–0.385, n = 8) as compared to those who did not (median 0.301 L/day, IQR: 0.234–0.435, n = 33) ($p = 0.68$).

Table 1. Patient characteristics. Results are expressed as median (IQR), as appropriate.

	Estimate
Gender (female)	46.3% (19/41)
Age (years)	43 (34–49)
CD Diagnosis (vs UC)	76% (31/41)
Concomitant Immunomodulators	20% (8/41)
Albumin (g/L)	42.6 (40.4–44.3)
IFX (µg/mL)	
Mid cycle	13.2 (6.2–20.5)
End cycle	3.9 (1.2–7.7)
ATI status	
Mid cycle	15% (6/41)
End cycle	19% (8/41)
CRP (mg/L)	
Mid cycle	2.4 (0.6–5.4)
End cycle	2.7 (0.1–8.8)

Table 1. Cont.

	Estimate
TNF-α (pg/mL)	
Mid cycle	4.6 (3.1–8.8)
End cycle	8.0 (4.8–12.0)
Disease activity	
HBI	2 (1–5)
Partial Mayo	0 (0–3)
Clinical & Biochemical Remission	44% (18/41)

Table 2. Montreal Classification criteria.

	n/N
Crohn's Disease	
Age:	
≤16 (A1)	2/31
17–40 (A2)	25/31
>40 (A3)	4/31
Location	
Terminal Ileum (L1)	2/31
Colon (L2)	6/31
Ileocolon (L3)	23/31
Behavior	
Non structuring, non-penetrating (B1)	15/31
Stricturing (B2)	12/31
Penetrating (B3)	3/31
Perianal	1/31
Ulcerative Colitis	
Proctitis (E1)	0/10
Left sided (E2)	3/10
Pancolitis (E3)	7/10

3.1. End of Cycle IFX Levels Can Be Forecasted Using Mid Cycle Determinations

A typical pK profile of patient under IFX is presented in Figure 1.

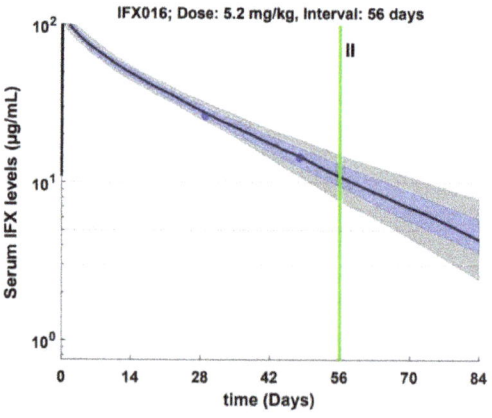

Figure 1. Performance of MIPD in forecasting Trough levels, PK profile. Solid line corresponds to the median IFX levels calculated from 100 random samples from the condition distribution of individual Pk parameters. Blue zone corresponds to interquartile range, grey zone corresponds to the 10th and 90th percentile.

The performance characteristics of the Bayesian method in forecasting end of cycle levels using mid-cycle determinations is presented in Figure 2. Median forecasted end of cycle IFX levels (at the time of specimen collection) were 4.2 µg/mL (IQR: 2.2–8.3 µg/mL) and yielded Demings slope of 0.90 CI95%: 0.78 to 1.02) with 0.87 regression coefficient (R^2). We also tested the performances of the MIPD in the group of patients with ($R^2 = 0.89$; slope = 0.91; n = 18) or without clinical and biochemical remission status achieved ($R^2 = 0.75$; slope = 0.92; n = 23). A total of 17/41 (41%) patient specimens presented with IFX levels greater than 5 µg/mL at end of cycle, of which 14 specimens were predicted by the forecasting method as being greater than 5 µg/mL (82%). Alternatively, 24/41 (59%) patients specimens presented with end of cycle levels below 5 µg/mL, of which 21 specimens were predicted by the forecasting method as being below 5 µg/mL (87.5%). Kappa statistics at cutoff of 5 µg/mL was 0.70 ± 0.11. Forecasted median trough IFX levels (at 56 days) were 3.0 µg/mL (IQR: 1.6–7.6); individualized probability to achieve Trough IFX levels above 5 µg/mL was 0.21 (median, IQR: 0.07–0.78). The forecast time to reach threshold within maintenance cycle was 48 days (median, IQR: 37–68 days). The probability to achieve trough levels above 10 µg/mL was very low in this cohort (median 0.05 IQR: 0.02–0.21).

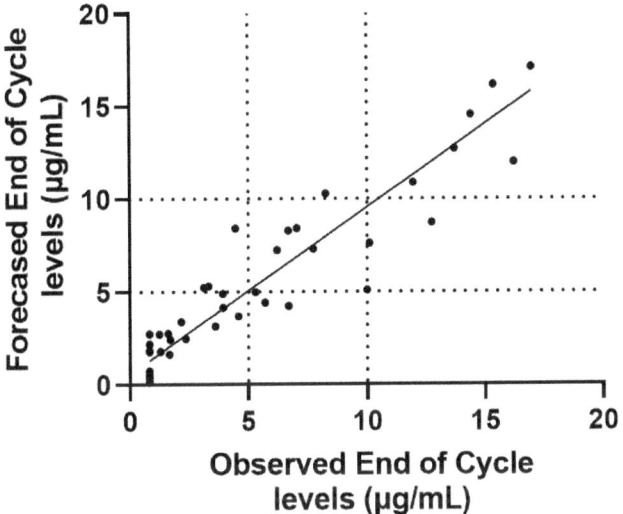

Figure 2. Comparison between observed and forecasted end of cycle IFX levels (Deming's slope = 0.90; slope = 0.87).

3.2. Forecasted IFX Levels Associate with Clinical and Biochemical Remission

The association between observed end of cycle and forecasted trough IFX levels with clinical and biochemical validation was tested in the 41 patients. Patients presenting with observed end of cycle IFX levels above 5 µg/mL were 7.2-fold (CI95%: 1.7–30.2) more likely to present with clinical and biochemical remission ($p < 0.001$) as compared to patients presenting with suboptimal exposure (below 5 µg/mL) ($p < 0.01$). Similarly, forecasted trough IFX levels above 5 µg/mL associated with clinical and biochemical remission (OR = 21.0 CI95%: 3.4–127.9) ($p < 0.001$). Results are summarized in Table 3.

As presented in Figure 3, the AUC under the ROC with clinical and biochemical remission was comparable between observed end of cycle IFX (AUC = 0.778; CI95%: 0.626–0.929) and forecasted trough (AUC= 0.766; CI95%: 0.599–0.933). The probability to achieve trough levels above target threshold of 5 µg/mL yielded an AUC of 0.761 (CI95%: 0.590–0.931) (OR range = 37.4; CI95%: 3.6–385.5) ($p < 0.001$). Median time to reach threshold exposure was 40.5 days (IQR: 28–50.5 days) among patients with active disease as compared to 65.5 days (IQR: 50–77) among patients with biochemical and clinical remission ($p < 0.01$).

Table 3. Performance of Observed and Forecasted IFX levels in associating with clinical and biochemical remission.

	Observed End of Cycle > 5 µg/mL			Forecasted Trough > 5 µg/mL		
	Estimate	−95CI	+95CI	Estimate	−95CI	+95CI
Sensitivity	0.67	0.44	0.84	0.67	0.44	0.84
Specificity	0.78	0.58	0.90	0.91	0.73	0.98
False positive	0.22	0.10	0.42	0.09	0.02	0.27
False Negative	0.33	0.16	0.56	0.33	0.16	0.56
Positive LR	3.1	1.4	7.2	7.7	2.3	28.4
Negative LR	0.4	0.2	0.8	0.36	0.2	0.6
Odds Ratio	7.2	1.8	30.2	21.0	3.9	109.0

LR: likelihood ratio.

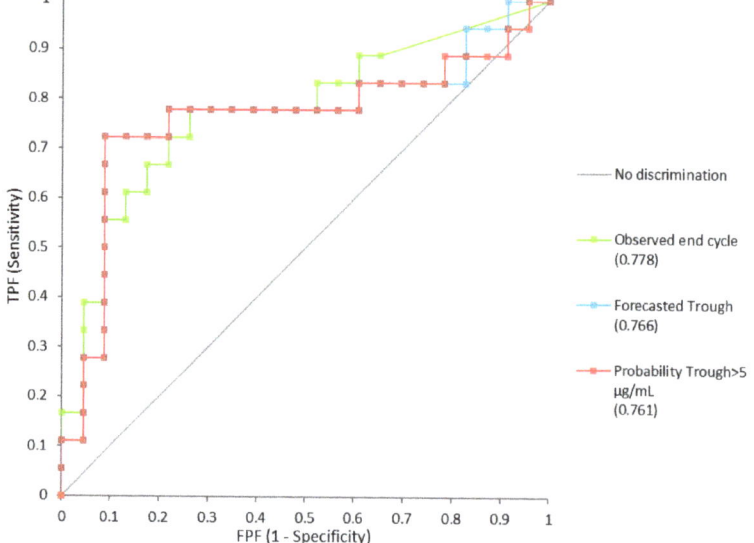

Figure 3. ROC of Observed and Forecasted IFX levels with clinical and biochemical remission. Measured endcycle IFX levels: AUC = 0.778 (CI95%: 0.626–0.929); Forecasted trough levels: AUC= 0.766 (CI95%: 0.599–0.936) (p = 0.89); Forecasted probability of trough level > 5 µg/mL: AUC= 0.756 (CI95%: 0.586–0.926).

3.3. Circulating TNF-α and CRP Levels Independently and Additively Impact IFX Clearance in IBD

There was significant increase in TNF-α levels from midcycle to end cycle ($p < 0.01$) (Table 1). In contrast the change in CRP level was not significant (p = 0.44). There was a directional trend between higher TNF-α levels and active disease that did not reach significance ($p > 0.10$; data not shown). Linear mixed effect models revealed that the change in TNF-α were independent of those from CRP (p = 0.67). In contrast the change in IFX levels from midcycle to end of cycle associated independently with CRP (marginal R^2 = 0.06; p = 0.047), TNF-α (marginal R2 = 0.21; $p < 0.01$). Multivariate analysis indicated that the impact of those inflammatory markers on IFX were additive (marginal R^2 = 0.27). Results are summarized in Table 4.

Table 4. Linear Mixed effect Model of IFX levels in relation to inflammatory markers. Each unit increase in TNF-α associated with 0.33 ± 0.08 μg/mL decrease in IFX levels.

	Intercept	Slope ± SEM	p Value	Marginal R^2
CRP	10.0 ±1.2	−0.13 ± 0.07	0.047	0.058
TNF-α	12.4 ± 1.2	−0.33 ± 0.08	<0.001	0.213
CRP + TNF-α	13.4 ± 1.3	−0.14 ± 0.06 −0.33 ± 0.07	0.022 <0.001	0.271

Finally, multivariate logistic regression analysis revealed that patients presenting with forecasted trough IFX levels above 5 μg/mL were 13.9-fold (adjusted OR, CI95%: 2.0–94.9; $p < 0.01$) and 7.3-fold (adjusted OR, CI95%: 1.3–40.4; $p < 0.01$) less likely to have end cycle CRP levels above 3 mg/L, and TNF-α above 8 pg/mL (median), respectively. The cumulative impact of the inflammatory burden on IFX exposure is presented in Table 5.

Table 5. IFX exposure in relation to Inflammatory burden.

End of Cycle	CRP ≤ 3 mg/L and TNF-α ≤ 8 pg/mL	CRP > 3 mg/L or TNF-α > 8 pg/mL	CRP > 3 mg/L and TNF-α > 8 pg/mL	p Value
Observed end cycle μg/mL	7.0 (4.6–14.4)	3.3 (0.8–7.7)	1.7 (0.8–3.9)	<0.01
Forecasted Trough μg/mL	6.7 (5.3–9.0)	3.7 (0.7–7.7)	2.0 (1.1–3.2)	<0.01
Probability Trough > 5 μg/mL	0.68 (0.47–0.90)	0.25 (0.05–0.70)	0.10 (0.04–0.19)	<0.01

4. Discussion

There is considerable interpatient variability in drug exposure following standard dosing of monoclonal antibodies such as IFX, and MIDP tools are poised to improved patient outcome by guiding dose and improving disease control [7,12]. These MIDP tools typically employ Bayesian forecasting methods for dose individualization and have been implemented for several therapies such as busulfan [13], vancomycin [14] and may be also helpful for controlling side effects in oncology [15]. In this report we have established the performance characteristics of MIPD in forecasting trough IFX concentrations by using prior information from a model that uses two compartment pharmacokinetics with weight, ATI and albumin as covariates [7]. In this study, the parameter estimates from the prior published models were tested in this validation cohort with specimens collected during the linear phase of elimination of IFX, and trough levels were forecasted by calculating the conditional distribution of individual parameters. Traditionally MIPD rely on the estimation of maximum a posteriori but as reported previously these methods provide limited information and no do not reflect the uncertainty of the measurement for decision making [15,16]. In this report, Bayesian assimilation techniques were employed by calculating the probability to achieve a certain pre-specified trough.

The forecasting method revealed generally good agreement between forecasted and observed end of cycle levels and thus suggests that collection of one specimen during mid cycle may be sufficient to ascertain and forecast of subsequent trough levels. While this validation cohort establishes the performances of the MIPD tool in fore-casting trough the number of patients enrolled was limited and additional data are currently collected to confirm these findings.

There are several clinical applications with the MIPD tool. First, the collection of patient specimen during the linear terminal phase of elimination of IFX may help identify early those patients who are likely to present with suboptimal exposure at trough and thus facilitate the implementation of countermeasures during this window of opportunity (i.e., dose intensification at the next scheduled dose). Second the MIPD tool can allow the most appropriate time for dosing where IFX levels reach suboptimal threshold and can inform on dose and dose interval combinations that can produce desired trough levels commensurate with target troughs (i.e., >5 or 10 μg/mL). While endoscopic assessments were not available in this study, we established a significant association between forecasted trough IFX levels and clinical and biochemical remission, and these data add the already existing large body of evidence supporting the value of PK measurements in association with disease control [1,4]. We also reported a significant association between the disease outcome variable with the probability of achieving trough concentration above 5 μg/mL. However, a very low number of patients achieved forecasted trough concentration above 10 μg/mL and thus suggest the opportunity to improve outcome by dosing intensification in a significant proportion of patients. These data illustrate the potential of MIPD in optimizing Infliximab therapy, and this premise could also be applied to other monoclonal antibodies such as adalimumab that is also prone to underexposure leading to poor disease control.

While anti-TNF therapy have been available for over two decades, there is paucity of data reporting the impact of antigenic inflammatory TNF-α levels on IFX exposure in IBD, and clinicians have traditionally relied on serum CRP as indicator of inflammation. This is primarily due to past constraints in that there were several limitations with the determination of TNF-α levels in the clinical practice setting, owing to significant pre-analytical variations associated with the stability of TNF-α during specimen transportation and processing and the challenge in determining pg quantities of the cytokine. In this report we used highly sensitive immunoassay to quantify TNF-α levels and our data suggest a strong association between IFX and TNF-α within maintenance cycle, whereby the decrease in IFX levels during the elimination phase parallels a rise in circulating TNF-α. Recent studies using drug tolerant assays have established that treatment with adalimumab associates with an increase TNF-α, most likely reflecting the formation of adalimumab and TNF-α complexes18. In our study, only free TNF-α levels were determined and thus it is not surprising that the decrease IFX levels associated with lower TNF-α neutralization and thus increase in free circulating levels of the cytokine. Whether these changes in the circulation also associate with tissue dynamics in inflamed gut is not known, but likely, and we speculate that inadequate exposure (as seen in most patients presenting with suboptimal IFX trough levels) may insufficiently provide TNF-α neutralizing capabilities as seen in patients with rheumatoid arthritis [9]. However, we acknowledge that perhaps due to the small size we were not able to detect a significant association between TNF-α levels and disease activity status in contrast to other studies and the levels detected in our assay may not be biologically active TNF-α [9,17,18].

Interestingly there was also no significant correlation between CRP and TNF-α and our analysis revealed that both CRP and TNF-α contributed independently and additively to IFX exposure. CRP is an acute phase reactant protein produced by the liver and most likely reflected the dynamics of inflammatory cytokine other than TNF-α such as Il-6 and IL-1 [19]. It follows that those multiple pathways can impact IFX exposure, and as already proposed, this inflammatory burden may sink IFX levels below threshold levels commensurate with disease control [8].

In conclusion, our data help support the implementation of MIPD to forecast IFX exposure in IBD and provide insights into the complex dynamics between IFX and antigenic TNF-α in IBD.

Author Contributions: Conceptualization, W.R., C.P., D.R.M., J.C.P., A.E. and T.D.; methodology, W.R., C.P., D.R.M., J.C.P. and T.D.; formal analysis, W.R., C.P., D.R.M. and T.D.; writing—original draft preparation, T.D.; writing—review and editing, W.R., C.P., D.R.M., J.C.P., A.E. and T.D. All authors have read and agreed to the published version of the manuscript.

Funding: This research received no external funding.

Institutional Review Board Statement: The study was conducted in accordance with the Declaration of Helsinki, and approved by the Institutional Review Board (or Ethics Committee) of University of Vienna (protocol 219/2011).

Informed Consent Statement: Informed consent was obtained from all subjects involved in the study.

Data Availability Statement: No data sharing.

Acknowledgments: We acknowledge the patients for their participation in the study.

Conflicts of Interest: CP: none; WR: none; A.E.: none; JCP: Prometheus Laboratories (consulting fees); D.R.M.: Prometheus Laboratories (consulting fees); TD: Prometheus Laboratories (employment).

References

1. Vande Casteele, N.; Herfarth, H.; Katz, J.; Flack-Ytter, Y.; Singh, S. American Gastroenterological Association Institute Technical Review on the Role of Therapeutic Drug Monitoring in the Management of Inflammatory Bowel Diseases. *Gastroenterology* **2017**, *153*, 835–857.e6. [CrossRef] [PubMed]
2. Feuerstein, J.D.; Nguyen, G.C.; Kupfer, S.S.; Falck-Ytter, Y.; Singh, S.; Gerson, L.; Hirano, I.; Rubenstein, J.H.; Smalley, W.E.; Stollman, N.; et al. American Gastroenterological Association Institute Guideline on Therapeutic Drug Monitoring in Inflammatory Bowel Disease. *Gastroenterology* **2017**, *153*, 827–834. [CrossRef] [PubMed]
3. Negoescu, D.M.; Enns, A.E.; Swanhorst, B.; Baumgartner, B.; Campbell, J.P.; Osterman, M.T.; Papamichael, K.; Cheifetz, A.S.; Vaughn, B.P. Proactive Vs Reactive Therapeutic Drug Monitoring of Infliximab in Crohn's Disease: A Cost-Effectiveness Analysis in a Simulated Cohort. *Inflamm. Bowel Dis.* **2019**, *26*, 103–111. [CrossRef] [PubMed]
4. Papamichael, K.; Vajravelu, R.K.; Vaughn, B.P.; Osterman, M.T.; Cheifetz, A.S. Proactive Infliximab Monitoring Following Reactive Testing is Associated with Better Clinical Outcomes Than Reactive Testing Alone in Patients With Inflammatory Bowel Disease. *J. Crohns Colitis* **2018**, *12*, 804–810. [CrossRef] [PubMed]
5. Dubinsky, M.C.; Phan, B.L.; Singh, N.; Rabizadeh, S.; Mould, D.R. Pharmacokinetic Dashboard-Recommended Dosing is Different than Standard of Care Dosing in Infliximab-Treated Pediatric IBD Patients. *AAPS J.* **2017**, *19*, 215–222. [CrossRef] [PubMed]
6. Strik, A.S.; Löwenberg, M.; Mould, D.R.; Berends, S.E.; Ponsioen, C.I.; Brande, J.M.H.V.D.; Jansen, J.M.; Hoekman, D.R.; Brandse, J.F.; Duijvestein, M.; et al. Efficacy of dashboard driven dosing of infliximab in inflammatory bowel disease patients; a randomized controlled trial. *Scand. J. Gastroenterol.* **2021**, *56*, 145–154. [CrossRef] [PubMed]
7. Xu, Z.; Mould, D.; Hu, C.; Ford, J.; Keen, M.; Davis, H.; Zhou, H. Population pharmacokinetic analysis of infliximab in pediatrics using integrated data from six clinical trials. *Clin. Pharmacol. Drug Dev.* **2012**, *1*, 203.
8. Yarur, A.J.; Jain, A.; Sussman, D.A.; Barkin, J.S.; Quintero, M.A.; Princen, F.; Kirkland, R.; Deshpande, A.R.; Singh, S.; Abreu, M.T. The association of tissue anti-TNF drug levels with serological and endoscopic disease activity in inflammatory bowel disease: The ATLAS study. *Gut* **2016**, *65*, 249–255. [CrossRef] [PubMed]
9. Takeuchi, T.; Miyasaka, N.; Tatsuki, Y.; Yano, T.; Yoshinari, T.; Abe, T.; Koike, T. Baseline tumour necrosis factor alpha levels predict the necessity for dose escalation of infliximab therapy in patients with rheumatoid arthritis. *Ann. Rheum. Dis.* **2011**, *70*, 1208–1215. [CrossRef] [PubMed]
10. Wang, S.-L.; Ohrmund, L.; Hauenstein, S.; Salbato, J.; Reddy, R.; Monk, P.; Lockton, S.; Ling, N.; Singh, S. Development and validation of a homogeneous mobility shift assay for the measurement of infliximab and antibodies-to-infliximab levels in patient serum. *J. Immunol. Methods* **2012**, *382*, 177–188. [CrossRef] [PubMed]
11. Todd, J.; Simpson, P.; Estis, J.; Torres, V.; Wub, A.H.B. Reference range and short- and long-term biological variation of interleukin (IL)-6, IL-17A and tissue necrosis factor-alpha using high sensitivity assays. *Cytokine* **2013**, *64*, 660–665. [CrossRef] [PubMed]
12. Xiong, Y.; Mizuno, T.; Colman, R.; Hyams, J.; Noe, J.D.; Boyle, B.; Tsai, Y.-T.; Dong, M.; Jackson, K.; Punt, N.; et al. Real-World Infliximab Pharmacokinetic Study Informs an Electronic Health Record-Embedded Dashboard to Guide Precision Dosing in Children with Crohn's Disease. *Clin. Pharmacol. Ther.* **2021**, *109*, 1639–1647. [CrossRef] [PubMed]
13. Shukla, P.; Goswami, S.; Keizer, R.J.; Winger, B.A.; Kharbanda, S.; Dvorak, C.; Long-Boyle, J. Assessment of a Model-Informed Precision Dosing Platform Use in Routine Clinical Care for Personalized Busulfan Therapy in the Pediatric Hematopoietic Cell Transplantation (HCT) Population. *Front. Pharmacol.* **2020**, *11*, 888. [CrossRef] [PubMed]
14. Hughes, J.H.; Tong, D.M.H.; Lucas, S.S.; Faldasz, J.D.; Goswami, S.; Keizer, R.J. Continuous Learning in Model-Informed Precision Dosing: A Case Study in Pediatric Dosing of Vancomycin. *Clin. Pharmacol. Ther.* **2021**, *109*, 233–242. [CrossRef] [PubMed]
15. Maier, C.; Hartung, N.; Kloft, C.; Huisinga, W.; de Wiljes, J. Reinforcement learning and Bayesian data assimilation for model-informed precision dosing in oncology. *CPT Pharmacomet. Syst. Pharmacol.* **2021**, *10*, 241–254. [CrossRef] [PubMed]
16. Maier, C.; Hartung, N.; de Wiljes, J.; Klots, C.; Huisinga, W. Bayesian Data Assimilation to Support Informed Decision Making in Individualized Chemotherapy. *CPT Pharmacomet. Syst. Pharmacol.* **2020**, *9*, 153–164. [CrossRef] [PubMed]
17. Berkhout, L.C.; L'Ami, M.J.; Ruwaard, J.; Hart, M.H.; Heer, P.O.-D.; Bloem, K.; Nurmohamed, M.T.; van Vollenhoven, R.F.; Boers, M.; Alvarez, D.F.; et al. Dynamics of circulating TNF during adalimumab treatment using a drug-tolerant TNF assay. *Sci. Transl. Med.* **2019**, *11*, eaat3356. [CrossRef] [PubMed]

18. Komatsu, M.; Kobayashi, D.; Saito, K.; Furuya, D.; Yagihashi, A.; Araake, H.; Tsuji, N.; Sakamaki, S.; Niitsu, Y.; Watanabe, N. Tumor necrosis factor-alpha in serum of patients with inflammatory bowel disease as measured by a highly sensitive immuno-PCR. *Clin. Chem.* **2001**, *47*, 1297–1301. [CrossRef] [PubMed]
19. Gross, V.; Andus, T.; Caesar, I.; Schölmerich, J. Evidence for continuous stimulation of interleukin-6 production in Crohn's disease. *Gastroenterology* **1992**, *102*, 514–519. [CrossRef]

MDPI
St. Alban-Anlage 66
4052 Basel
Switzerland
www.mdpi.com

Journal of Clinical Medicine Editorial Office
E-mail: jcm@mdpi.com
www.mdpi.com/journal/jcm

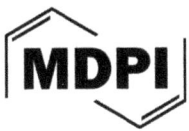

Disclaimer/Publisher's Note: The statements, opinions and data contained in all publications are solely those of the individual author(s) and contributor(s) and not of MDPI and/or the editor(s). MDPI and/or the editor(s) disclaim responsibility for any injury to people or property resulting from any ideas, methods, instructions or products referred to in the content.

www.ingramcontent.com/pod-product-compliance
Lightning Source LLC
LaVergne TN
LVHW070640100526
838202LV00013B/848